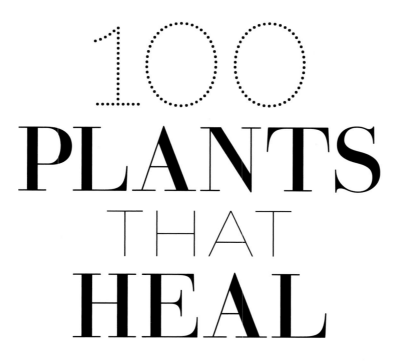

100 PLANTS THAT HEAL

*The Illustrated Herbarium
of Medicinal Plants*

Text by Gérard Debuigne
& François Couplan

Photos by Pierre Vigne
& Délia Vigne

DAVID & CHARLES

www.davidandcharles.com

THE 100 PLANTS THAT HEAL

PRECAUTIONS FOR USE AND WARNINGS

The publisher and authors bear no liability for any inappropriate use of the remedies suggested in this book. The plants described in this book should not be consumed in excessive quantities or for longer than recommended. This book should not be a substitute for medical treatment. Under no circumstances should you stop treatment without medical advice. Always seek your doctor's opinion before following the recommendations set out in this book. If you are suffering any chronic illness, ask your doctor or pharmacist for advice before using medicinal plants.

INTRODUCTION

This book of *100 Plants that Heal* seeks to cast a spotlight on a selection of common healing plants. Most of the examples given are indigenous to Europe, although some are naturalized (such as Garden Nasturtium), and harmless if used properly. It is not an exhaustive collection.

The aim of this book is to teach you to recognize these healing plants, magnified by the remarkable botanical photographs by Pierre and Délia Vignes, learn a little of their history, and try out the traditional recipes that use them. No "deadly" plants have been included, even those with widely recognized healing powers (such as Foxglove, Henbane, Hellebore, Naked Ladies and Deadly Nightshade).

Humankind has always had a close relationship with the plant world. Plants have been part of our food since time immemorial as it is not physiologically possible for us to live entirely on animal products. However, in addition to this fundamentally nutritional approach, humans learnt early on that specific plants, in a wide variety of forms, could be used to treat ailments. Excavations in Iraq have uncovered a 60,000-year-old tomb containing the remains of eight medicinal plants. There is little doubt that the medicinal use of plants is as old as the human race itself. Observations of chimpanzees in West Africa indicate that it may even be older. These studies revealed the apes were using many plants with as-yet-unexplored medicinal properties.

There have been many changes in the relationship between plants and humans since the days when our great-great-grandmothers used healing plants from jars on the kitchen shelves to make infusions with boiling water and to treat family ailments. Our knowledge of plants has grown considerably and a genuine upheaval could be said to have taken place in the field of medicinal plants. Analysis has become much more widespread and active elements have been isolated. This has led to a better understanding of how many (but far from all) plants react with the body.

Numerous clinical studies have enabled reliable results to be obtained on the effects of several dozen plants. Some hazards have also come to light. While the most poisonous plants tend to be widely known, recent research has indicated that others may demonstrate a more subtle toxicity and that their regular use over a prolonged period can cause major problems, sometimes even resulting in death.

Work has also begun on exploring exotic plants boasting medicinal properties, some of which have quickly come into common use. In some cases, such as Ginkgo, Devil's Claw and Echinacea, they have effectively dethroned their European equivalents. In addition to the classic infusions, other means of using plants for medicinal purposes have been developed, such as gels or integrated fresh plant suspensions. Other therapeutic techniques, such as aromatherapy, have also become widespread. In the light of the profusion of new data, combined with a significant expansion in the medicinal plants market and an increased interest in self-treatment, the law has had to adapt, becoming more relaxed in some areas while tightening up in others.

We have moved far from the medicinal plants and beneficial infusions of yesteryear. For pharmacologists, plants are simply a medium of support for the active elements they contain. If it is possible to synthesize these elements, so much the better, as plant matter itself is often regarded with suspicion. On the other hand, users often prefer to take responsibility for their own healthcare, and look for advice in books or on the internet rather than visiting a doctor. However, the occasional accidents that result from this approach provoke an immediate reaction from the medical profession and the authorities who are always keen to retain control over the therapeutic use of plants. The commercial successes of some plants, such as St. John's-wort and Stevia, have even provoked vigorous reactions from the chemical- and sugar-industry lobbies, who are concerned about losing market share.

Despite the enormous advances in modern medicine, the use of healing plants still offers multiple advantages. Indeed, it is easy to forget that it is only within the last 150 years that humans have had anything other than plants to cure their ailments.

Nowadays, plant-based treatments are once again taking centre stage, as the efficacy of medications, such as antibiotics (considered the almost universal solution to serious infections), is on the decline. Bacteria and viruses are continually adapting and learning to resist the drugs that target them. Herbal medicine, which offers natural remedies that are well accepted by the human body, is often associated with classic treatments. It is currently undergoing an exceptional renaissance, especially for the treatment of chronic illnesses, such as asthma or arthritis.

Botany has also seen a significant evolution. The old medieval plant names have drifted out of use. Who still remembers that Celandine, Valerian and Convulvulus were once known as Pilewort, All-heal and Granny Pop Out of Bed? Family names have been rationalized: Compositae replaced with Asteraceae, Cruciferae with Brassicaceae, Umbelliferae with Apiaceae. The scientific names of many plants have been changed by application of the principle of anteriority, which stipulates that the name used at the time of the first valid description of a species must be used; while, following the study of plant genomes, some plants have been moved from one family to another.

A medicinal plant is a plant that has a therapeutic effect on the body without being toxic at a normal dosage: *primum non nocere* (first, do no harm). It is important above all else that reasonable use aimed at healing a given illness does not cause any ill effects. Naturally, it is also desirable that it should fulfil the aim of effectively treating a health problem or injury. The general term "medicinal plant" covers a wide range of flora, from those that are entirely edible (in the form of food or condiments) to those that are genuinely deadly, and should be treated with the utmost caution. At the former end of the spectrum is the wide variety of wild, edible fruits and vegetables, some of which are included in this book (such as Blackcurrant and Leek). Even if at first glance their medicinal properties are not particularly powerful, they generally have remarkable nutritional qualities. Regular consumption of these sorts of plants is beneficial to the body and represents a genuine form of preventive medicine. While plants are easy to use, some of them may also produce side effects. Like all medicines, medicinal plants should be used with caution. Even Comfrey, a plant that was widely used in the past, can have fatal effects in certain circumstances; it has been restricted or prohibited for oral use in Europe and several countries including the United States. However, when a herbal remedy is used correctly, the risk of side effects is very limited.

And if we started refusing to eat a plant because it contained a toxic substance, we would find a large number of fruits and vegetables missing from our plates: celery is a photosensitizer; grapefruit reduces the elimination of active substances by the liver and therefore makes the effects of drugs more powerful, which in turn may potentially lead to an overdose; cabbage and black radish, meanwhile, reduce the effectiveness of drugs— as does St. John's-wort which has come under such scrutiny.

THE PUBLISHER

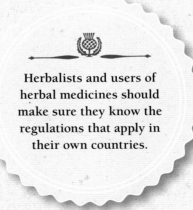

Herbalists and users of herbal medicines should make sure they know the regulations that apply in their own countries.

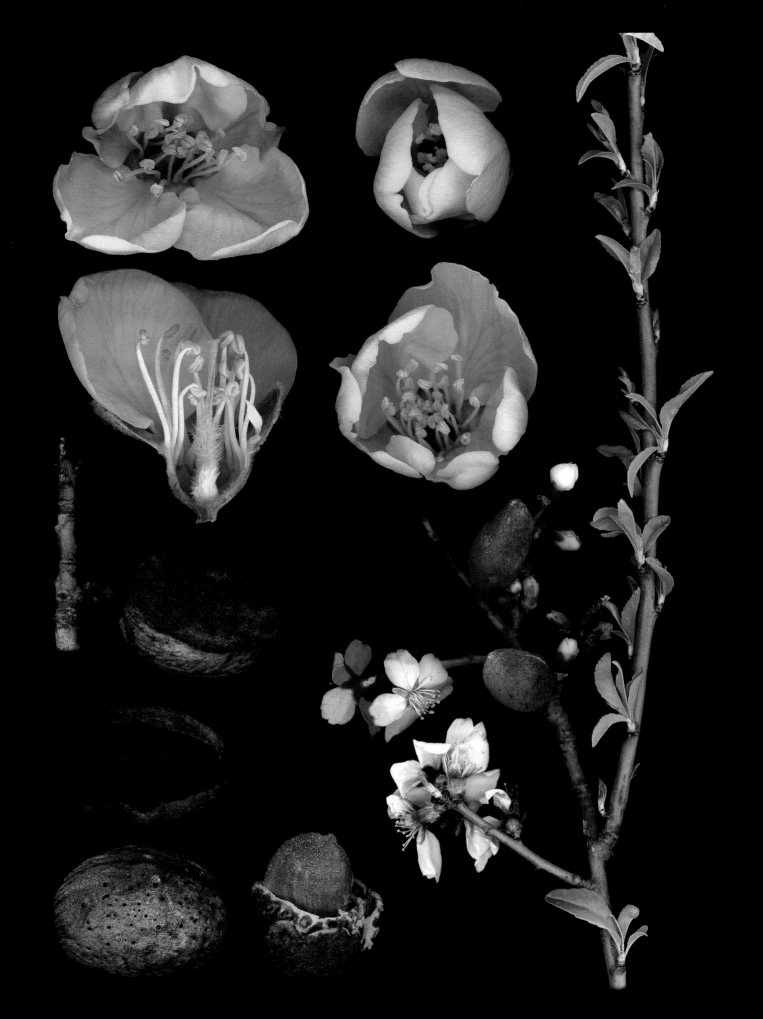

Almond

Prunus dulcis (=Amygdalus communis)

FAMILY: ROSACEAE

Active elements:
Almonds: fatty oil, rich in oleic and linoleic acids.
The bitter variety (var. *amara*) also contains
a cyanogenic heteroside, amygdalin.

More than 3,000 years ago, the Almond was highly prized by the ancient Egyptians for the cosmetic properties of sweet almond oil to soften and hydrate the skin.

The most potent softener

- Almond leaves **relieve coughs**. The shells do the same; their decoction makes a soothing pectoral infusion that tastes very pleasant, and is strongly indicated for whooping cough.
- Sweet almond oil is an **excellent laxative for newborns**.
- **Highly softening**, it is the basis for numerous beauty products.
- Bitter almond paste can be used instead of soap **for eczema on the hands**. It is alleged to remove freckles.
- Eating almonds, which contain monounsaturated fatty acids, **helps lower cholesterol**. Their antioxidant compounds make them effective in reducing cardiovascular risk and are said to have anti-cancerous properties.
- They are also rich in proteins, vitamins and minerals, very **nutritious** and, because of their high fibre content, they are very **beneficial for bowel movement**.

OTHER USES: Sweet almond is used to make orgeat syrup for a refreshing and calmative cordial. Industrially extracted bitter almond oil is used as a food flavouring.

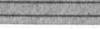
DID YOU KNOW? A Greek myth tells how princess Phyllis turns into a bare almond tree when she dies of a broken-heart believing she will never see her lover Demophon again. When Demophon, the son of Theseus, returns, he embraces the tree trunk and it blooms, covering itself in flowers and leaves. The flowers can be used to make a wine.

MAIN BENEFITS

- ★ Softening
- ★ Laxative for babies
- ★ Skincare
- ★ Cholesterol-lowering
- ★ Nutritional, remineralizing

PARTS USED

- ★ Roots, leaves, whole plant

Description

An elegant shrub, originating in western and central Asia. Its leaves are oblong and serrated. Its white or pinkish blossom is often exposed to frost as it flowers so early (February). The drupes have a light green, velvety skin containing a dry outer hull around the sweet or bitter almond.

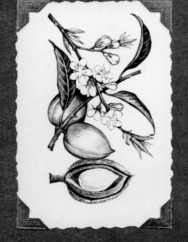

METHOD OF USE

- **INTERNAL: Infusion.** A small tablespoonful of leaves per cup. Infuse for 10 minutes. Drink 4 cups a day between meals. To relieve coughing.
  Decoction. 50g (1¾oz) of hulls boiled for 20 minutes in a litre (quart) of water. Drink throughout the day for the same purpose.
  Orgeat syrup. Add ½kg (1lb) of sweet almonds and 150g (5¼oz) of blanched bitter almonds to 125g (4½oz) of cold water and 750g (1½lb) of sugar and reduce to a paste. Dilute the paste obtained with 1½ litres of cold water and pass through a sieve. Add 2½kg (5½lb) of sugar and stir to dissolve in a *bain-marie*. When the sugar has fully dissolved, flavour with 250g (9oz) of orange blossom water.
- **EXTERNAL: Almond milk.** Soak 100g (3½oz) of sweet almonds in warm water to remove their skin, then crush with a little cold water. Dissolve 100g (3½oz) of sugar in 2 litres of water and pass it all through a sieve to strain. A wonderful skincare product that also relieves itchiness.
  Gargles. Use strongly sweetened almond oil after accidentally swallowing a fish bone or something similarly sharp, to soothe pain and prevent ulceration.

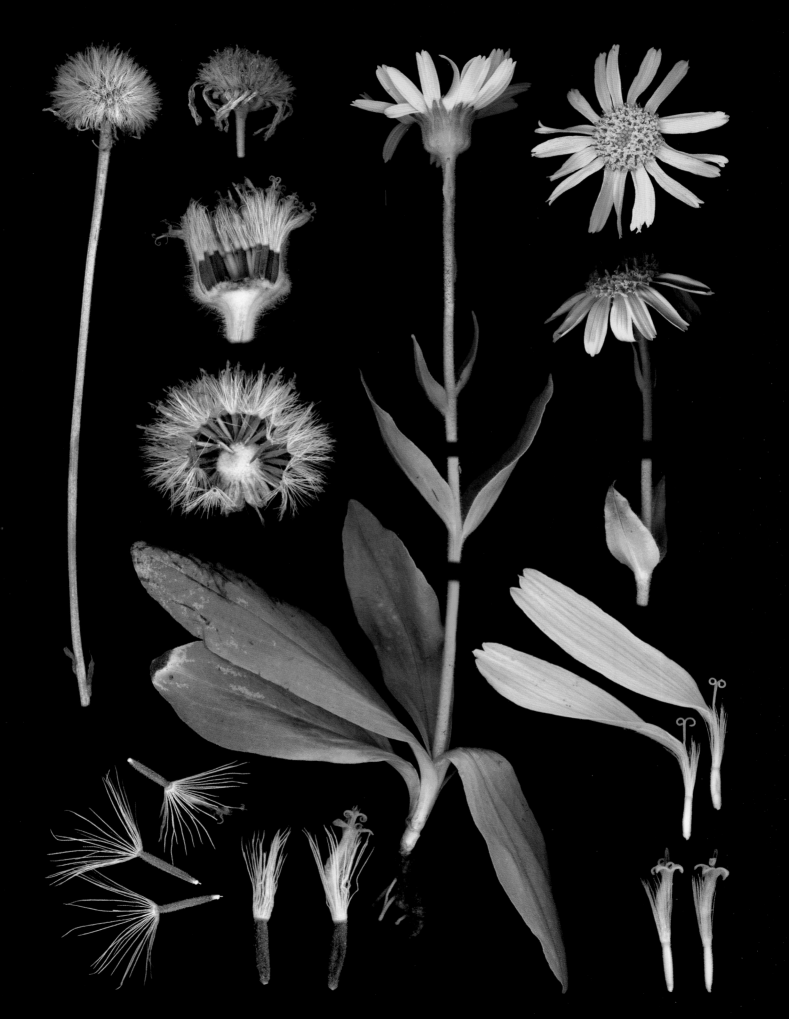

Arnica

Arnica montana
FAMILY: ASTERACEAE

Active elements:
Carotenoid pigments, sesquiterpene lactones (including helenalin), flavonoids, coumarins, aromatic essence rich in thymol.

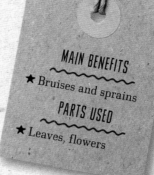

MAIN BENEFITS
★ Bruises and sprains

PARTS USED
★ Leaves, flowers

OTHER SPECIES: Given the growing demand from the herbal therapy industry, the plant's relative rarity and the difficulties in growing it, the European and German Pharmacopoeia have authorized the use of the American Arnica, *Arnica chamissonis*, which has equivalent properties, and can be cultivated more easily.

Saint Hildegard, the abbess of Rupertsberg, near Bingen, Germany, was the first to describe the effectiveness of Arnica in the treatment of bruises in the Middle Ages. Mattioli, a renowned Italian botanist and physician of Renaissance times, also helped popularize this remedy for knocks and falls. The Marquise de Sevigne, a 17th-century French aristocrat, famed for her letters, who also dabbled in herbal remedies, recommended "Arquebusade Water", a remedy made of Arnica, Common Hedgenettle and Spurge. But it was not until the 18th century that the preparation of Arnica tincture, as it is still used today, was perfected.

The best remedy for bruises

• Arnica is widely advocated for external use to treat **bruises, sprains, muscle and joint pain**. It speeds up the reabsorption of haematoma. **Note:** It can be used in the form of a tincture, ointment, oil or gel or, if home-made, as a decoction or poultice.
• It is also a widely used homoeopathic remedy for concussion, general injuries and pain.

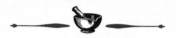

METHOD OF USE

• **EXTERNAL:** Leaves and flowers can be crushed to make a **poultice** for application after knocks or falls.
A **decoction** made with boiling water, using 5 to 10g (¼oz) of flowers per litre (quart) of water, to be used as very hot compresses to treat bruises and sprains (the same decoction is also good for getting rid of lice).
Tincture. Steep 200g (7oz) of flowers in 1 litre of alcohol (60% by volume) for 10 days. This tincture should never be used neat, but always diluted with water. The most effective formula is that set down by the botanists of Liège, Belgium: mix 20g (¾oz) of tincture of Arnica with 50g (1¾oz) of glycerine and 60g (2oz) of water. Use the mixture in compresses to treat contusions, bumps and bruises, but never on or near open wounds, the eyes, or the mouth.

TOXICITY

Arnica is far too dangerous to be recommended for internal use. Above 4 to 8g per litre(quart), it can trigger a profound alteration in the nervous system, leading to cold sweats, headaches, abdominal pain, palpitations and breathing problems. There are occasional cases of allergies to Arnica, as well as to other plants in the Asteraceae family. Varieties from the Iberian Peninsula do not contain the allergenic helenalin and are therefore better tolerated.

Description

A perennial found in sub-Alpine meadows, growing to a height of 40 to 60cm (16 to 24in) on acid soil at an altitude of 800 to 2,400m (2,600 to 7,870ft). Its single stem emerges from a rosette of pale green leaves and bears two small opposite leaves towards the middle. The stem terminates in one or more bright yellow flower heads, with a heart of tubular florets and a crown of tongues, all the same warm colour. The flowers have an aromatic scent and pungent taste.

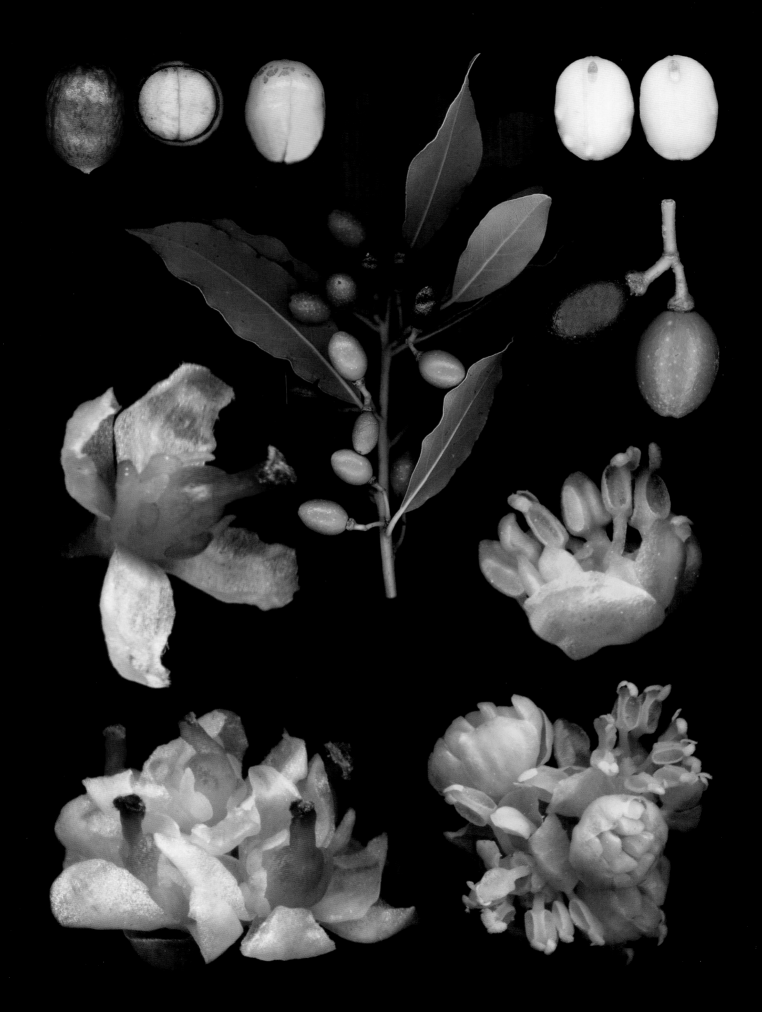

Bay Laurel

Laurus nobilis

FAMILY: LAURACEAE

Active elements:
Aromatic oil rich in cineole, sesquiterpene lactones, isoquinoline alkaloids. The pulp of the fruit contains a significant proportion of lipids.

The physicians of ancient Greece used the leaves and berries of the Bay Laurel extensively, advocating them for their invigorating effects on the stomach and bladder. Dioscorides used the bark to treat kidney stones and relieve liver ailments. During the Renaissance, the Bay Laurel was considered by Thibault Lespleigney, a 16th-century apothecary, to be a true panacea.

The famous Bay Laurel

• Bay Laurel has digestive properties. It **stimulates sluggish stomachs**, whets the appetite and combats fermentation. Its **antiseptic** properties are one reason why it is used in marinades.

• It is also advocated as an expectorant, and is used to **treat colds and bronchitis**.
• Laurel leaf powder has **febrifuge properties** (it reduces fever).
• Used externally, the Bay Laurel can **relieve rheumatic pain**. It can be made into a salve, or used in in the form of essential oil distilled from the leaves, diluted in olive oil or sweet almond oil.

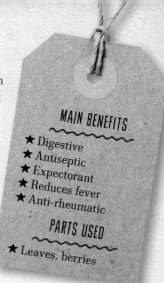

MAIN BENEFITS

★ Digestive
★ Antiseptic
★ Expectorant
★ Reduces fever
★ Anti-rheumatic

PARTS USED

★ Leaves, berries

OTHER USES: Bay leaves are a classic condiment for flavouring sauces, stews, fish and marinades. They are indispensable for making stock and *bouquets garnis*. Other less familiar dishes include omelette or polenta with bay leaf that come from Italy. The Bedouins of North Africa use them to flavour coffee.

DID YOU KNOW? Many other plants are called "laurels", such as Rose Laurel, Cherry Laurel, Californian Bay Laurel, Spotted Laurel and Alexandrian Laurel. Not one belongs to the genus *Laurus*, and most of them are not even in the family Lauraceae. Only the Bay Laurel is edible. The magnificent Rose Laurel, commonly known as Oleander (*Nerium oleander*) is one of the most poisonous plants in the world.

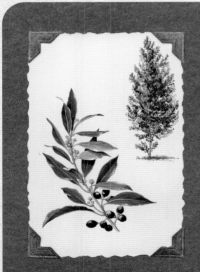

Description

A small tree reaching up to 10m (33ft) in height, native to the Mediterranean basin, where it occurs naturally in woodland or on rocky ground, usually not far from the coast. The dark bark of its trunk bears tough, spear-shaped, evergreen leaves with slightly undulating margins, which give off a balsamic smell when torn. Its white flowers, tinged with yellow, bloom from February to April in small clusters in the leaf axils. The female flowers, on separate stems, produce blackish oval fruits the size of a small cherry, with a highly aromatic, green, fatty pulp.

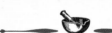

METHOD OF USE

• **INTERNAL:** *Bouquet garni.* Laurel (or bay) is the king of *bouquet garni*. It is widely used, particularly in sauces and marinades, for its antiseptic and digestive properties.
Infusion. 16 to 30g (½ to 1oz) of leaves per litre (quart) of water. Promotes digestion.
• **EXTERNAL: Laurel leaf oil** is used to treat the symptoms of rheumatism. Steep 100g (3½oz) of dried leaves in 100g (3½oz) of alcohol in a well-sealed jar for 24 hours. Then add a litre of olive oil and heat in a *bain-marie* for 6 hours (never boil). Strain and store in a cool place.
Anti-rheumatic balm is made with the "fatty oil" of Laurel berries. Crush the berries and boil for quarter of an hour. Strain the juice through a muslin cloth. Leave to cool. The brown, strong-smelling oil floats to the surface. Scoop it off carefully and keep in small, well-stoppered bottles. Mix two parts Laurel berry oil with one part lard to make the balm.

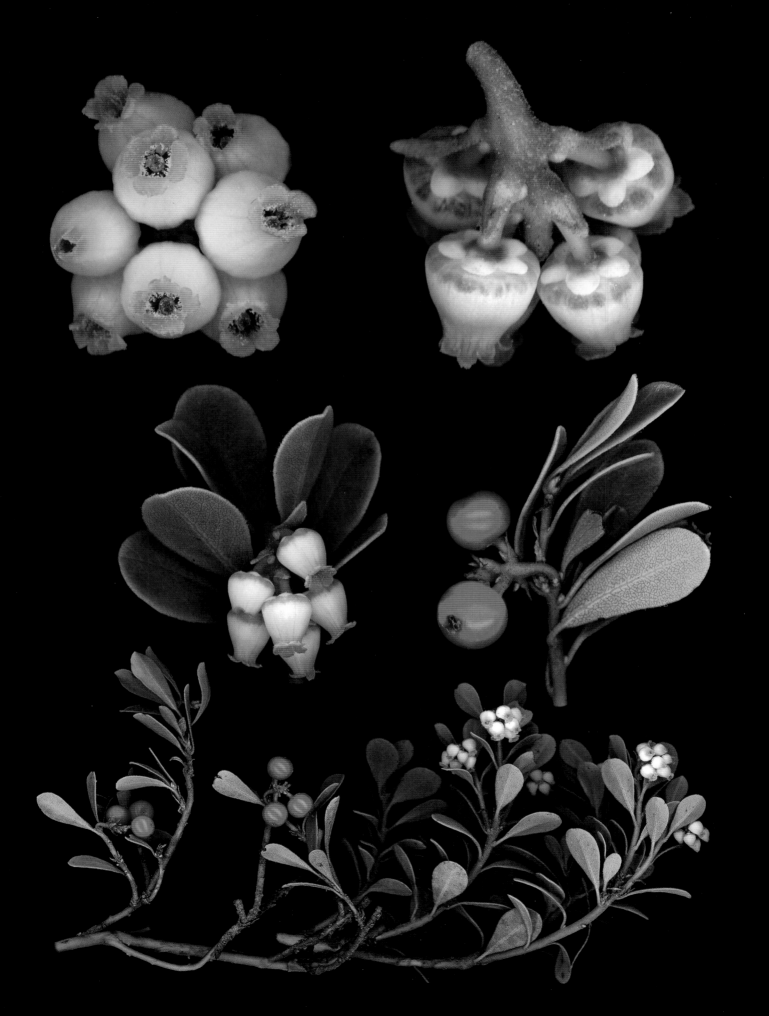

Bearberry

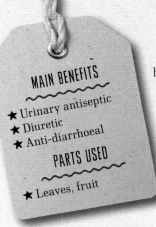

Arctostaphylos uva-ursi

FAMILY: ERICACEAE

Active elements:

Phenolic heterosides (including arbutoside, which transforms into hydroquinone), flavonoids (including hyperoside), triterpenes, iridoids, tannins.

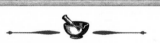

Rabelais, the 15th-century French satirical writer and physician, highlighted the diuretic properties of Bearberry and its use as an effective treatment of bladder stones and even gonorrhoea, when it cured Pantagruel: "he had got also the hot piss, which tormented him more than you would believe. His physicians, nevertheless, helped him very well, and, with store of lenitives and diuretic drugs, made him piss away his pain". Although highly advocated by 17th-century doctors, Bearberry fell into disregard in the following century, under the influence of the 18th-century French physician, Jean-Charles Desessartz, who claimed it was inert. It did not come back into use until 1857. Since then, various modern works confirm its indisputable medicinal powers.

The virtuous Bearberry

• The leaves are a **powerful urinary antiseptic** due to their high hydroquinone content. They are recommended for the **treatment of urinary tract infections**. They are especially used in the treatment of cystitis and urethritis, if the kidneys are not affected. For it to have maximum effect, it is important for the urine to be alkaline, therefore foods or medications that could acidify it should be avoided.

• Bearberry is rich in tannins, making it an **excellent astringent**, recommended for the treatment of enteritis with diarrhoea, leucorrhoea (white discharge) and uterine bleeding.

OTHER USES: The fruits are edible and have a tart, floury, astringent pulp. In centuries past, they were mashed and mixed with flour to make cakes or bread. American Indians mixed them with animal fat to make pemmican. The pulp of Bearberry fruit is rich in carbohydrates and nutritious.

DID YOU KNOW? Bearberry is so called because of the love bears have for its fruit. The name of the genus *Arctostaphylos*, which means "bears' grapes" suggests the same thing in Greek.

METHOD OF USE

• **INTERNAL: Infusion.** 20g (¾oz) of dried leaves per litre (quart) of water. Drink 2 or 3 cups per day for urinary tract infections.
Concentrated decoction. 30g (1oz) of dried leaves per litre of water. Simmer until reduced to a quarter. Take throughout the day as an anti-diarrhoeal.

Description

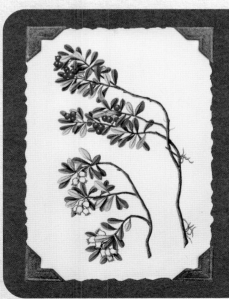

This evergreen dwarf shrub carpets the ground in dry pine or larch forests, especially in the mountains. It is widespread throughout the northern hemisphere. Its trailing, reddish-brown twigs, with smooth bark, grow haphazardly, bearing shiny, leathery leaves evoking those of boxwood. The clusters of pinkish-white, bell-shaped flowers, narrowing towards the tip, are succeeded by large, round, bright-red berries which ripen in late summer.

TOXICITY

Tannins can cause constipation as well as nausea and vomiting in people who are particularly sensitive. Plants containing arbutoside should not be used for more than one week, a maximum of five times a year. They should not be used by pregnant or breastfeeding women or by children under the age of twelve.

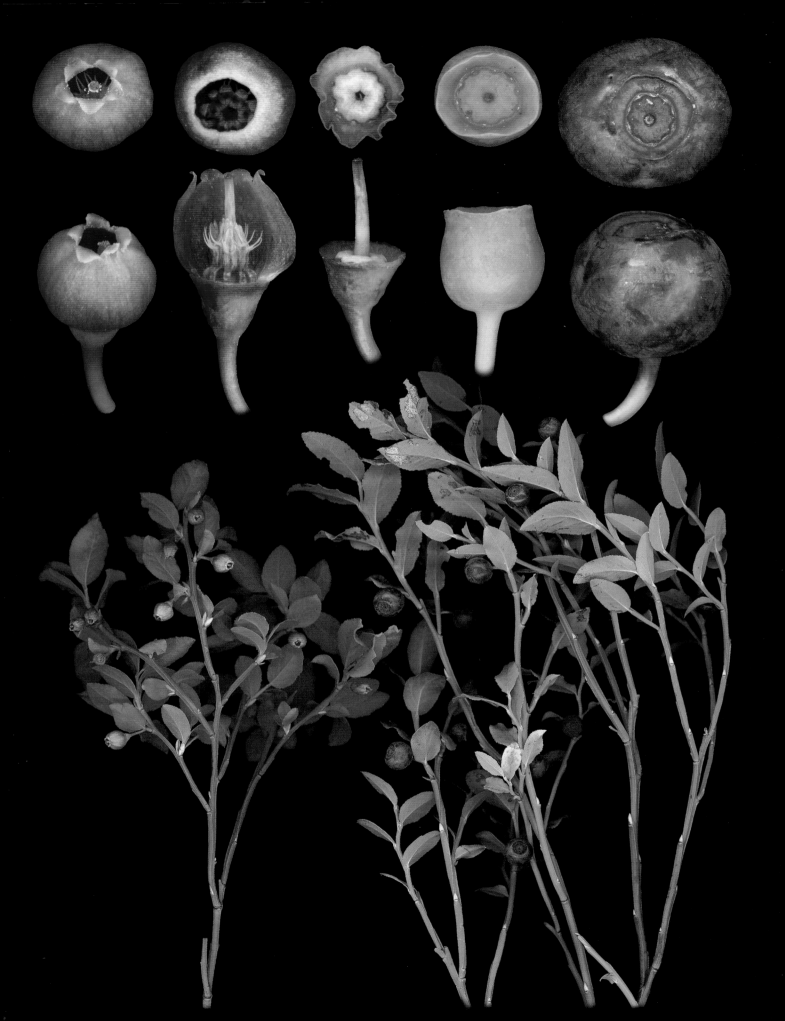

Bilberry

Vaccinium myrtillus

FAMILY: ERICACEAE

Active elements:

Leaves: phenolic acids, flavonoids, traces of quinolizidinic alkaloids, proanthocyanidins, catechol. Fruit: rich in carbohydrates, organic acids, tannins, vitamins B1 and C and proanthocyanidins.

Dioscorides was the first to vaunt the properties of Bilberry, which he recommended for treatment of dysentery. Arnaldus de Villa Nova, the 13th-century Catalan physician, advised haemorrhoid-sufferers to sit on a cushion of boiled bilberry and rose leaves. Later, it was advocated to treat stomatitis, mouth ulcers and infant thrush. However, its main use has continued to be for enteritis.

Anti-diarrhoeal

• The dried fruits are **antiseptic and astringent**. When fresh, they have a **slightly laxative** effect.

• The decoction of the berries is a **powerful antibacterial**, which is very effective against colibacillosis (infection of the digestive or urinary tracts by *Escherichia coli*) or acute enteritis.

• **Excellent results have been obtained in treating isolated bouts of diarrhoea**, including in children.

• Bilberry is recommended for **irritation of the oral mucosae**.

• It is also effective against digestive problems caused by certain antibiotics (Aureomycine, Terramycine).

• The anthocyanins in Bilberry explain why it is so effective in tonifying **blood vessels**, and relieving **heavy legs, varicose veins, haemorrhoids** and fragile capillaries.

• It is likewise the anthocyanins that **enable Bilberry to treat certain visual problems**. The pigments extracted from it are used for retinal vascular problems such as glaucoma. They also **significantly improve visual acuity** in low light.

OTHER SPECIES: The Lingonberry (*Vaccinium vitis-idaea*), which grows in mountainous woodland and the Cranberry (*V. oxycoccus*) on boggy ground, produce edible, red fruit. Cranberries have historically been renowned as a bacteriostatic agent that prevents and relieves cystitis, but results of recent research dispute this property.

METHOD OF USE

• **INTERNAL:** To treat diarrhoea of different origins, or to improve visual acuity; for once a remedy that tastes delicious! **Ripe bilberries can be eaten** in compotes, jellies and syrups.
Decoction. 50g (1¾oz) of berries per ¼ litre of water, boil for 10 minutes. Drink 4 cups per day. As an antidiabetic, drink an infusion of a large handful of leaves per litre (quart) of boiling water over 24 hours.

• **EXTERNAL: Decoction.** A handful of berries per litre of water, reduce by half by boiling. Use as an enema or compress for haemorrhoids; use as a mouthwash to treat ulcers and oral thrush (fungal infection).

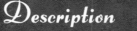

Description

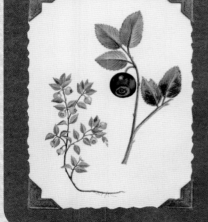

Sub-shrub growing to a height of 20 to 60cm (8 to 24in), forming dense carpets in woodland and on siliceous soil, particularly mountains and northern regions. Found in central and northern Europe, Asia and North America. Its many upright, angular, green branches bear small glossy, oval leaves, with finely serrated margins and green and red bell-shaped flowers which grow singly or in pairs in the leaf axils, producing the dark blue berries that are so eagerly harvested.

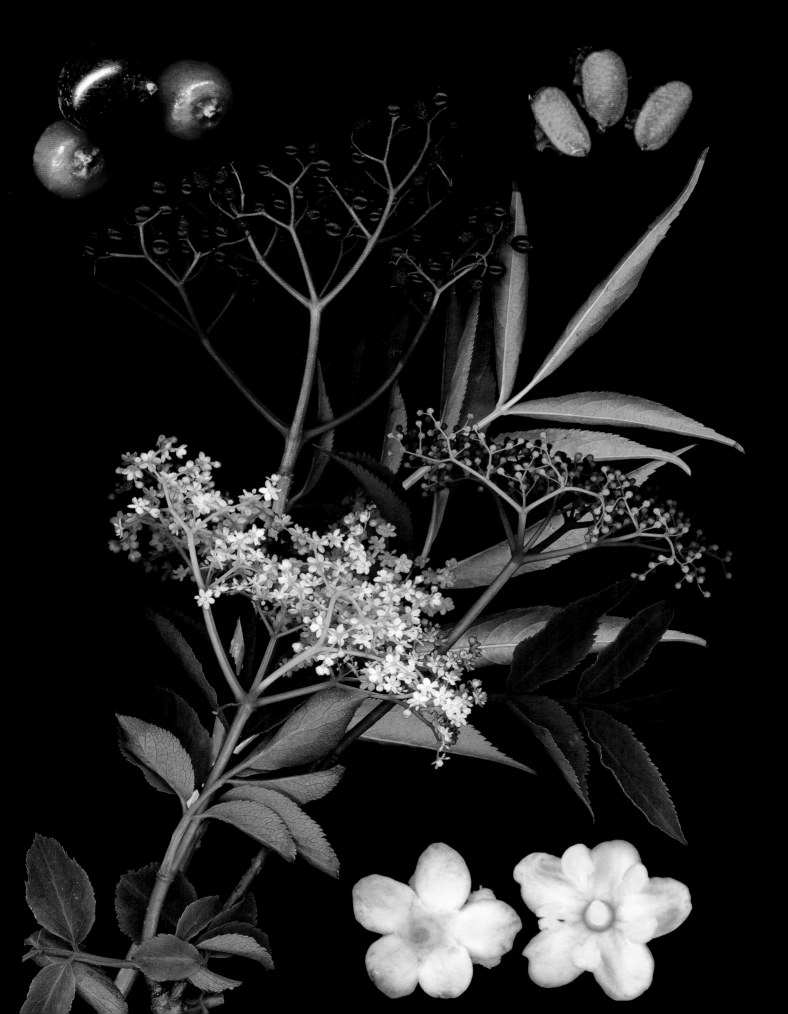

Black Elder

Sambucus nigra

FAMILY: CAPRIFOLIACEAE

Active elements:
Berries: phenolic components (including cyanidin), flavonoids, vitamins A and C. Flowers: flavonoids, phenolic acids, sterols, mucilage, tannins.

Ancient Greek physicians, including Hippocrates and Galen, were among the first to laud the virtues of the Elder. The latter recommended it for catarrh and excessive mucus. In the Middle Ages, Elder Water (water in which flowers had been macerated) was used to lighten the complexion and remove freckles. The flowers and fruit have long been the basis for refreshing drinks. In springtime, great quantities were drunk to purify the body of the toxins accumulated over the winter.

All parts a laxative

- The second bark, which has a strong, nauseous odour, is **diuretic and laxative**.
- The leaves appear to have the **same properties as the bark**, but are rarely used internally. They are **widely advocated for haemorrhoids and burns**.
- The fresh flowers are also laxative. The dried flowers can be used to **stimulate perspiration** (sudorific) in various ailments, such as colds, flu, chronic bronchitis and bouts of rheumatism.
- The flowers' **softening, restorative and anti-inflammatory** properties mean they are used externally to treat chilblains, attacks of gout and eye inflammations.
- The **sudorific** berries are advocated for the alleviation of rheumatism and generalized oedema.

PRECAUTION FOR USE: respect the dose of 4 to 8g of berries per day, whatever form they are in. Above this dose, they become purgative.

OTHER USES: Elder flowers are used to flavour wine, vinegar and soft drinks and to make delicious tarts. Elderberry jams and jellies are slightly bland.

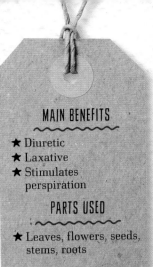

MAIN BENEFITS

★ Diuretic
★ Laxative
★ Stimulates perspiration

PARTS USED

★ Leaves, flowers, seeds, stems, roots

TOXICITY

If you collect the berries in the wild, make sure you do not confuse Black Elder with Dwarf Elder (*Sambucus ebulus*), which has poisonous berries.

METHOD OF USE

- **INTERNAL: Second bark decoction.** 45 to 60g (1½ to 2oz) per litre (quart) of water. Reduce to half and drink throughout the day as a diuretic.
Wine. Pour a litre of boiling wine over 150g (5¼oz) of the second bark. Steep for 48 hours and drink 2 small glasses (100g (3½oz)) per day for the same purpose.
Infusion. 50g (1¾oz) of dried flowers per litre of boiling water. Infuse for 10 minutes. Drink 4 or 5 cups daily as a sudorific and for rheumatism.
Juice of the pressed berries. 20 to 30g (¾ to 1oz) to be taken in the morning as a purgative.
Elderberry rob. Crush the berries and leave in an uncovered bowl for 24 hours. Press to extract the juice. Allow the juice to evaporate in a *bain-marie*, until it reaches the consistency of honey. Take 4 to 8g as a sudorific.
- **EXTERNAL: Concentrated infusion.** 100g (3½oz) of flowers per litre of water. Use to soak compresses for gum and cheek inflammations, eczema and dry skin. Excellent for puffy eyes.

Description

A shrub growing to a few metres in height, native to Europe and Asia, common in hedgerows and on rubble. Its light-coloured bark has numerous, characteristic corky lenticels. The large opposite, composite leaves have five to seven broad, pointed leaflets, which exude an unpleasant smell when crushed. The small, creamy-white flowers are grouped in large terminal corymbs, and have an intense, musky scent. The fruit are small, glossy black berries, filled with purple juice and multiple seeds.

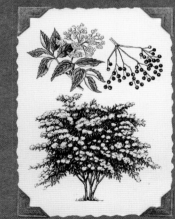

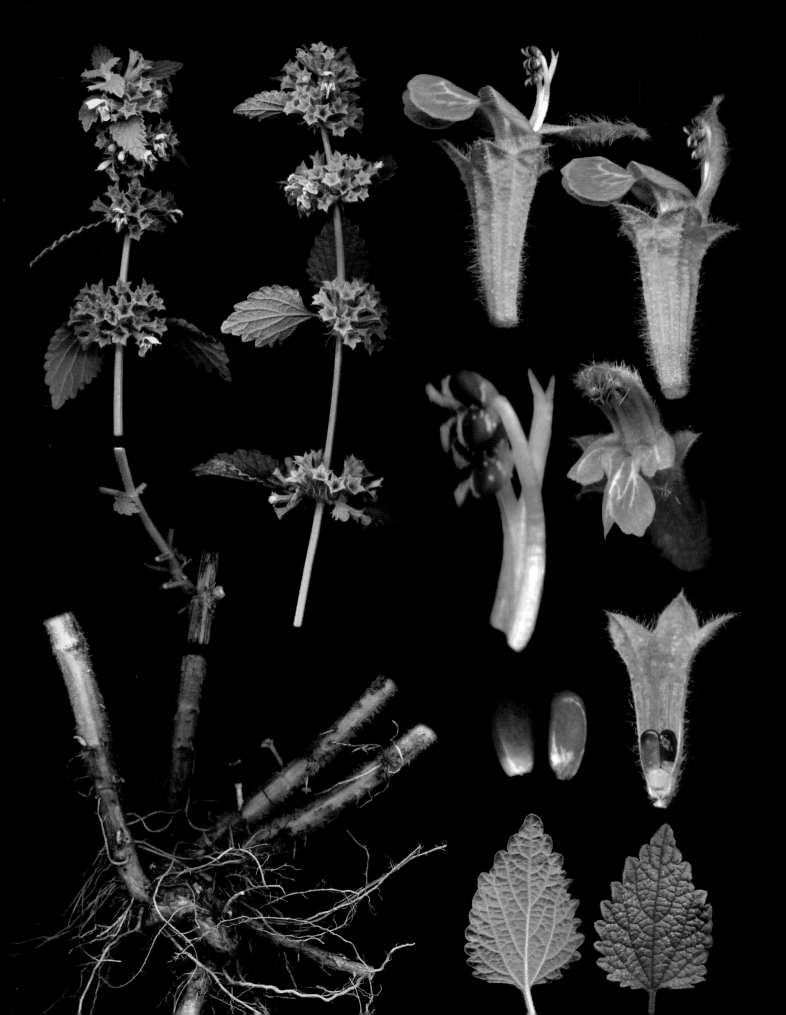

Black Horehound

Ballota nigra
FAMILY: LAMIACEAE

Active elements:
Polyphenols: flavonoids, phenylpropanoid heterosides (including verbascoside); diterpenoid lactones (including marrubiin), vitamin C.

In the first century AD, Dioscorides used a mixture of Black Horehound leaves and honey to disinfect wounds and skin ulcers. He also advocated its use for dog bites.

For all ailments of nervous origin

• The flowering tops have proven **antispasmodic properties**. Black Horehound works as a successful **sedative** for all nervous disorders and is included in some pharmaceutical products.
• Although it is almost exclusively used as a sedative, it can also be taken as **a diuretic, antihelminthic and emmenagogue** (stimulates menstruation). Not only does it induce sleep and provide a better quality of rest for people who are anxious or tired, it is also used to treat various nervous disorders: anxiety, dizziness, hot flushes, palpitations, oesophageal spasms, urine incontinence in nervous children and hysteria. It also reduces whooping cough attacks.

• In the United States, it is used to **treat nausea and vomiting**, especially in infants.
• It also has an **antioxidant** effect because of its high level of polyphenols, and may contribute to the protection of the cardiovascular system.

DID YOU KNOW?
Studies have confirmed the sedative and anxiety-reducing effects of Black Horehound, which works on the central nervous system in the same way as benzodiazepines.

MAIN BENEFITS
★ Antispasmodic
★ Calming

PARTS USED
★ Whole plant

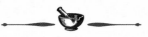

METHOD OF USE

• **INTERNAL: Infusion.** Prepared with 30 to 60g (1 to 2oz) of plant per litre (quart) of water, however it has a particularly unpleasant smell and taste. Drink 2 or 3 cups per day, including one just before bed, as a sedative.
Tincture. Tastes nicer than the infusion. Made with one tightly packed glass of the plant steeped for at least 15 days in 2 glasses of a colourless spirit. Strain, filter and store in a capped bottle. Take a teaspoonful 3 or 4 times a day, depending on the intensity of the ailment.
Black Horehound **wine** (tastes almost as bad as the infusion). Add 50g (1¾oz) of dry plant to a litre of boiling white wine and steep for 6 hours. After filtering, drink half a glass before meals.

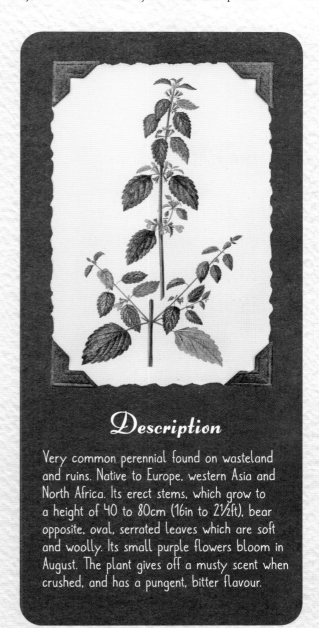

Description

Very common perennial found on wasteland and ruins. Native to Europe, western Asia and North Africa. Its erect stems, which grow to a height of 40 to 80cm (16in to 2½ft), bear opposite, oval, serrated leaves which are soft and woolly. Its small purple flowers bloom in August. The plant gives off a musty scent when crushed, and has a pungent, bitter flavour.

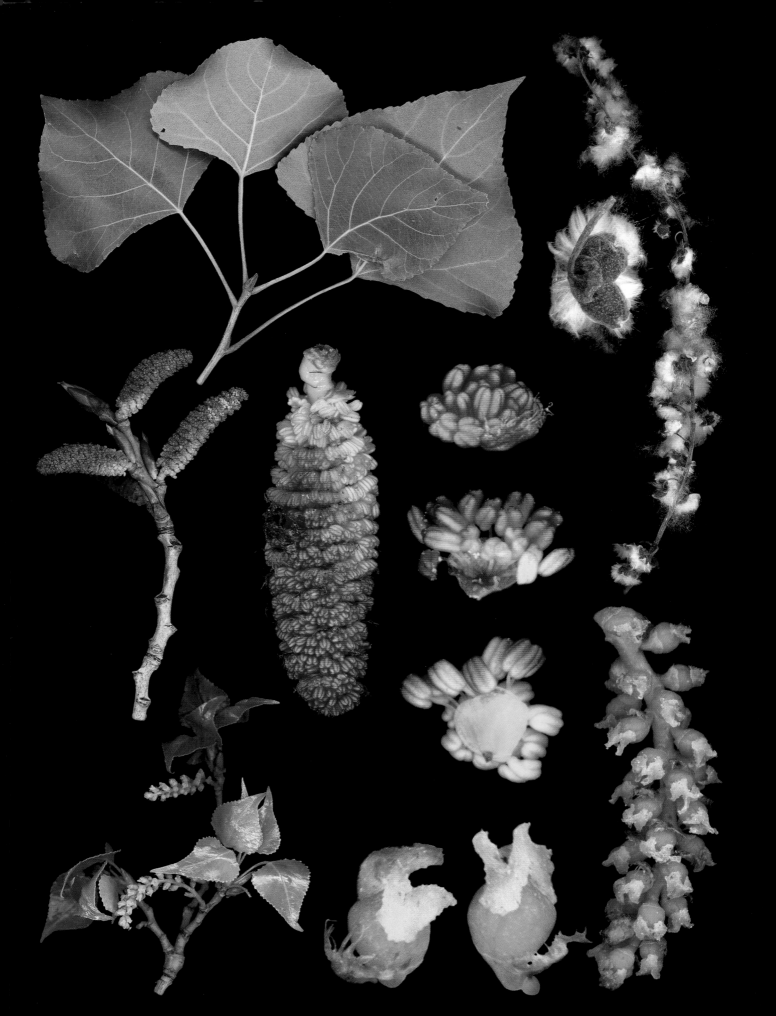

Black Poplar

Populus nigra

FAMILY: SALICACEAE

Active elements:

Buds, bark of the young branches: phenolic glucosides (including salicin), fatty acids, flavonoids, tannins, salicylates, an aromatic oil rich in alpha- and beta-caryophyllene.

MAIN BENEFITS

★ Diuretic
★ Anti-rheumatic
★ Bacterial infections
★ Haemorrhoids
★ Healing

PARTS USED

★ Buds, bark

Poplar unguent (*unguentum populeum*) was a widely used Renaissance herbal medicine, made with a few leaves of Belladonna, Henbane, Nightshade and Poppy, with the addition of Poplar buds. It was lauded in 1538 by the French apothecary and poet, Thibault Lespleigney. This soothing ointment was widely used, especially for haemorrhoids and rheumatic pains. However, Poplar buds were actually the only thing in it that did not present a danger to humans.

Super buds

• It is mainly the buds of the Black Poplar that are used in herbal medicine. They have **diuretic and anti-rheumatic** properties (they increase the volume of urine and eliminate uric acid) and also have a sedative effect on joint pains. They can be used to relieve **muscle aches** following sporting exertions.

• Their **expectorant and antiseptic** properties make them useful for treating coughs and bronchial congestion. Their resin, akin to the propolis compound produced by bees, with proven antibiotic action, is effective on bacterial infections and fungal diseases.

• Externally, Poplar buds are used to **treat superficial wounds**.

• They are well known for their ability to **cure haemorrhoids**, and their healing power extends to **chilblains and chapped and cracked skin**.

• The charcoal obtained by burning the Poplar is good at **absorbing intestinal gases**.

• Bark from young branches that are 2 to 3 years old has **astringent, tonic and febrifugal** properties.

OTHER SPECIES: Bark of the Aspen (*Populus tremula*) contains higher levels of salicin and populin than Black Poplar and has the same antipyretic and anti-inflammatory properties as Willow. It is advocated for rheumatic pain and to reduce fever.

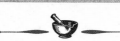

METHOD OF USE

• **INTERNAL: Infusion.** 15 to 30g (½ to 1oz) of buds per litre (quart) of boiling water or sweetened wine. Steep for 30 minutes; drink 3 glasses per day for rheumatism and muscle aches, **Poplar charcoal** should be used at a dose of 2g per day, to treat gut fermentation.

• **EXTERNAL: Macerate** 100g (3½oz) of crushed buds in a litre of colourless spirits. Wait at least one month before using. Massage into joints or muscles to relieve aches and pains.

Oil. Place 200g (7oz) of crushed buds in half a litre of olive oil in a *bain-marie* over boiling water and cook for 1 or 2 hours. Strain. Use in ointments to treat wounds and cracks.

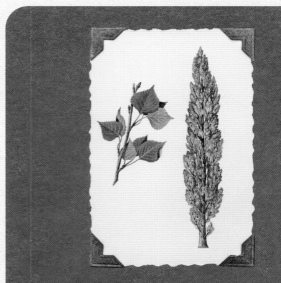

Description

A common tree on riverbanks and in wet places, reaching 25m (82ft) in height. It is widely cultivated, especially the columnar form known as the Italian Poplar. The bark of the trunk is deeply furrowed. Its broad, almost triangular leaves are glossy on both sides. The buds are covered with a yellow resinous substance that exudes a strong balsamic fragrance. The flowers take the form of reddish, pendulous male catkins and smaller, green female catkins. The flowers produce seeds covered in a fluffy down.

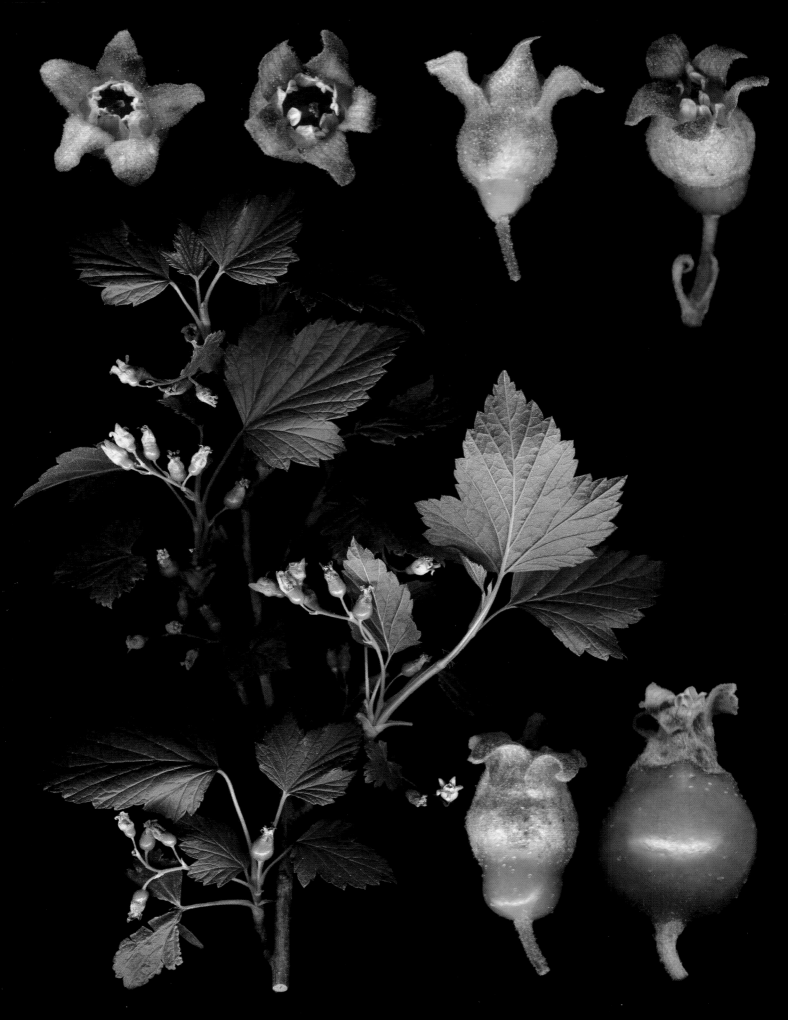

Blackcurrant

Ribes nigrum

FAMILY: GROSSULARIACEAE

Active elements:
Leaves: flavonoids, tannins, aromatic oil.
Fruit: sugars, organic acids, pectin, flavonoids, anthocyanosides, high level of vitamin C.

Native to northern and central Europe, Blackcurrant has only been consumed since the 16th century. In the 18th century, people attributed it with a wide range of properties. It was said to be effective "against fevers, plague, smallpox, worms, all bites and stings.... It cures jaundice, gravel, and alleviates the trying vapours of melancholy". Praise indeed! In 1757, a J. B. P. de Beaumont even published a *Traité du Cassis* ("Blackcurrant Treaty"), in which he emphasized that blackcurrant could ensure a youthful old age.

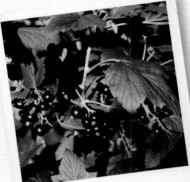

Blackcurrant berries are a popular fruit.

They are used both internally and externally to **relieve joint pains**.

• According to recent research, they stimulate the production of cortisol by the adrenal glands and consequently the **sympathetic activity of the nervous system**. As a result, they contribute to **decreasing the symptoms of stress**.

• They can be used, as gargles, to **soothe sore throats and mouth ulcers**.

• The berries contain around 200mg of vitamin C per 100g. In addition, the vitamin C in Blackcurrant is remarkably stable and is preserved, unlike that of citrus fruit for example. As a result of this vitamin C, Blackcurrant fruit and juice has a **general tonic** effect during infectious processes and **stimulates resistance to infections**.

• The berries are also said to **contribute to eye health** on a day-to-day basis because of their high anthocyanoside content.

Multiple benefits

• Blackcurrant leaves have **diuretic and anti-rheumatic** properties. They help eliminate uric acid and purines, so are indicated for the general treatment of arthritis and arthrosclerosis.

Description

A bush, growing to a height of 1m (3¼ft), native to central and northern Europe, as well as Asia. It is often cultivated in gardens along with other Grossulariaceae. Blackcurrants have three- or five-lobed leaves and greenish or reddish flowers in hanging clusters. The black berries have an aromatic, musky and very fruity flavour. The leaves give off a pleasant smell when crushed.

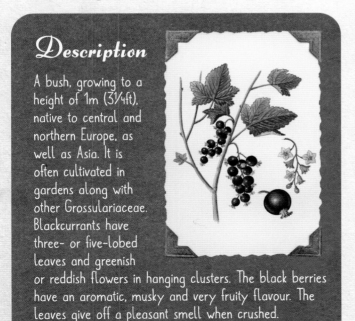

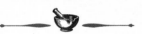

METHOD OF USE

• **INTERNAL: Juice, syrup, jelly.** Prepared with the berries, all of these are not only therapeutic but also taste delicious, and can be consumed whenever the properties of Blackcurrant are required. **Blackcurrant wine.** Steep 500g (17½oz) of berries in a litre (quart) of red wine for 3 days. Strain and add sugar syrup. Drink a glass before each meal to alleviate lymphatism, nutritional disorders and symptoms of ageing.

Crème de cassis. Put dry berries in a bottle, alternating a layer of fruit with a layer of granulated sugar. Seal and leave to steep for several months, shaking from time to time. Filter the liqueur obtained.

Infusion. 50g (1¾oz) of Blackcurrant leaves per litre of boiling water. Infuse for 10 minutes. Drink 3 cups a day between meals for rheumatism. The treatment should be followed for at least 6 months.

• **EXTERNAL:** For insect bites (wasp, hornet), crush Blackcurrant leaves and squeeze the juice onto the painful area. The pain is drawn out very quickly and the swelling reabsorbed.

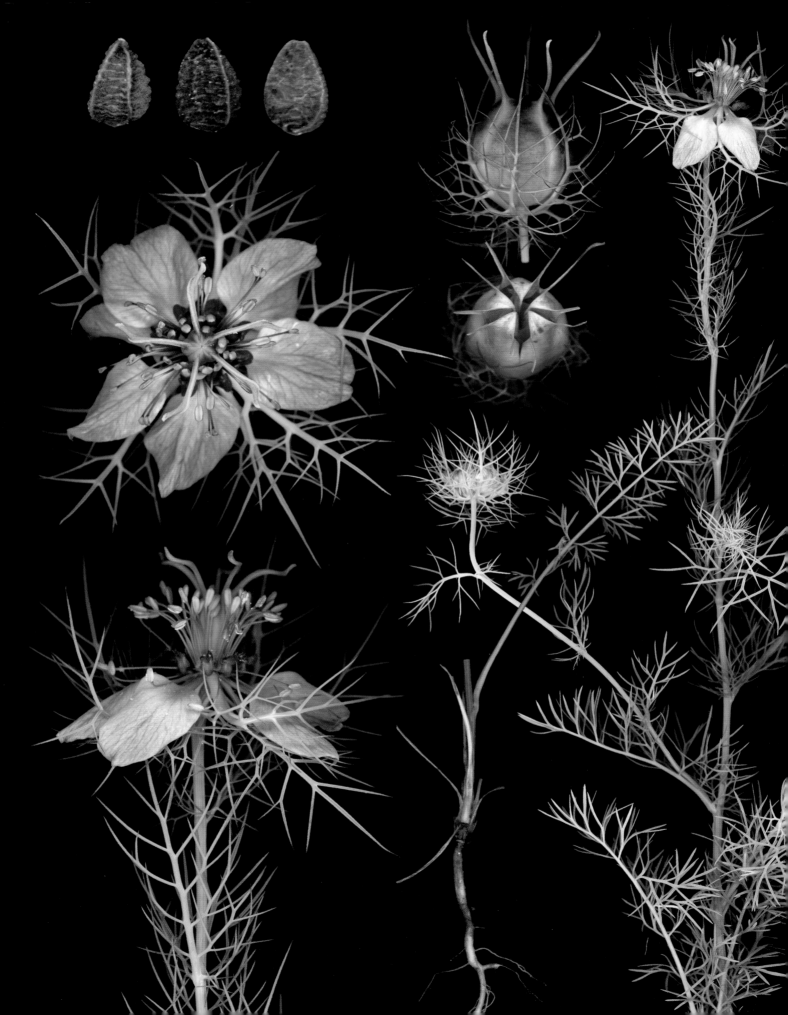

Blackseed

Nigella sativa

FAMILY: RANUNCULACEAE

Active elements:
Seeds: around 40% fatty oil, a saponoside (melanthin), aromatic oil.

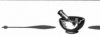

Also widely known as Black Caraway and Black Cumin, Blackseed has a history as a medicinal plant going right back to ancient times; some of its seeds were even found in Tutankhamen's tomb. Dioscorides, the Green physician, lauded its virtues in treating headaches and toothaches. It is widely used in Africa, the Middle East and Asia. Its traditional uses, which are associated with the treatment of numerous ailments, have often been validated by scientific research.

Miracle oil

- Blackseed (often known as Nigella seeds) **promotes digestion** and expels gas from the intestines.
- It is an anthelmintic (vermifuge), successfully ridding the body of various parasitic worms.
- Blackseed **relieves respiratory tract inflammations** and alleviates menstrual pains.
- In India, it is prescribed to nursing mothers to **increase milk production**.
- An amber, **aromatic oil** can be extracted using a press, and is considered a panacea in North Africa. It is especially used topically to **treat skin problems** (irritation, eczema, acne), rheumatic pains and asthma.
- Blackseed continues to be the subject of studies seeking to confirm its properties. These have demonstrated that it is **antibacterial and antifungal**. It also **stimulates the immune system**. Blackseed oil has also shown anti-tumoural activity in the laboratory, but it is not yet known whether it could be successfully used in treating or preventing cancer.

OTHER SPECIES: A close relation, Love-in-a-Mist (*Nigella damascena*), a native of the Mediterranean basin, is grown in ornamental gardens for its beautiful blue or white flowers and attractive, finely dissected leaves. Its small black seeds have an unusual smell, reminiscent of artificial strawberry flavouring. They were highly regarded as a spice in Europe up until the 17th century.

OTHER USES: Nigella seeds are used with vegetables and pulses. They are used in Indian cooking in different spice blends, such as Five Spice (*Panch Phorton*) with cumin, fennel, mustard and fenugreek. Blackseed is sprinkled on breads such as nan.

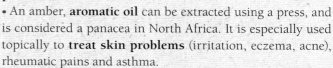

MAIN BENEFITS
- ★ Digestive
- ★ Anthelmintic
- ★ Promotes lactation

PARTS USED
- ★ Seeds

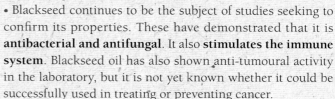

METHOD OF USE

Blackseed is most often used in the form of the oil that can be pressed from its seeds. This can also be found in capsule form (follow the dosage given on the packet).
- **INTERNAL:** 1 to 3 teaspoonsful per meal, or 1 large tablespoonful in the evening. For children, ½ to 1 teaspoonful per day.
- **EXTERNAL:** Pure oil for topical use, to nourish the skin and for a beautiful complexion.

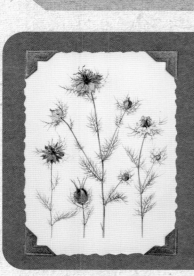

Description

Small annual plant growing to between 10 and 50cm (4in to 1½ft), growing wild in North Africa and western Asia. It has long been grown in the gardens and fields of the Mediterranean basin. Its upright stems bear finely dissected leaves and pale blue flowers with numerous stamens. The fruits are capsules containing a multitude of small, black, aromatic seeds.

TOXICITY
The use of Blackseed during pregnancy is strongly discouraged. The consumption of just 20g (¾oz) can trigger miscarriage.

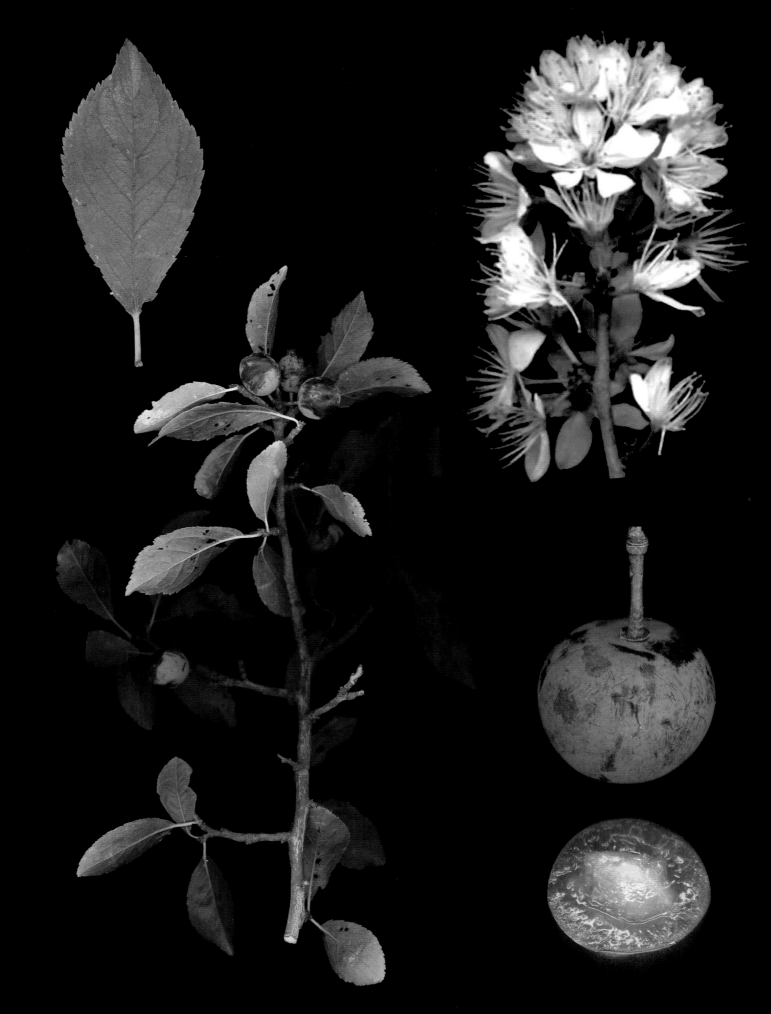

Blackthorn

Prunus spinosa
FAMILY: ROSACEAE

Active elements:
Bark: rich in tannins. Flowers: cyanogenic heteroside (produced by hydrolysis of hydrogen cyanide and benzoic aldehyde, with a smell of bitter almond). Fruit: tannins, organic acids, anthocyanosides and vitamins.

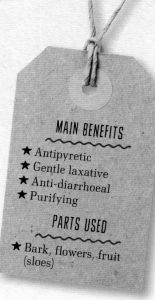

In days gone by, every part of this shrub was used for medical purposes. The bark contains numerous tannins and is astringent: it was used in the past as an antipyretic. The flowers, which taste of bitter almonds, were recommended as laxatives. However, they were also used as calmatives, diuretics and depuratives (purifiers), and enjoyed a certain renown as treatments to drain off fluid from serous ailments.

OTHER USES: An excellent way of preserving sloes is to pickle them, a traditional French countryside practice. Simply place them in an airtight jar, cover with brine (salt water) and store at room temperature. A process of lactic fermentation, as used in making sauerkraut, takes place and after three weeks the sloes can be eaten like olives. They are salty, acidulous and very aromatic, without the slightest bitterness. On the tree, sloes soften when the icy weather arrives. They can then be made into jams, compotes, tarts and syrups. Sloe berries are sometimes distilled into a fragrant alcohol, which is particularly popular in Romania and the countries of the former Yugoslavia. Blackthorn blossoms perfume the liqueurs, imparting a light, bitter almond scent.

Each part has its benefits

• The bark can be used to **reduce fevers (antipyretic)**.
• The flowers have a **gentle laxative power**. They are also expectorant, tonic, diuretic and sudorific (sweat inducing), which gives them **detoxifying** properties.
• The leaves are indicated for **relieving inflammation of the ear, nose and throat**. Like the flowers, they are antispasmodic and anti-inflammatory.
• The fruit (sloe) gathered before maturity is highly astringent and consequently a great natural **cure for diarrhoea**. A gargle of the fresh juice soothes **inflammation of the oral mucosa** (ulcers, gingivitis) and throat.

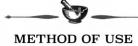

METHOD OF USE

• **INTERNAL: Decoction.** 30 to 60g (1 to 2oz) of bark per litre (quart) of water. Boil for 15 minutes and drink half a litre over 24 hours for fever.
Infusion. 60 to 80g (2 to 3oz) of flowers per litre of boiling water. Drink 2 cups per day between meals as a gentle laxative.
Decoction of sloes. 50g (1¾oz) of fresh or dried fruit per litre of water. Boil for a few minutes. Drink throughout the day until the diarrhoea has passed.

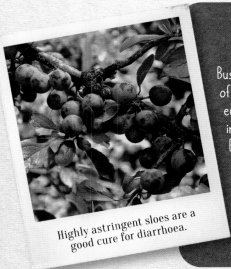

Highly astringent sloes are a good cure for diarrhoea.

Description

Bushy, very thorny shrub growing up to a height of 2m (6½ft), very common in hedgerows, on the edge of woodland and on uncultivated land. Found in Europe, western Asia and North Africa. The Blackthorn is sometimes used to make defensive barriers. It has small, serrated leaves and clusters of white flowers, each with five petals. Its fruit, sloes, are the size of blueberries and turn a bluish black on maturity. Their tart pulp is both acidic and astringent.

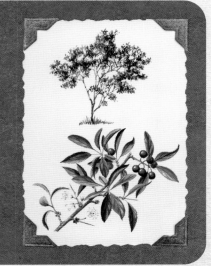

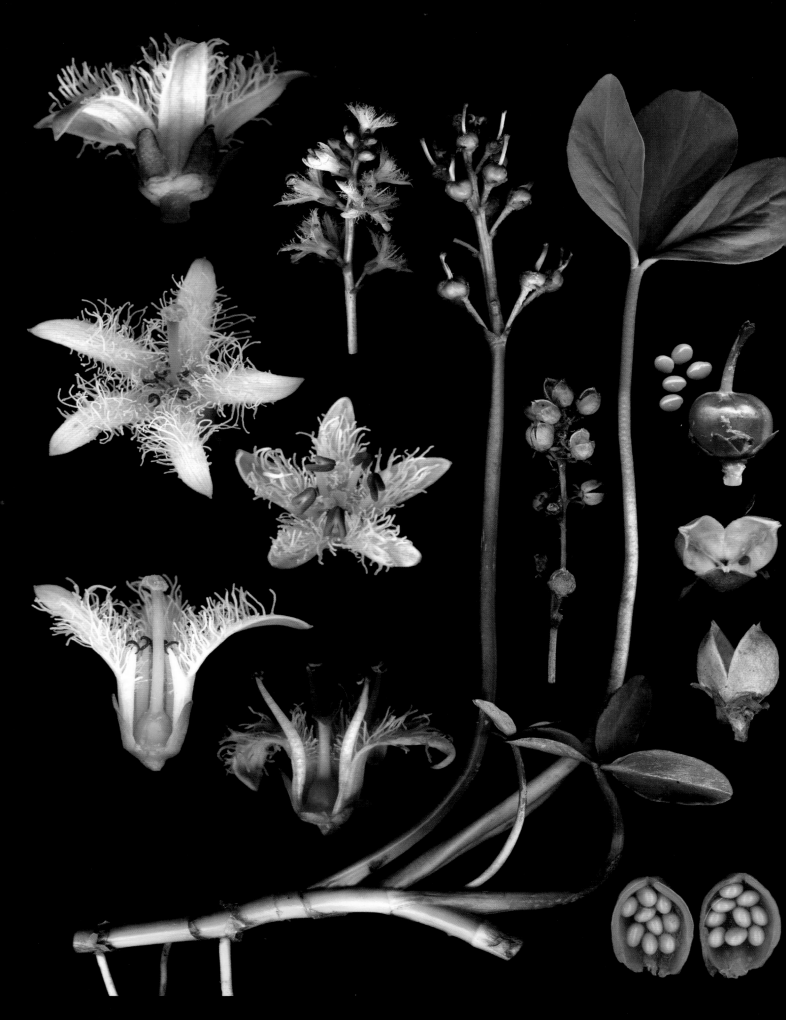

Bogbean

Menyanthes trifoliata

FAMILY: MENYANTHACEAE

Active elements:

Tannins, flavonoids, phenol acids, phytosterols, iridoids (responsible for the plant's bitterness).

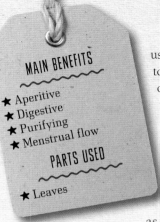
In the 17th century, Simon Paulli, the Danish physician and naturalist, used vitamin C-rich Bogbean to cure scurvy. Physicians of the renowned Liège medical school and Leclerc, the French physician and medical herbalist, likewise advocated its use for this purpose. It was considered to be a febrifuge, as suggested by its old French and German common name, "Fever Clover" (Bogbean is still used to bring down fever in some regions). Jean-François Cazin, the 19th-century French doctor and botanist used it to treat rickets, scrofula, sluggish stomach and skin complaints as well as gout, rheumatism and arthritis. In Swedish traditional medicine it is used to treat inflammatory ailments affecting the kidney and in Britain to relieve rheumatism. In the 19th century, the German-Swiss botanist, Ferdinand Otto Wolf, noted that according to traditional belief, "a cup of Bogbean tea, taken every day, [can] prolong life".

A bitter aperitive and digestive

• Generally speaking, the properties of Bogbean are similar to those of Gentian. Like Gentian, it is a **bitter tonic with aperitive qualities** (it stimulates salivary and gastric secretions), which are also beneficial in cases of dyspeptic complaints (slow and difficult digestion). Consequently, it helps **treat headaches linked to poor digestion**. By aiding digestion, it has a tonic effect on the body.

• Bogbean is also a **depurative** (it helps to 'flush' toxins from the body), which explains why it is used in the **treatment of skin problems** such as eczema or acne. It is an anthelmintic and emmenagogue (stimulating and increasing menstrual flow).

• Studies have shown that Bogbean has **anti-inflammatory properties**. It also stimulates the immune system, helping to ward off infection. In the laboratory, Bogbean has demonstrated anti-cancer properties on several tumour cells lines.

OTHER USES: Bogbean has been used instead of Hop to flavour beer.

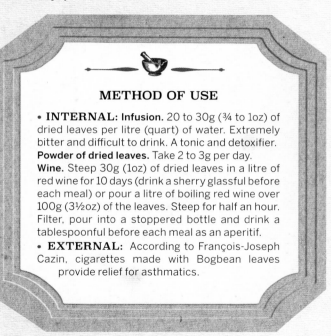

METHOD OF USE

• **INTERNAL: Infusion.** 20 to 30g (¾ to 1oz) of dried leaves per litre (quart) of water. Extremely bitter and difficult to drink. A tonic and detoxifier.
Powder of dried leaves. Take 2 to 3g per day.
Wine. Steep 30g (1oz) of dried leaves in a litre of red wine for 10 days (drink a sherry glassful before each meal) or pour a litre of boiling red wine over 100g (3½oz) of the leaves. Steep for half an hour. Filter, pour into a stoppered bottle and drink a tablespoonful before each meal as an aperitif.

• **EXTERNAL:** According to François-Joseph Cazin, cigarettes made with Bogbean leaves provide relief for asthmatics.

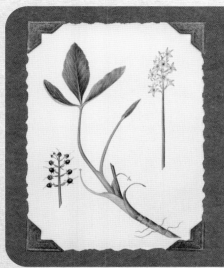

Description

Aquatic perennial found in swamps and bogs in the north and the mountains of Europe, Asia and America. Occasionally grown to decorate water features. The stem is a thick, spongy rhizome bearing trifoliate leaves with a long, sheathed petiole, reminiscent of clover. Its pretty pinkish-white flowers bloom in spikes, at the end of a long, bare stem, from April to June. The whole plant is very bitter.

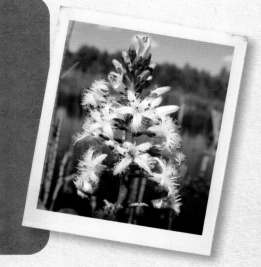

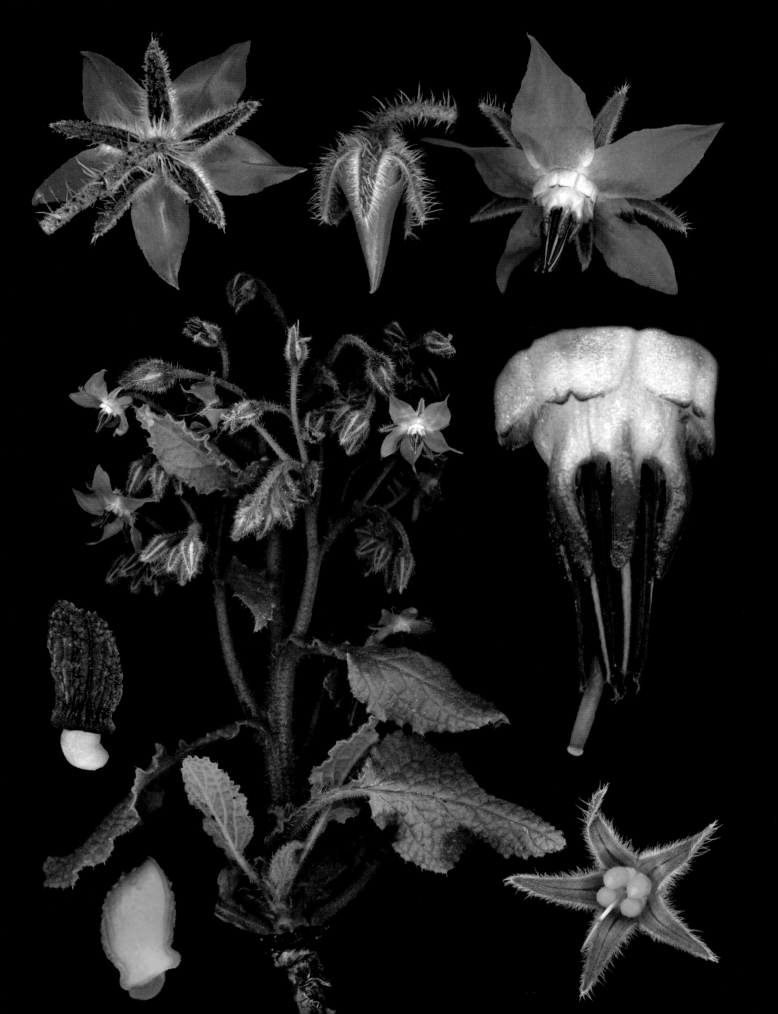

Borage

Borago officinalis

FAMILY: BORAGINACEAE

Active elements:

Mucilage, tannins, potassium nitrate, pyrrolizidine alkaloids. The seeds contain a fatty oil rich in gamma-linolenic acid (omega-6).

The ancient Greeks used Borage flowers to perfume salads and wines. They named it *euphrosyne* meaning "cheerful". The plant is believed to have been introduced to southern Spain by the Arabs in the Middle Ages. Moreover, its name derives from the Arabic *abou er-rach* ("father of sweat"), an allusion to its sudorific properties. References to Borage appear in poems of the Schola Medica Salernitana (9–13th century): *Ego Borago, Gaudia semper ago* ("I, Borage, always bring courage").

Wonderful oil of Borage

• The flowers are used as a **sudorific** (sweat inducer) for chills, colds, bronchitis and rheumatism.
• The high mucilage content in Borage makes it an **effective emollient**. It relieves respiratory disorders.
• Its significant potassium nitrate content makes Borage an **excellent diuretic**. It is advocated as a treatment for eruptive fevers (measles, scarlet fever, smallpox) and a purifier for skin diseases, particularly herpes.
• A poultice made from the leaves **soothes skin irritations**.
• Borage oil, generally taken in the form of capsules, has an effect akin to evening primrose oil on disorders as wide-ranging as **premenstrual tension (PMT), atherosclerosis, diabetes, liver problems, arthritis and schizophrenia**.
• It is used to **maintain skin elasticity** and prevent the appearance of wrinkles.

OTHER USES: The young leaves taste of cucumber. They are good in salads. The older leaves can be cooked in the same way as spinach or deep fried in batter. In Greece they are stuffed with rice or bulgur wheat and herbs to make dolmades, instead of vine leaves. In Spain, a variety with white flowers is cultivated and sold in the markets. This variety has thick petioles and is eaten like Chard. The flowers have an unusual taste, reminiscent of oysters. Borage's bright blue corollas can be added to salads or used to decorate *canapés*.

MAIN BENEFITS

★ Acute bronchitis
★ Diuretic
★ Anti-inflammatory
★ Skincare

PARTS USED

★ Flowers
★ Parts of plant above the ground
★ Seeds

METHOD OF USE

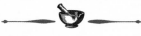

• **INTERNAL: Infusion.** Infuse 20 to 40g (¾ to 1½oz) of flowers per litre (quart) of boiling water. Drink 3 or 4 cups per day to bring on a healthy perspiration.
Decoction of flowers, leaves and young branches (about 15g (½oz) of each per litre of water), as a purifier and for respiratory ailments.

Description

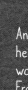

An annual that grows in clumps to a height of 30 to 50cm (1 to 1½ft) on wasteland, especially in the South of France. It is native to the Mediterranean basin. Its thick stem and large, slightly fleshy, wavy, dull green leaves are covered with coarse hairs. Borage can be easily identified by its attractive, sky-blue flowers (occasionally pink or white) formed of five petals in a star shape around a protruding heart, which bloom in May–June.

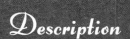

TOXICITY

Administered in high doses on a regular basis, some pyrrolizidine alkaloids have been shown to be toxic in experiments on laboratory animals, causing liver tumours. Borage leaves and flowers contain a small amount, but no problems subsequent to their use have ever been recorded.

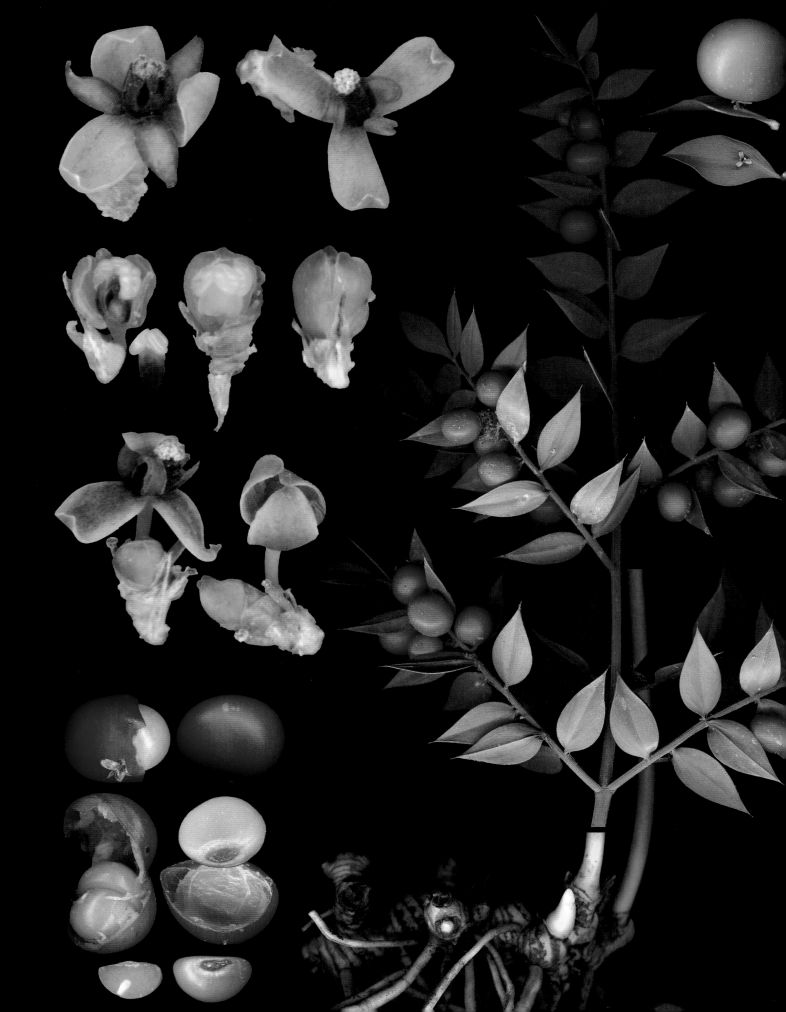

Butcher's Broom

For the circulation and as treatment for haemorrhoids

Ruscus aculeatus

FAMILY: ASPARAGACEAE

Active elements:
Rhizome: sterols, flavonoids, benzofuran, steroid saponosides, giving ruscogenin and neoruscogenin.

Highly praised by Dioscorides, Butcher's Broom is one of the traditional five "opening roots" that are aperitive and diuretic. It has been prescribed for gout-sufferers since time immemorial. It was also used to treat oedema, calculi, ailments of the urinary tract, tissue inflammation, jaundice and iron-deficiency.

TOXICITY

The attractive red fruit should be treated as slightly toxic because of its high saponin content.

• Butcher's Broom is a **vasoconstrictor and venotonic**. It fortifies vein walls, alleviating heavy legs, nocturnal calf cramps and itching, and wards off thrombosis.

• It also helps **improve lymphatic circulation** and tackle swelling (oedema) of the lower limbs. It is effective against post-surgical lymphoedema.

• Butcher's Broom is also advocated for the **treatment of fragile capillaries** that cause the tiny red dots known as petechiae and the larger bruised areas of ecchymoses.

• Butcher's Broom can boast remarkable success in **treating haemorrhoid flare-ups**.

• It **prevents inflammation and exudation** of damage-related fluid build-ups so is recommended whenever there is a vein-related inflammatory reaction, in particular following chronic venous insufficiency.

• According to some studies, ruscogenin can be used to **treat orthostatic hypotension** (a sudden drop in blood pressure on standing up, accompanied by nausea) which is common among people who are bedridden for significant periods of time, without increasing their blood pressure when supine, unlike classic blood-pressure medication.

• Butcher's broom invigorates the skin and **lessens the appearance of wrinkles**.

OTHER USES: Butcher's Broom is a cousin of asparagus and is likewise edible. In springtime, young shoots of a beautiful, glossy purple appear, fragile as glass, in the midst of the spiny tufts. They can be eaten raw or cooked.

METHOD OF USE

• **INTERNAL:** Decoction. 20 to 40g (¾ to 1½oz) of root per litre (quart) of water, boil for 15 minutes. Use for vein problems.

• **EXTERNAL:** Sold as **suppositories** or **ointment**, Butcher's Broom is a proven remedy for haemorrhoids. It is also used in ointments as the refining active ingredient for treating wrinkles or bags under the eyes.

Description

A bushy, evergreen sub-shrub, growing to a height of 30 to 80cm (1 to 2½ft), found on rocky, uncultivated ground and in dry woodland. Its upright stems are bare at the base, with multiplying branches towards the top, forming compact tufts. The flat, dark-green "cladodes", or new stems, look like stiff, spine-tipped leaves. The real leaves are barely visible, membranous scales. The small, greenish flowers have six petals and appear in winter in the middle of the cladodes. These produce the large, bright red berries.

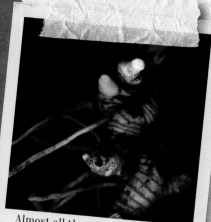

Almost all the active principles of Butcher's Broom are concentrated in its rhizome.

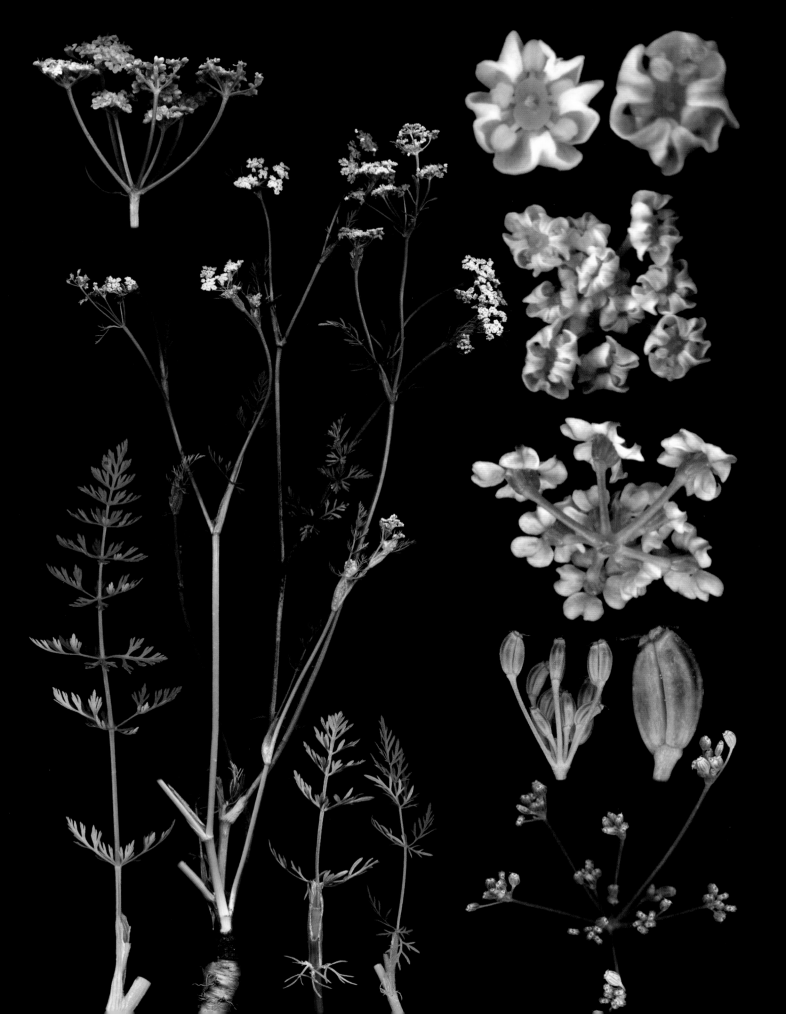

Caraway

Carum carvi

FAMILY: APIACEAE

Active elements:

Aromatic oil rich in carvone and limonene, polyphenols, petroselinic acid, polysaccharides.

northern Europe. It is used to flavour sauerkraut, bread (Pumpernickel), as well as Münster and Gouda cheese. In German, it is called Kümmel, and is distilled into an alcohol of the same name. The dried seeds are generally used, but when fresh, their flavour provides delicious citrus notes. They are used successfully by some creative cooks. Caraway can be given to both horses and dogs, especially as a stimulant.

In the 17th century, Caraway was advocated as a remedy for colds and flatulence, as well to increase "urine emissions". Caraway counted along with Cumin, Aniseed and Fennel as one of the traditional "four hot seeds" in French herbalism.

DID YOU KNOW? The Dutch claim that eating Caraway hones the memory and helps students to pass exams. Artists used to consume Caraway seeds to help them find inspiration.

An excellent digestive

• Caraway is a great carminative, and **relieves digestive problems**, such as a sluggish stomach or flatulence (carminative). It is **especially advocated for aerophagia** (excessive swallowing of air), as it is effective in clearing gas from the stomach.
• The seeds can be used as **stimulants, diuretics, anthelmintics and to promote milk flow (galactogenous) and menstruation (emmenagogues)**.

OTHER USES: Caraway, often confused with Cumin (*Cuminum cyminum*, which is also a digestive), is a typical condiment of

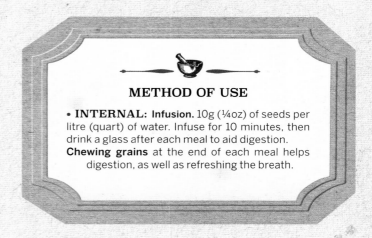

METHOD OF USE

• **INTERNAL: Infusion.** 10g (¼oz) of seeds per litre (quart) of water. Infuse for 10 minutes, then drink a glass after each meal to aid digestion. **Chewing grains** at the end of each meal helps digestion, as well as refreshing the breath.

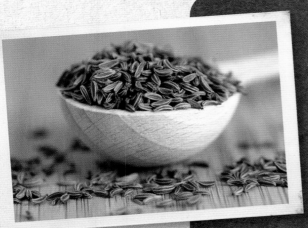

Caraway seeds are aromatic, and are commonly used to flavour cheeses, particularly the famous Leyden, or "Caraway Gouda".

Description

A perennial plant, growing to a height of 30 to 80cm (1 to 2½ft), common on mountain pastures throughout Europe and Asia. The Caraway looks like carrot, with its thin, smooth leaves growing at widely spaced intervals along the stem, ending abruptly in a small pointed tip, but it is not hairy. The white flowers cluster at the top of the stems in compound umbels with unequal rays. The berries, ripe in late summer, are very fragrant. They have a strongly aromatic flavour, with a slight spiciness.

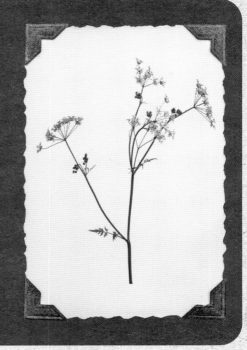

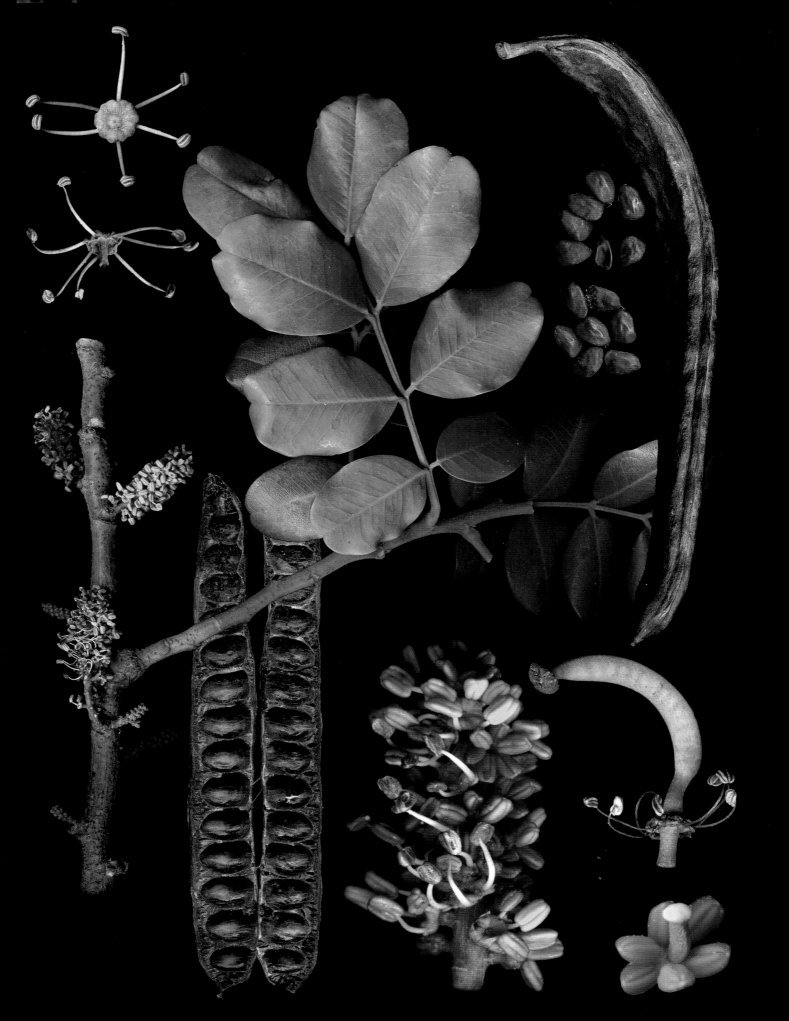

Carob

Ceratonia siliqua

FAMILY: FABACEAE

Active elements:
Pod: 40 to 50% soluble sugars, cyclitol, around 20% tannins. Seeds: gum made almost entirely of a complex sugar, galactomannan.

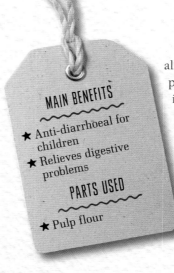

MAIN BENEFITS

★ Anti-diarrhoeal for children
★ Relieves digestive problems

PARTS USED

★ Pulp flour

Carob pods—also widely known as locust beans— have been consumed since earliest antiquity in the Mediterranean region, and their anti-diarrhoeal properties are well recorded. The Arabs considered the Carob an excellent expectorant softener and prescribed it for sufferers of chronic bronchitis.

A cocoa-flavoured anti-diarrhoeal agent

• Carob pulp flour is advocated for the **treatment of diarrhoea** in infants, children and adults. It has a general, positive effect on digestive disorders.

OTHER USES: The pods are very sweet and are delicious eaten raw. Some cultivated varieties release a juice as thick as honey when broken. The flavour of Carob pods is reminiscent of chocolate, to the extent that in the United States, Carob pod powder is a common substitute for cocoa. In Greece, a chocolate loaf is made with half ground Carob and half wheat flour. It is also used to make liqueurs. Carob pods reduced to flour, are used in the food industry, under the code E410, as a thickener in ice cream, pastries and in powdered milk for babies. Carob flour is also used in health food because, unlike wheat flour, it is gluten-free. Carob gum from the beans is used in the manufacture of paper, textiles, medicines and cosmetics.

DID YOU KNOW? Carob is also known as "St. John's Bread", as he is said to have eaten it during his life of abstinence in the desert. The seeds were the first "carats" of the jewellers of antiquity, who used them as a standard due to their uniform weight (one carat = 0.2g).

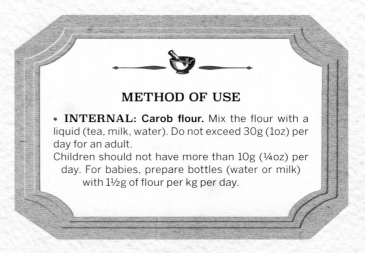

METHOD OF USE

• **INTERNAL: Carob flour.** Mix the flour with a liquid (tea, milk, water). Do not exceed 30g (1oz) per day for an adult.
Children should not have more than 10g (¼oz) per day. For babies, prepare bottles (water or milk) with 1½g of flour per kg per day.

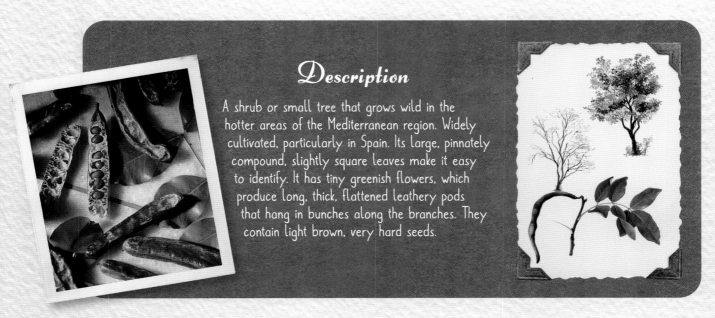

Description

A shrub or small tree that grows wild in the hotter areas of the Mediterranean region. Widely cultivated, particularly in Spain. Its large, pinnately compound, slightly square leaves make it easy to identify. It has tiny greenish flowers, which produce long, thick, flattened leathery pods that hang in bunches along the branches. They contain light brown, very hard seeds.

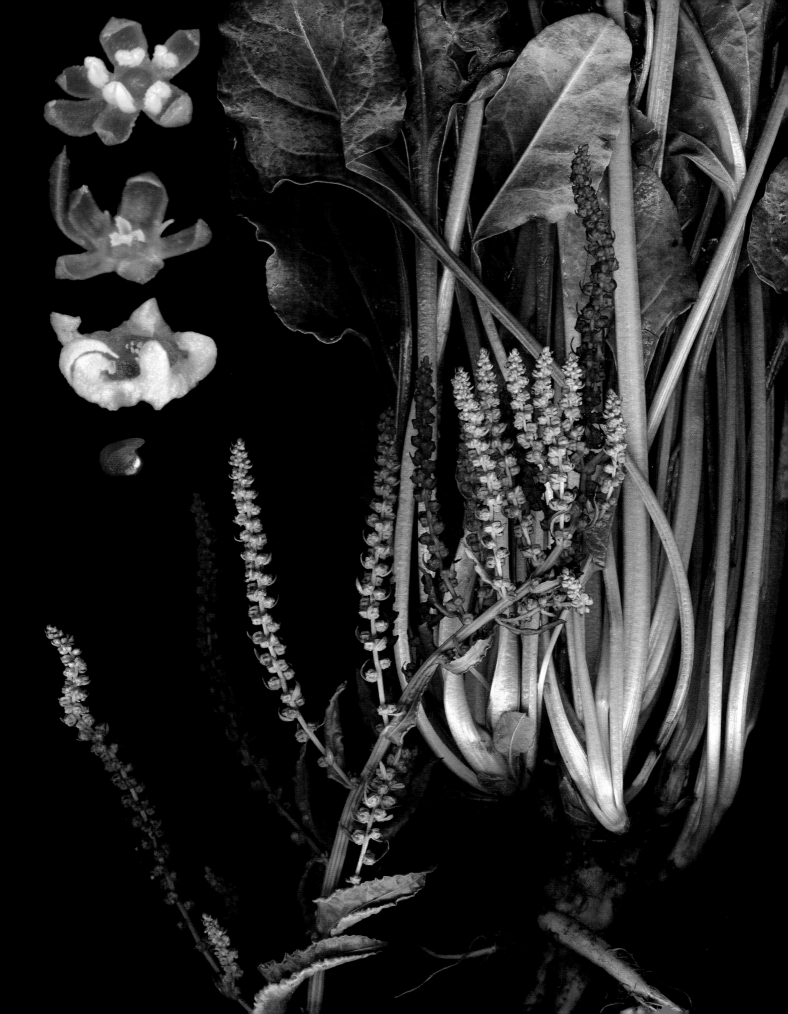

Chard

Beta vulgaris
FAMILY: AMARANTHACEAE

Active elements:
Betaine, betanin.
Roots: rich in saccharose.

The Romans ate Chard as a vegetable, but it was not held in high regard. Pliny, Cicero and Galen saw it as unhealthy, only to be tolerated by the robust stomachs of the poor. By contrast, it was very popular in the Middle Ages when Charlemagne recommended it be grown in his own gardens and those of the monasteries. The recipe for the French soup known as *potée*, in which Chard is a key ingredient and for which Arras is still famous, dates back to this period. The majority of towns in the north of France still have their *rue à la poirée* (a French name for the plant), which was historically the site of the vegetable market. Although Chard fell somewhat out of favour in the 19th century, it has a number of medicinal properties. The Arabs were the first to record the use of Chard for medicinal purposes, squirting the juice into the nostrils to treat epilepsy. In Lemery's 18th-century "Treatise on Drugs", he recommends this same therapeutic procedure, "to dissolve the nasal mucus, make people sneeze and unburden the brain". Joseph Roques and Jean-François Cazin, two great French medical herbalists of the 19th century advocated the use of Chard for calculi (stones) and constipation.

From leaves to roots

- Chard has **refreshing, emollient and laxative properties** and is also effective in reducing urinary tract inflammation.
- Betaine **encourages the regeneration of liver cells** and has a positive effect on fat metabolism.
- Beetroot, another variety of *Beta vulgaris*, is rich in betanin, which is said to **stimulate the immune system**.
- When used externally, Chard leaves are a soothing poultice for treating areas of **dry skin and cradle cap**.

DID YOU KNOW? The Creole word *brèdes* designates various leafy vegetables and a way of cooking them using onions, tomatoes and chilli pepper. This comes from the southern French term *blettes* referring to Chard leaves, which in turn comes from a vegetable highly prized by the Romans and known as the *blite*, an amaranth (*Amaranthus blitum*), today relegated to the rank of "weed".

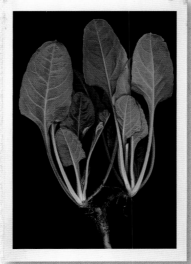

Chard leaves are a nice garnish on soup.

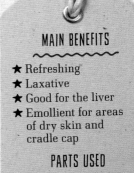
METHOD OF USE

- **INTERNAL:** Chard is a tasty addition to broths and soups or can just be puréed. It will relieve the liver and encourage healthy bowel movement. It can also be cooked *au gratin*, or Provençal style, with olive oil and garlic, then simmered with tomatoes.
- **EXTERNAL**: **Poultice** of crushed leaves, with maybe the addition of a little sweet almond oil. Use to treat skin ailments.

Description

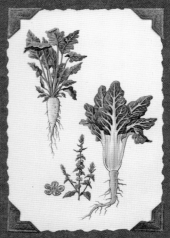

Sea Beet (*Beta vulgaris* subspecies *maritima*), is a wild ancestor of Chard and Beetroot. It is common along sea coasts from the Mediterranean to the Baltic. Like its wild cousin, Chard has large, fleshy leaves that are rubbery to the touch. The Swiss Chard variety, whose leaves are also used as a vegetable, is the closest in horticultural terms to the natural state. The enlarged petiole gives the fleshy ribs that are used in *gratins*. The Beetroot, as its name suggests, is the root, which is full of sugar and in some varieties, takes on a rich purple colour.

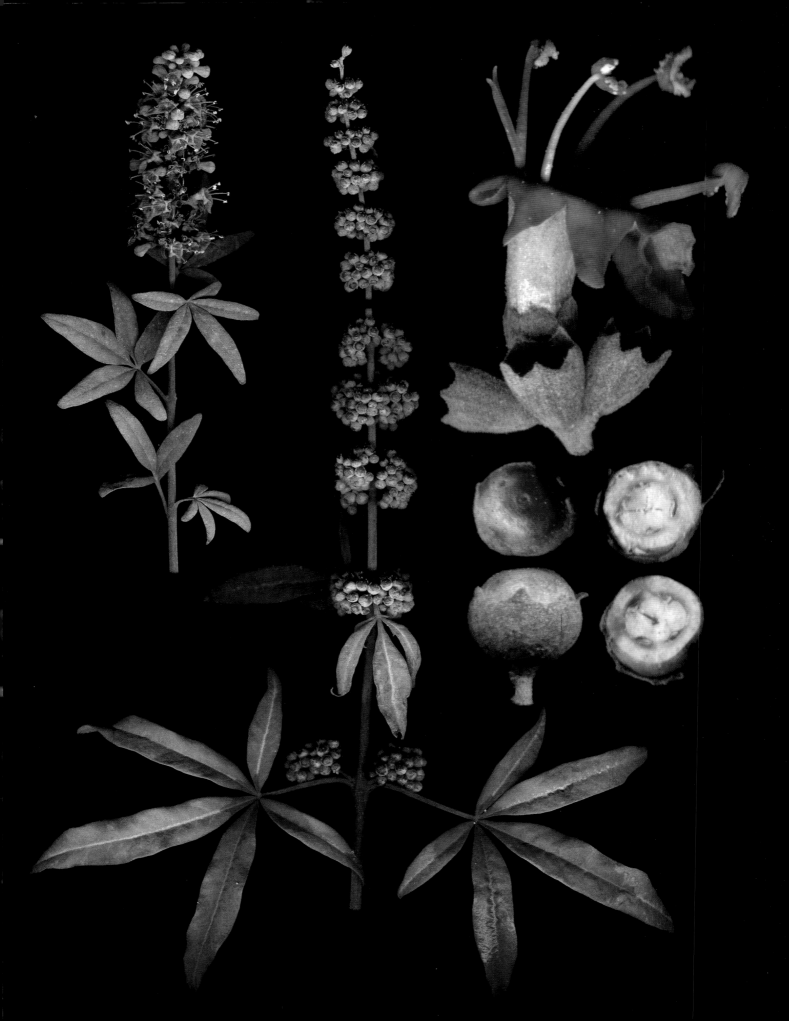

Chaste Tree

Vitex agnus-castus

FAMILY: LAMIACEAE

Active elements:
Flowering tops, fruit: aromatic oil rich in cineol, flavonoids, iridoids, maybe also steroids.

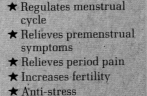

MAIN BENEFITS

★ Regulates menstrual cycle
★ Relieves premenstrual symptoms
★ Relieves period pain
★ Increases fertility
★ Anti-stress

PARTS USED

★ Dried fruit

Renowned since the times of the ancient Greeks and Romans for its anaphrodisiac properties, the Chaste Tree is thought to have been scattered on the floor of sacred places to protect them from pleasures of the flesh. For the same reasons, priestesses would sleep on mattresses made of Chaste Tree to ensure they remained pure. Unsurprisingly, the plant became a symbol of chastity, from whence its name. In the Middle Ages, monks chewed its fruit to decrease sexual desire. As a result it also became known as "monk's pepper". In the same era, the fresh fruit were sometimes used to treat paralysis and painful limbs.

The plant of the female cycle

• The fruit acts on the pituitary gland to **reduce premenstrual symptoms and regulate the cycle** (increasing the secretion of luteinizing hormone and decreasing those of follicle-stimulating hormone and prolactin), balancing the production of female hormones (progesterone and oestrogen). At the same time, it blocks the action of androgens.

• The resultant regulation of hormonal balance can contribute to **increasing fertility**.

• Chaste Tree is also used in **cases of stress**, **anxiety** and minor cases of insomnia.

• It can be used as part of **acne treatment**.

• Popular medicine continues to recommend it as an **anaphrodisiac** (reduces libido); however, this property has never been demonstrated.

DID YOU KNOW? The flexible stems of the Chaste Tree were used in times gone by as ties. According to legend, it was Chaste Tree stems that Ulysses used to tie his companions under the stomachs of the sheep belonging to the Cyclops, Polyphemus, in order to enable them to escape from his cave.

OTHER SPECIES: The Chinese Chaste Tree (*Vitex negundo*) is widely used in India for its medicinal properties. Its leaves and seeds can be applied topically to relieve rheumatism and joint inflammation. Internally the leaves are said to be diuretic, expectorant, anthelmintic, tonic and antipyretic. The Chinese Chaste Tree is also antifungal and an insecticide.

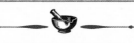

METHOD OF USE

• **INTERNAL:** 2 to 4g (1 to 2 flat teaspoonsful) of dried, crushed fruit per day, on its own or in an infusion. Used to tackle premenstrual syndrome and painful periods. Start treatment a week before menstruation is due to begin and stop 2 days after it comes to an end. This can be repeated for each cycle, decreasing the dose when an improvement is noted. Standardized extracts are also available commercially.

TOXICITY

The Chaste Tree should be avoided during pregnancy and while breastfeeding, and by women who have a history or risk of breast cancer, or are undergoing IVF.

Description

A bushy shrub growing to a height of 1½ to 2m (3¼ to 5ft), frequently found growing around the mouths of rivers and streams in Mediterranean areas. The Chaste Tree has long, palmate leaves, which look a little like hemp but the margins are not serrated. They exude a spicy fragrance, which is both floral and animal, slightly reminiscent of leather. Long elegant spikes of lightly fragranced lavender-coloured flowers adorn the ends of the flexible branches. They are followed by tiny, round, grey, crunchy seeds.

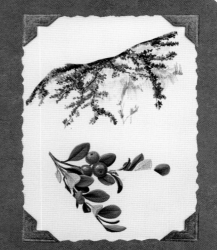

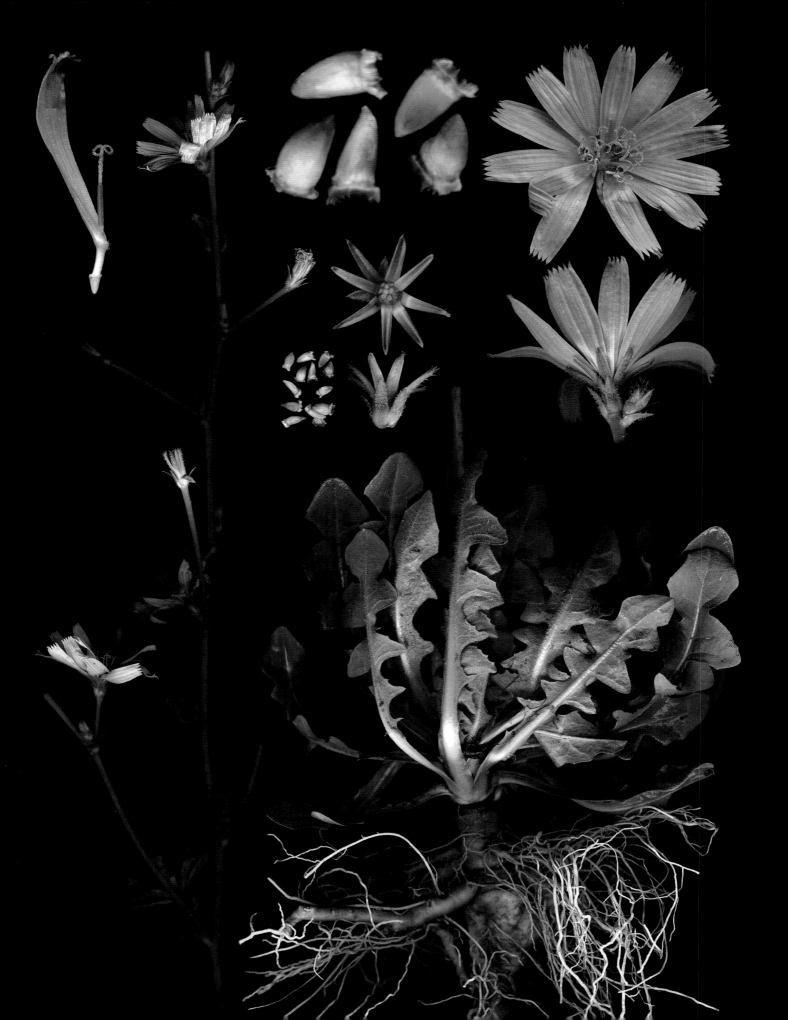

Chicory

Cichorium intybus

FAMILY: ASTERACEAE

Active elements:
Roots: rich in inulin.
Leaves: vitamins and mineral salts.
Bitterness is due to sesquiterpene lactones.

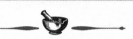

MAIN BENEFITS
★ Tonic for the liver and digestive system
★ Diuretic

PARTS USED
★ Leaves, roots, juice, whole plant

OTHER USES: Chicory is cultivated for its roots, a classic mild coffee substitute. They are cut into "chips" and then roasted. Other varieties are grown for their leaves (known as endives), which can be blanched as a salad ingredient (known in France as *barbe de capucin* or the red-leafed Radicchio). Chicory is one of the most commonly harvested wild salad leaves in the Mediterranean region.

The first records of Chicory are from 4,000 BC when it is mentioned in the Egyptian Ebers Papyrus, and it has been used ever since, either for its undeniable curative powers or simply as a vegetable. Renowned physicians have attested to its medical properties throughout history. Dioscorides advocated its use to fortify the stomach. Pliny attributed it with refreshing properties and St. Hildegard noted its use as an excellent digestive in the Middle Ages. Galen called it the "friend of the liver", and all the ancient authors attested to its aperitive, digestive, cholagogic (promotes bile flow), diuretic and purifying qualities, for which it is still used today.

Friend of the liver

• Chicory root and leaves increase bile production and promote its discharge. They are diuretic, stomachic and **boost the liver and the digestive system**.
• Chicory is also recommended in cases of **rheumatism or gout**.
• Chicory infusion **calms the thirst of diabetics**, without causing secondary sweating, and also regulates diuresis (elimination of urine).

METHOD OF USE

• **INTERNAL: Salad of young leaves.** When eaten at the beginning of a meal, it is an aperitive, diuretic and stimulates bowel movement. Its bitter flavour is really rather pleasant.
Infusion. 8 to 15g (½oz) of dried leaves per litre (quart) of water or 15 to 40g (½ to 1½oz) of the dried root, not roasted, per litre of water. To stimulate the liver and the digestive system. Likewise as a thirst-quencher. **Decoction.** 100g (3½oz) of fresh plant, root and leaves. Boil in a litre of water. For the same purposes.
Syrup. Mash and press leaves and root to obtain a ½ litre of juice. Mix with 500g (17½oz) of sugar. Reduce at a low heat, without boiling, to a syrup. Recommended for children as a laxative and purifier. Administer 2 to 4 teaspoonfuls daily, on an empty stomach, depending on age.

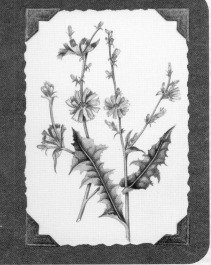

Description

This annual, biennial or perennial plant can reach 1m (3¼ft) in height. Common in meadowland, on uncultivated land and on roadsides, it is widespread in the northern hemisphere. It is cultivated for its roots and salad leaves or endives. Its leaves grow in a rosette and look like those of Dandelion. They are deeply divided into widely spread or inverted lobes. The stem bears thin, rigid shoots growing off at an obtuse angle. It blooms in late summer with elegant flower heads composed of tender, pale blue, flowers with strap-like petals. When cut, the plant exudes a very bitter, white latex.

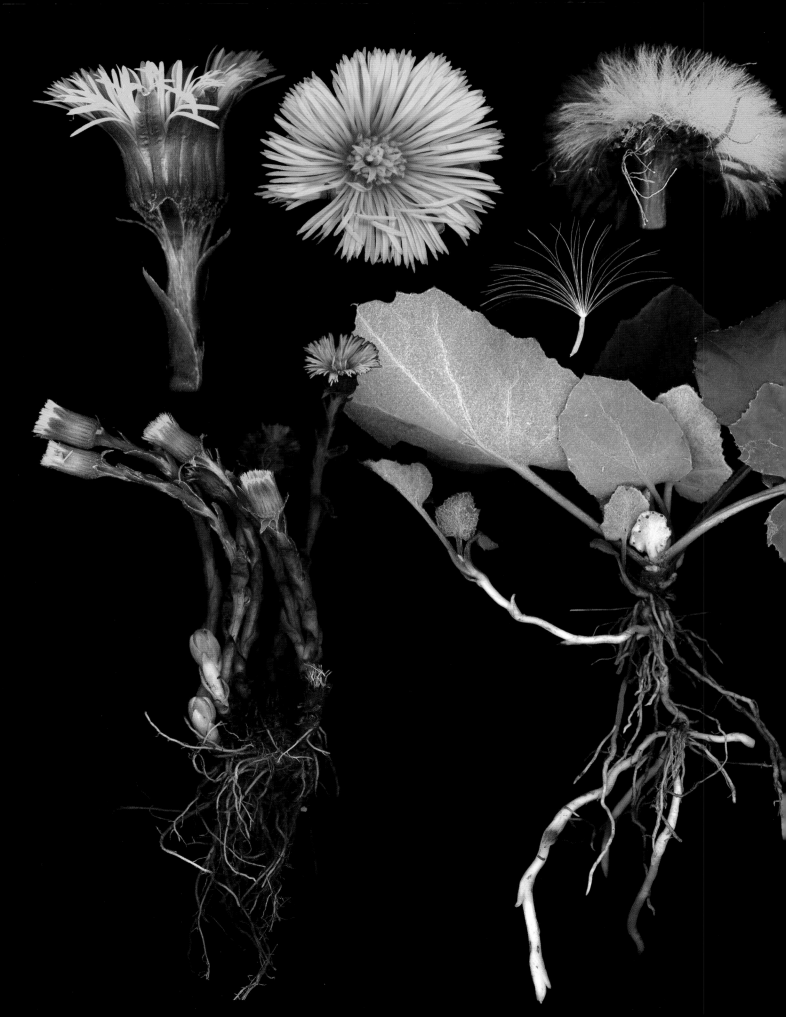

Colt's-foot

Tussilago farfara

FAMILY: ASTERACEAE

Active elements:

Flower heads: mucilage, triterpenes, flavonoids, carotenoids, pyrrolizidine alkaloids (including senkirkine and senecionine). The content of the last is lower in the European plants than in their Asiatic counterparts. The leaves also contain tannins, mineral salts and vitamins.

• The plant is also soothing **in cases of inflammation of oral mucosae**.

• The flowers **tighten skin** and decrease the appearance of wrinkles.

• Studies conducted in China have highlighted the **anti-inflammatory effects** of the plant extracts, which also seem to **strengthen the body's immune defences**.

OTHER USES: The flowers, stems and young leaves can be eaten raw in salad. Older leaves can be cooked.

I t is not difficult to guess the properties of this plant from its scientific name, since the word *tussilago* comes from the Latin *tussis*, meaning "cough", and *agere* "to chase". The flowers are indeed an old cough remedy. People in ancient times even used them to treat consumption (pulmonary tuberculosis). The Colt's-foot flower is the yellow note in the poetic and effective "infusion of four pectoral flowers". The leaves and roots are perspiration-inducing and were renowned cures for scrofulous ailments. The root was used in the past to treat flu.

Cough suppressant

• Colt's-foot flowers and leaves are **pectoral, calmative and soothing** and can be used for inflammations of the respiratory tract, to relieve persistent coughs, colds, bronchitis and flu. In times gone by, the leaves were sometimes smoked in cigarettes to treat asthma.

• Colt's-foot infusions are **expectorant and soothing** for the bronchial tubes.

• The leaves are applied externally as restorative poultices to treat abscesses. They have **healing** properties and can be applied to wounds and burns.

METHOD OF USE

• **INTERNAL: Infusion.** 50g (1¾oz) of flowers per litre (quart) of boiling water. Drink 3 cups per day for coughs.

Syrup. 250g (9oz) of flowers per litre of boiling water. Infuse for 8 to 10 minutes. Strain. Add the same weight in sugar, and cook on a low heat until it has the consistency of syrup. Take 4 or 5 tablespoonsful per day for coughs.

• **EXTERNAL:** Poultice of cooked leaves, to treat abscesses, or compresses soaked in a concentrated decoction of these leaves, allowing 50 to 100g (1¾ to 3½oz) per litre of boiling water.

Infusion of flowers. In hot compresses, it is slightly astringent and good for greasy, open-pored skin. It reduces the appearance of fine lines.

TOXICITY

In laboratory experiments, pyrrolizidine alkaloids have caused liver tumours. Although no classified disorders are associated with the plant, its regular use as an infusion is not recommended. It should not be used for more than one month at a stretch. It should not be taken by pregnant women or young children.

Description

This small perennial grows from rhizomes to 10 to 30cm (4 to 12in) on damp clay soil throughout the northern hemisphere. The flowers bloom in single, bright-yellow capitula at the top of stems covered in reddish, fluffy scales. The basal leaves appear when the flowers wither. The leaves are as wide as they are long, with serrated margins: green and rubbery on top, white and fluffy on the underside. The feathery fruit is an achene, similar to that of the Dandelion.

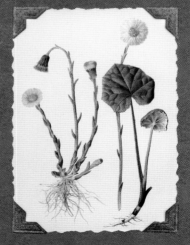

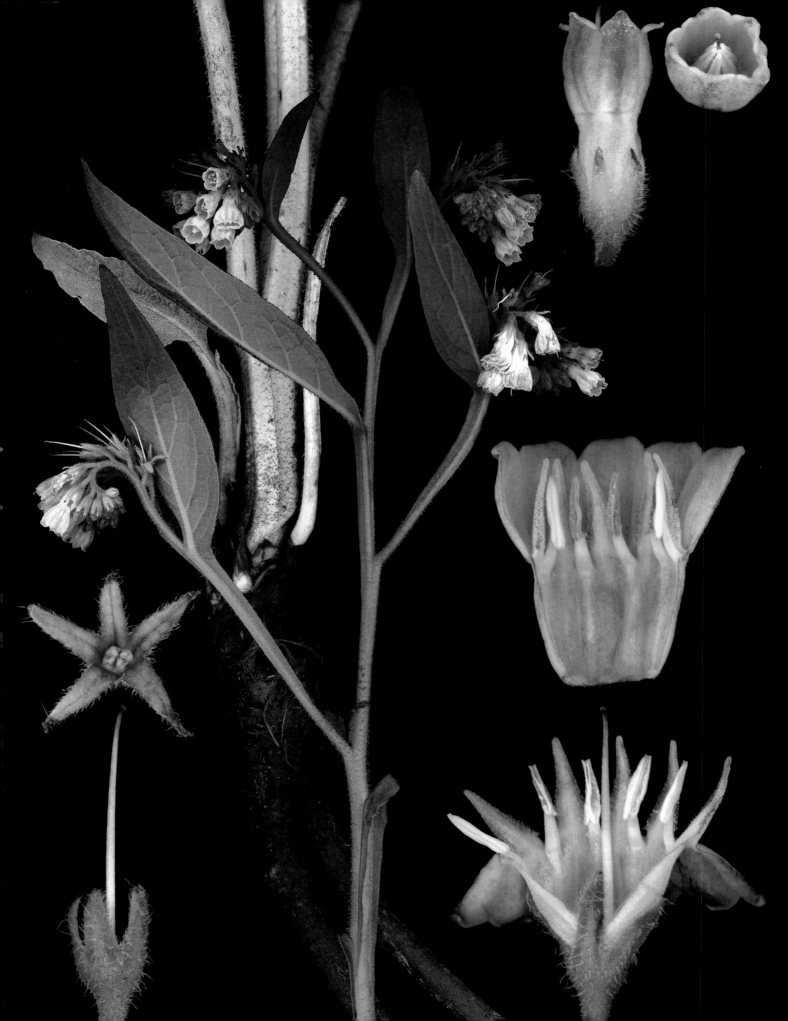

Comfrey

Symphytum officinale
FAMILY: BORAGINACEAE

Active elements:

Plant: tannins, mucilage, allantoin, asparagine, choline, triterpenes, phenolic acids and pyrrolizidine alkaloids (including lycopsamine and symphytine), especially in the root. The leaves are also said to contain cobalamin (vitamin B12).

The name Comfrey comes from the medieval Latin *confervere*, "to grow together" as it was believed to help heal bone fractures. In the Renaissance, Jean Fernel, the famous French physiologist, advocated its use by surgeons for the treatment of injuries involving fractures. As Comfrey's tannin-content makes it slightly astringent it was recommended to relieve haemoptysis (coughing up blood), minor uterine haemorrhages and benign diarrhoea. A century ago, Henri Leclerc, the French physician and renowned medical herbalist, used it to relieve tubercular enteritis and stomach ulcers. He also found it good for drying out the bronchial tubes in cases of bronchitis and pulmonary infections.

Healing and analgesic

• Comfrey is used externally to bring **rapid relief to the pain of burns**, **stimulate healing** of wounds and relieve venous ulcers, cracked nipples and anal fissures. Allantoin accelerates the formation of new tissue, while choline promotes irrigation.

• It can be applied topically to relieve the pain of **bruises, contusions and sprains**. It is likewise **good for backache** and joint pain.

• Comfrey ointment preparations **treat skin complaints**.

OTHER USES: Traditionally, Comfrey leaves have been eaten raw or cooked in a variety of ways. They contain between ten and one hundred times more alkaloids than the roots. Many gardeners grow it because it makes an excellent compost. It can also be made into a liquid manure which stimulates vegetable growth.

METHOD OF USE

• **EXTERNAL:** Concentrated **maceration**, in lotions and compresses for all skin complaints. **Poultices** made of the fresh crushed root. Particularly good for burns and cracked nipples that breast-feeding women may suffer.

TOXICITY

At high doses, the alkaloids in Comfrey have been shown to be toxic to laboratory animals, causing liver tumours. In humans, veno-occlusive syndromes have been reported with regular and prolonged consumption over several months of Comfrey infusions or capsules. However, it seems that reasonable consumption is safe: in England and the United States, many people have taken them on an occasional basis over a 30-year period without experiencing any health problems. By way of caution, it is best not to use Comfrey internally for medical purposes.

Description

An attractive perennial covered with stiff, prickly hairs, growing to a height of 40cm to 1m (16in to 3¼ft), native to Europe and Asia, common in damp meadows, ditches and on banks. The leaves grow along the tall, thick stem. Its pretty flowers, which bloom from May to July, have a bell-shaped corolla which may be white, yellow, pink or purple. The root is black outside, and white inside.

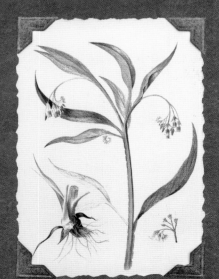

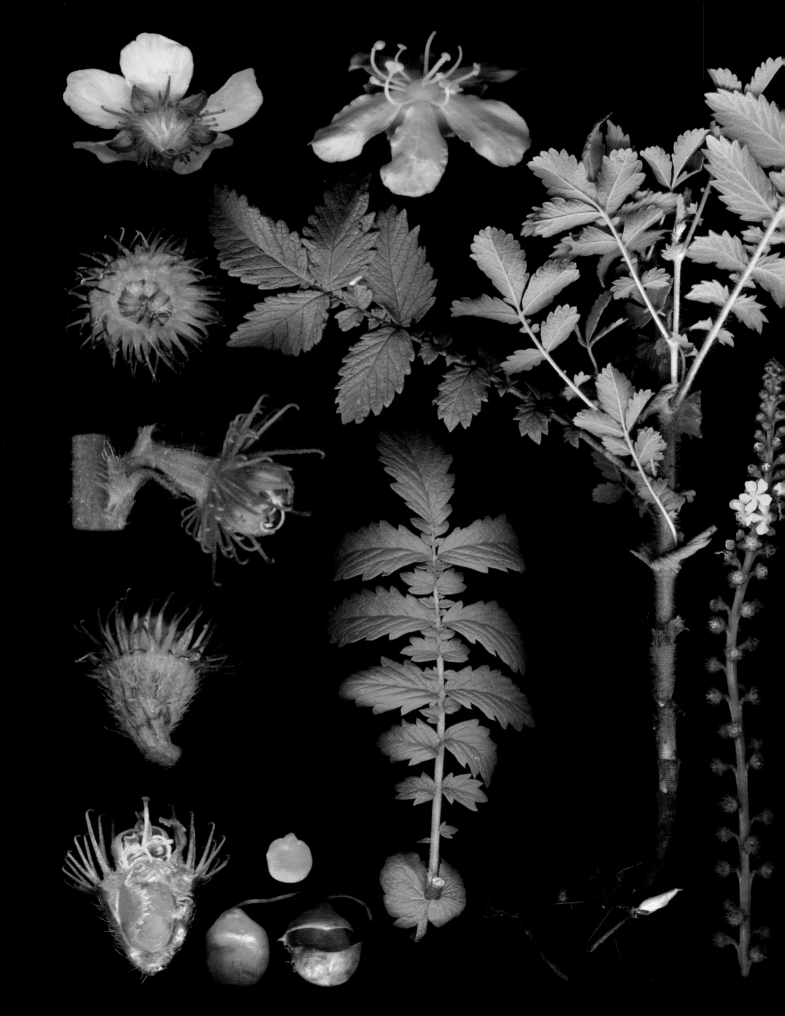

Common Agrimony

Agrimonia eupatoria

FAMILY: ROSACEAE

Active elements:
Tannins (including catechins) and flavonoids (including luteolin). Catechins have an astringent and antibacterial effect, while flavonoids have an anti-inflammatory effect.

MAIN BENEFITS

★ Anti-diarrhoeal
★ Ailments of the throat and mouth
★ Anti-diabetic

PARTS USED

★ Leaves, flowers, whole plant

sore throats and hoarseness, and boasts especially good results in **treating chronic pharyngitis** (lingering sore throat) suffered by singers or public speakers. It is renowned for its ability to **relieve inflammations and ulcerations of the mouth** (ulcers, gingivitis caused by the friction of dentures or orthodontic braces).

OTHER SPECIES: Fragrant Agrimony (*Agrimonia procera*) is commonly found in hedges and woodland. It is slightly larger in all aspects and gives off a subtle smell when crushed due to the aromatic essence it contains. Same uses as Common Agrimony.

Common Agrimony was believed to cure ailments such as cataracts, jaundice and snake bites in antiquity. Dioscorides used it to treat ulcers. It then became one of the ingredients of "Arquebusade Water". Its high tannin content makes it a good astringent, recommended by Dr Reutter in cases where tuberculosis caused patients to cough up blood.

The singer's friend

- Common Agrimony is still used to **reduce urinary sugar and quench the thirst of diabetics**, while stimulating digestion.
- Thanks to its high tannin content, the plant is also **a remarkable anti-diarrhoeal**, and is effective in treating digestive disorders as accompanied by diarrhoea, enteritis and chronic liver diseases. Note that tannins can also cause constipation.
- It is also valuable and **beneficial for throat and mouth ailments**. It relieves

METHOD OF USE

- **INTERNAL: Infusion.** 10 to 30g (¼ to 1oz) per litre (quart). Drink 3 or 4 cups per day.
- **EXTERNAL: Decoction.** 100g (3½oz) of plant per litre. Boil until reduced to one-third. Use as a prolonged, regular mouthwash or gargle (five to six times per day) for all ailments of the mouth. Can be sweetened with honey or blackberry juice. The same decoction, applied on a poultice, relieves sprains and dislocations.

Description

A plant reaching a height of around 40cm (16in), common in hedgerows, along paths, at the edge of woodland and in shady locations. Widespread in Europe, Asia Minor and North Africa. A hairy, often reddish stem from a thick base, with leaves divided into serrated segments with a greenish-white underside. The flowers have five yellow petals and grow in spikes. They produce elongated fruit covered with small hooks designed to catch in the hair of animals and allow the plant to spread.

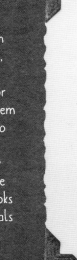

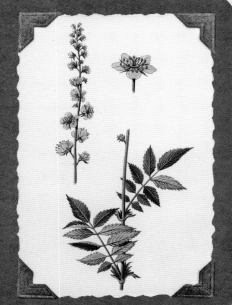

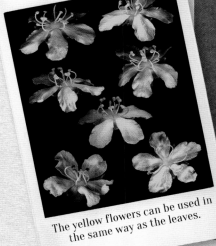

The yellow flowers can be used in the same way as the leaves.

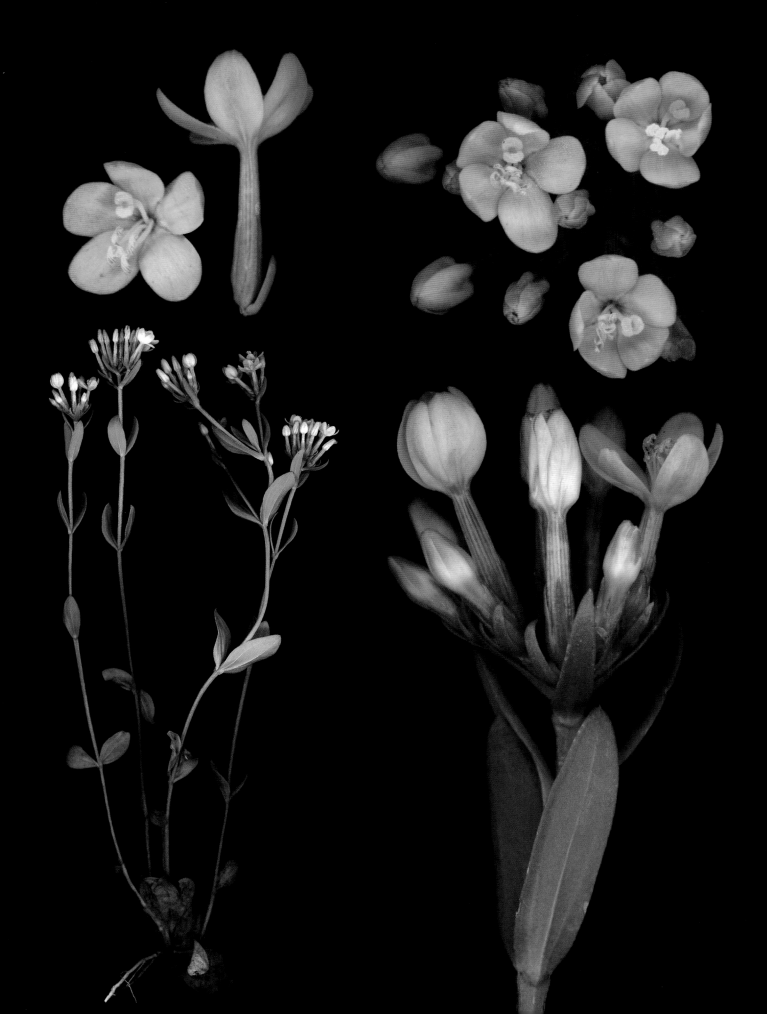

Common Centaury

Centaurium erythraea

FAMILY: GENTIANACEAE

Active elements:

Phenolic acids, flavonoids, xanthines and heterosides (centauroside, gentiopicroside, sweroside and swertiamarin).

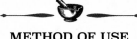

• It is used as a **remedy for heartburn and sluggish digestion**. It is effective against stomach pain in people suffering from gout. Its properties are similar to those of Gentian, but are less powerful.

• The Common Centaury has a confirmed **antipyretic effect**.

• It is also attributed with **anti-inflammatory and antibacterial effects**, and its infusion serves as an antioxidant.

C ommon Centaury has been around since antiquity, when it was widely used by the druids to treat snake bites and scorpion stings. They also recognized its fever-reducing (antipyretic) properties, hence its name, in Late Latin, *Febrefugium*. Its power to reduce fevers, almost equal to that of Cinchona, means it has long been used against intermittent fevers and malaria attacks. The genus of Common Centaury, *Centaurium*, should not be confused with that of Brown Knapweed for example, *Centaurea jacea*. They do not belong to the same family and do not have the same medicinal properties.

Fortifies and protects the liver

• Common Centaury is an **excellent tonic**. Its bitter taste stimulates appetite and bile secretion. It is used for convalescents, to alleviate anaemia, general weakness and liver disorders.

METHOD OF USE

• **INTERNAL: Infusion.** 10 to 30g (¼ to 1oz) per litre (quart) of boiling water. Drink 3 cups per day, before or between meals. Very bitter. As a general tonic and to stimulate digestion.
Wine. 50 to 60g (1¾ to 2oz) per litre of liquid. Allow to infuse for 48 hours, then strain. Drink the equivalent of 2 small glasses (100g (3½oz)) per day, as an aperitive, before each meal.

• **EXTERNAL: Decoction.** 50 to 60g per litre of water. Used in lotions to treat sores, sprains and scrofulous ulcers. It is said to achieve good results in preventing hair loss.

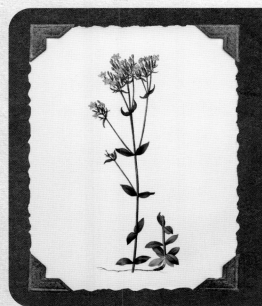

Description

A small biennial, growing to a height of 20 to 30cm (8 to 12in) found in wet meadows, dune grassland and woodland. Native to Europe, Asia, North Africa and North America. Its long, oval leaves form a rosette at the base of the plant and are opposite on the single stem. The pretty pink flowers grow in dense clusters at the top of the stem, and bloom in July and August. All parts of the plant are very bitter.

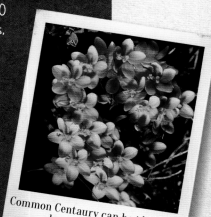

Common Centaury can be identified by its pink flowers.

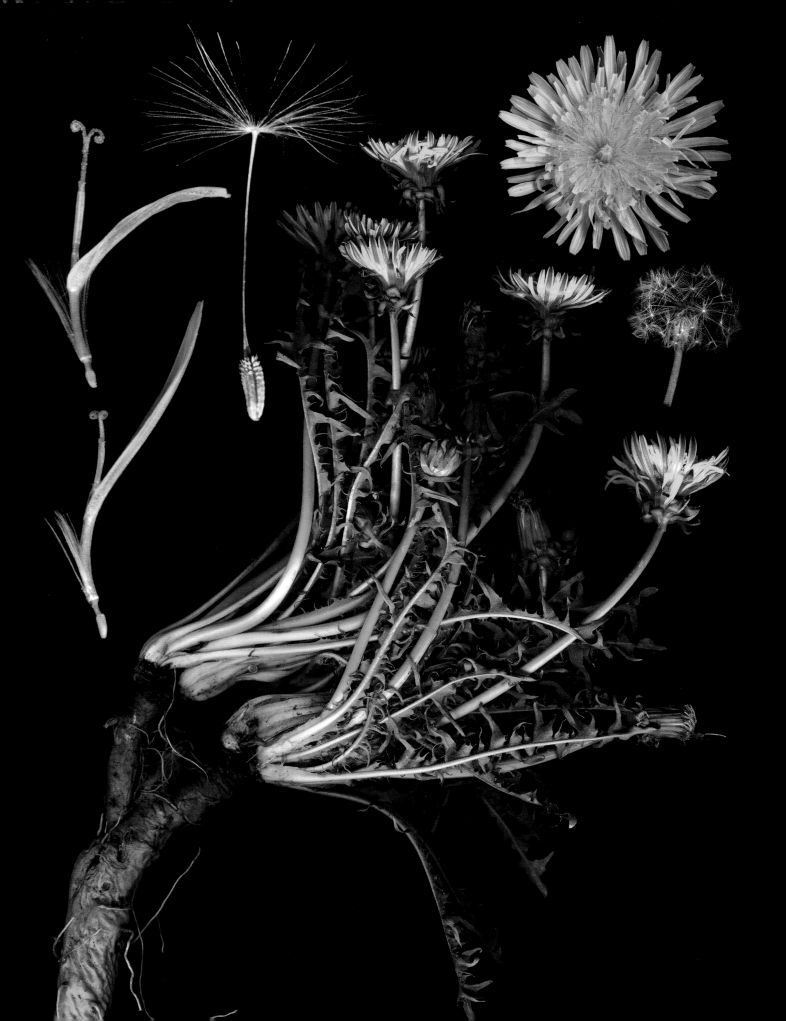

Common Dandelion

Taraxacum officinale

FAMILY: ASTERACEAE

Active elements:

Roots: inulin, fructose, potassium.
Plant: sesquiterpene lactones (which give it its bitterness), including germacranolide, triterpenic alcohols, sterols. Leaves: rich in flavonoids, provitamin A, vitamin C, mineral salts and complete proteins.

I n times gone by, Dandelion juice was held to be a specific remedy for vision problems (its scientific name *Taraxacum* comes from the Greek *taraxis* "eye trouble"). However, this property has not been demonstrated. From the 11th century onwards, the Dandelion was recommended by Arab physicians. Before that, however, Dandelion root was widely used in popular medicine to stimulate liver function.

The thousand benefits of Dandelion

• Dandelion **stimulates the gall-bladder**. It increases the quantity of bile produced while increasing the power of the gall-bladder to contract. It also works on the liver itself. It is advocated for the **treatment of liver failure**, painful liver attacks and jaundice.

• Dandelion **regulates intestinal function** and combats constipation remarkably effectively.

• It works well on **cellulite**, which is often related to liver disease. It is also **used to lower cholesterol**, and as a result, to treat atherosclerosis.

• It is renowned for its impressive **diuretic properties**, such that its popular name in French is *pissenlit* ("wet-the-bed").

• An **excellent natural purifier**, it helps flush toxins of infectious origin and those originating in food and the environment (pollution) from the liver and kidneys. It is effective on **skin problems**, such as acne, eczema and psoriasis, as well as rheumatic ailments (gout arthritis).

• The plant also has **aperitive and tonic properties**. Its bitter principles stimulate digestive secretions.

• In terms of cosmetic treatments, Dandelion juice is said to lighten the complexion.

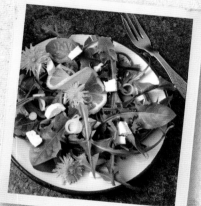

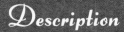

Description

A perennial growing from a tap-root, common in meadows. Its smooth leaves grow in rosettes and are generally divided into sharp downward-pointing or slightly serrated lobes. Each hollow, flowering stem has a single flower head of golden rays. The seeds, which fly at the slightest wind, have pappi as parachutes. Elisée Reclus, the 19th-century French geographer said, "This flower that is a sun becomes a milky way, a world of stars, after it flowers."

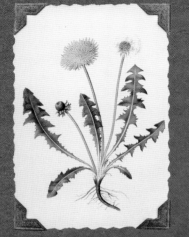

METHOD OF USE

• **INTERNAL: Dandelion leaf salad** is highly recommended for people with liver or over-eating problems, gout or anaemia.
Decoction. Boil 30 to 60g (1 to 2oz) of fresh roots and leaves per litre (quart) of water for 30 minutes, then leave to infuse for 4 hours. Drink 2 glasses per day between meals for liver problems and constipation.

• **EXTERNAL: Root decoction.** Cleans and firms the skin.
Fresh Dandelion juice. The beautiful ladies of the Renaissance would use a mixture of equal parts dandelion juice and cream. They would rub it on the face to remove impurities and obtain a radiant complexion.

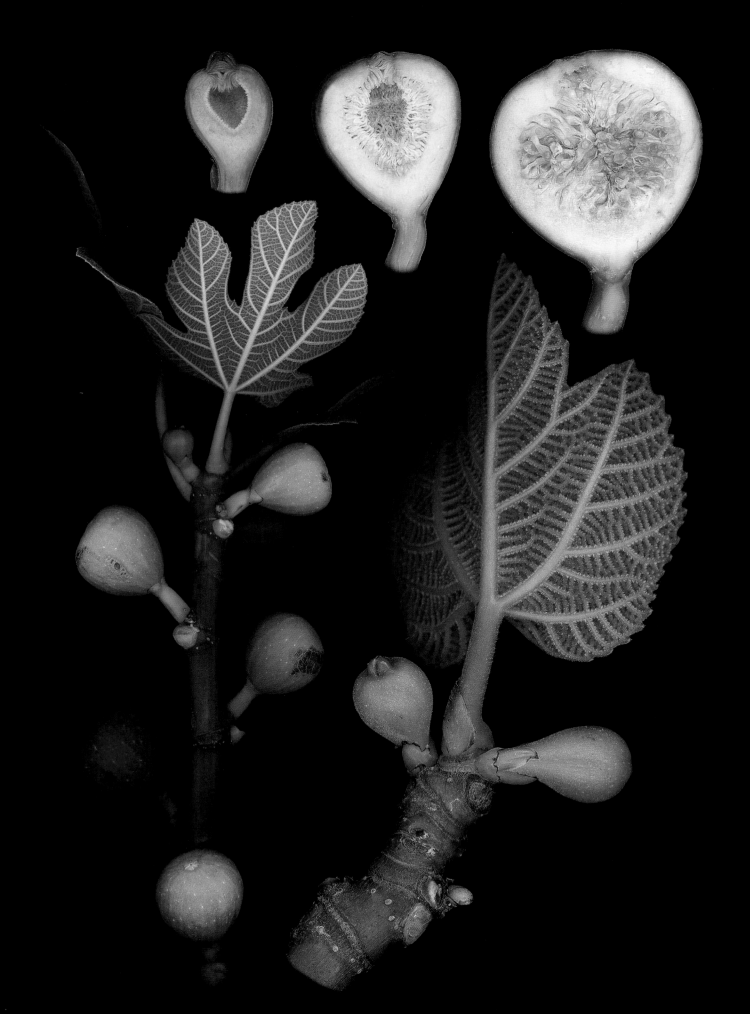

Common Fig

Ficus carica
FAMILY: MORACEAE

Active elements:
Fig: sugars (~50%), flavonoids, enzymes and furanocoumarins.

The Fig appeared regularly in writings of antiquity and according to Horace, gave its name to the liver in Latin because of Apicius, who used figs to fatten geese and obtain *iecur ficatum*, (literally, "figged liver" or *foie gras*). Renaissance physicians believed that the Fig "made for a good stomach and engendered good and praiseworthy blood".

The fig, fresh or dry

• Highly nutritious, the Fig is also easy to digest and has **laxative qualities**, so is useful as a treatment for constipation.
• Dried Fig has **emollient and softening properties** and is one of the traditional four "pectoral fruits", along with the raisin, jujube and date; however it can also be used on its own to treat stubborn colds, bronchitis, whooping cough and pneumonia.

• Used externally, a decoction of Fig is excellent for gargling **against throat irritations**, coughs, hoarseness and painful inflammation of the gums or cheeks.
• A hot Fig on a **dental abscess** also encourages maturation.
• The milky juice (latex) secreted by the Fig tree contains an enzyme that is active **against corns and warts**.

OTHER USES: Fig latex can be used as rennet to curdle milk in cheese production.

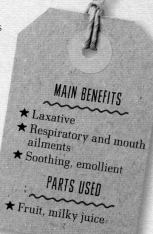

MAIN BENEFITS
★ Laxative
★ Respiratory and mouth ailments
★ Soothing, emollient

PARTS USED
★ Fruit, milky juice

TOXICITY
The Common Fig's milky juice, as well as its leaves, can cause allergies.

METHOD OF USE

• **INTERNAL: Pectoral decoction.** 80 to 100g (3 to 3½oz) of dried figs per litre (quart) of water.
Syrup. Boil 500g (17½oz) of figs per litre of water until reduced by half. Strain and mix with 250g (9oz) of honey. Shake before use and take a tablespoonful at a time. For sore throats.
Fig coffee. This infusion is prepared like real coffee, using roasted fig powder and is good for the chest, lungs and airways.
• **EXTERNAL: Decoction.** Use as a highly soothing gargle. For dental abscesses, apply half a warm fig between the cheek and the gum.
Poultices of figs cooked in water or milk encourage the maturation of abscesses and boils.
Fig juice. Apply twice a day to corns and warts.

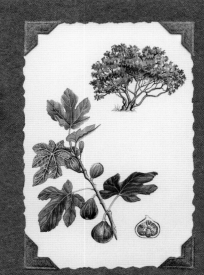

Description

A shrub growing to 2 to 5m (6½ to 16½ft) in height, native to the Mediterranean basin, where it grows in rocky places. Widely cultivated in many countries outside its area of origin, although it requires a fairly warm climate for the figs to ripen fully. The smooth grey bark bears thick, broad, lobed leaves that are rough to the touch. When cut, it exudes an abundant white latex which is very caustic if it comes into contact with mucous membranes. The flowers bloom inside a fleshy, cup-like structure. This is incorrectly referred to as the "fruit" and produces the fig after fertilization. When ripe, figs may be purple or green (the latter are known as "white figs") and can be eaten fresh or dried.

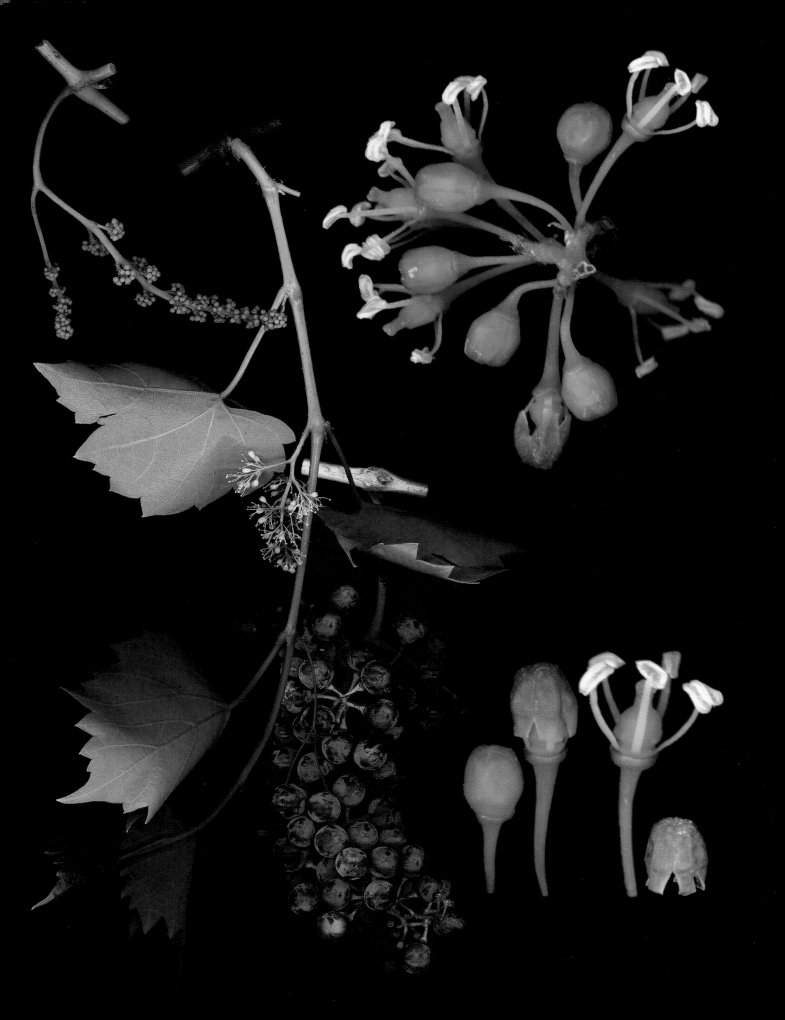

Common Grape Vine

Vitis vinifera

FAMILY: VITACEAE

Active elements:

Red vine leaves: many anthocyanosides, as well as tannins, flavonoids, phenolic compounds. Fruit: sugar, pectin, tartaric and malic acid, flavones, vitamins. Grape skin: rich in OPCs (powerful antioxidants). Pips: rich in resveratrol.

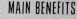

In the times of the ancient Greeks, the Common Grape Vine was the object of veneration, dedicated to Dionysus and dispensing its fruit to humans so they could make wine. Wine has been widely used in medicine for its antiseptic qualities and as the basis for a wide variety of remedies. In the Middle Ages, Montpellier had a famous medical school which was renowned for its production of these medicinal wines, some of which are still used today.

Multiple benefits

• Vine leaves and extracts from the pips are good at **relieving the symptoms of venous insufficiency** (heavy legs) and varicose veins, and treating problems linked to fragile capillaries (haemorrhages and nosebleeds but also bruises and petechiae, small red or purple spots).

• Red vine leaves can sometimes help relieve **menopause-related complaints**; they restore good blood circulation and tackle uterine haemorrhages.

• Their high tannin content makes them **very astringent**, so they are also used to treat chronic diarrhoea.

METHOD OF USE

• **INTERNAL: Decoction of leaves.** 50g (1¾oz) per litre (quart) of boiling water Take 3 cups per day, before each meal, including one in the morning on an empty stomach for menopause-related problems and venous complaints.

Verjuice (green juice). 200g (7oz) of juice per litre of water. Used to aid weight-loss.

Grape cure. Drink the juice of 500g to 1kg (2lb) of grapes (organic, as conventional grape farming is heavy on pesticide), Drink 1 hour before each of the three meals, throughout the season to cleanse the body.

• The abundant clear sap that flows from the branches when vines are pruned in spring ("tears of the vine") is effective in **treating eye ailments**. Its tonic, healing and anti-haemorrhagic properties makes it perfect for congestive conjunctival and ocular problems.

• Grapes are **refreshing, diuretic and laxative**. The Grape cure is advocated for constipation, arthritis, rheumatism, gout, obesity, high blood pressure, arthrosclerosis and conditions related to the liver and urinary tract.

• Verjuice, the acid, astringent juice of the unripened green grape is **diuretic** and recommended for the treatment of obesity.

• Results of animal testing indicate that the resveratrol extracted from grape skins is an antioxidant which may help **prevent cataracts**.

OTHER USES: Verjuice is used in the preparation of some mustards and a condiment in some typical cuisine of the vine-growing regions.

DID YOU KNOW? The first traces of cultivated vine stocks were found on the slopes of the Caucasus mountains, in present-day Georgia, and date back more than 7,000 years.

Description

A plant whose history is intertwined with that of humans. The numerous varieties (*cépages*) are widespread in warm and temperate regions. It is a climbing plant with toothed leaves whose fruit grow in characteristic bunches. The small, white or pale green flowers are grouped in clusters. The "red vine" is most commonly used in medicine; these cultivars have black fruit with a crimson pulp and attractive red foliage in autumn.

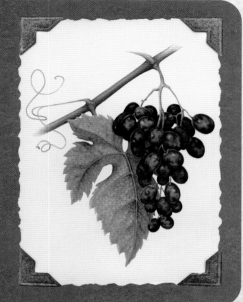

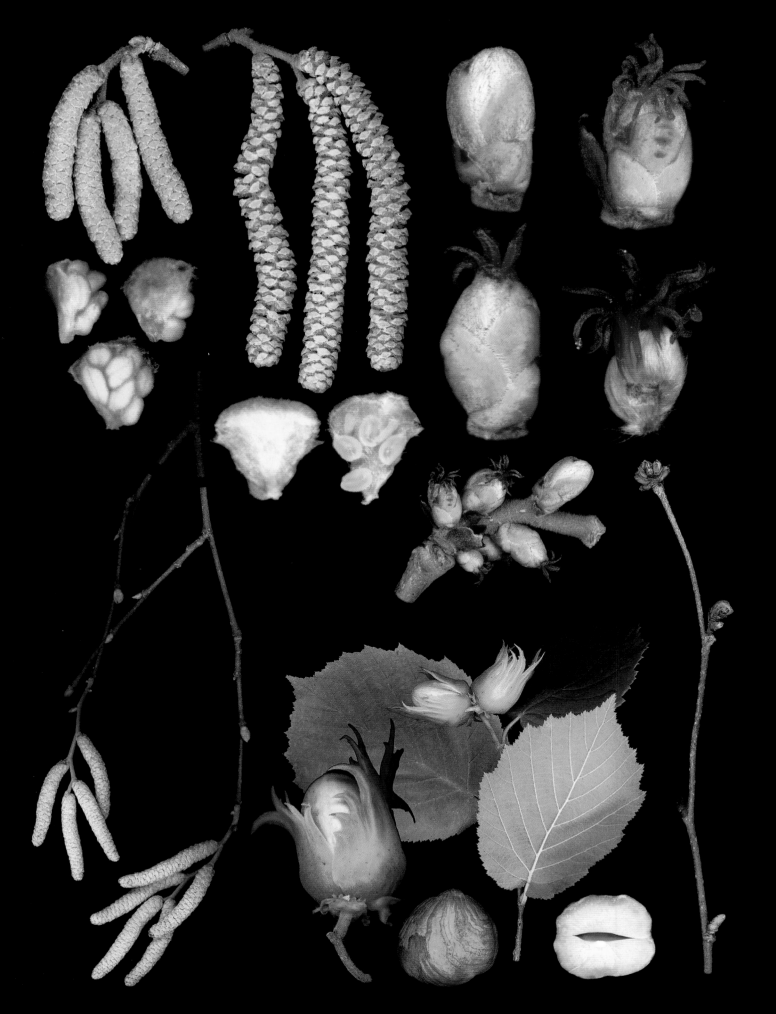

Common Hazel

Corylus avellana

FAMILY: BETULACEAE

Active elements:
Leaves: tannins, proanthocyanidins and a flavonoid, myricitrin. Seeds: protides and a fatty oil containing oleic acid, linoleic acid and palmitic acid.

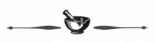

Nuts as food go back to the dawn of time. Fossilized remains have been discovered on archaeological sites dating back more than 10,000 years. Hazelnuts were traditionally held to have diuretic powers when infused in white wine. Some writers claimed that its flower pollen and Mistletoe gathered from its branches, were remedies for epilepsy. The bark of the root was used to regulate heavy periods and according to François-Joseph Cazin, the 19th-century French doctor and botanist, to treat intermittent malarial fevers.

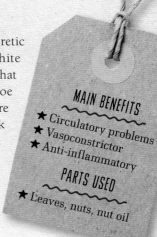

METHOD OF USE

- **INTERNAL: Decoction.** 30g (1oz) of leaves per litre (quart) of water. Boil for 15 minutes. Use for venous problems and diarrhoea.
- **EXTERNAL: Decoction.** 30g (1oz) of bark per litre of water. Boil for 15 minutes. Use for haemorrhoids. Add half a litre of alcohol (40% by volume) and use this solution to soak compresses. **Wine decoction.** Boil 50g (1¾oz) of bark in a half a litre of wine and half a litre of water, for the treatment of varicose ulcers. Use this decoction as a lotion and a dressing.

Tonic for the venous system

- Hazelnut leaves have **vasoconstrictive and anti-inflammatory properties** similar to Witch Hazel. They are prescribed for venous system ailments, such as varicose veins, haemorrhoids and the after-effects of phlebitis (inflammation of veins).
- The leaves are astringent, which makes them useful in **treating diarrhoea**.
- Hazelnut oil can be used as a **gentle anthelmintic**, suitable for children.
- When used externally, the bark of the branches is an excellent local sedative for haemorrhoids and helps to heal varicose ulcers.

OTHER USES: Hazelnuts are nutritious and have the highest protide and lipid content of all oleaginous fruit. They can be eaten raw or roasted, made into a nut butter and used in cakes. A fine nut oil can be extracted.

DID YOU KNOW? Hazelnuts are known as 'cobnuts' in Kent, where they are traditionally cultivated. The plant's scientific name *Corylus*, from the Greek word *korus*, means helmet, a reference to the nut shell's shape.

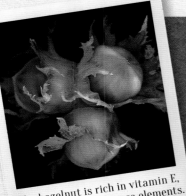

The hazelnut is rich in vitamin E, fibre, minerals and trace elements.

Description

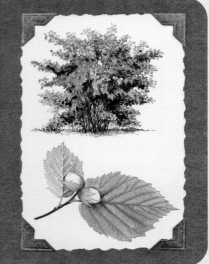

An easily identifiable shrub, growing to a height of 2 to 5m (6½ to 16½ft), common in hedgerows and woodland through Europe and western Asia. Straight, flexible Common Hazel saplings have given generations of children the pleasure of playing with bows, arrows and spears. Its leaves are large with a double-serrated margin. The flowers, which bloom long before the leaves come out, are of two kinds. The males are pendulous yellow, cylindrical catkins, seen from late winter. The female flowers, on the same twigs slowly swell to the recognizable hazelnut shape, protected by their shells, nestled in a collar of light green bracts.

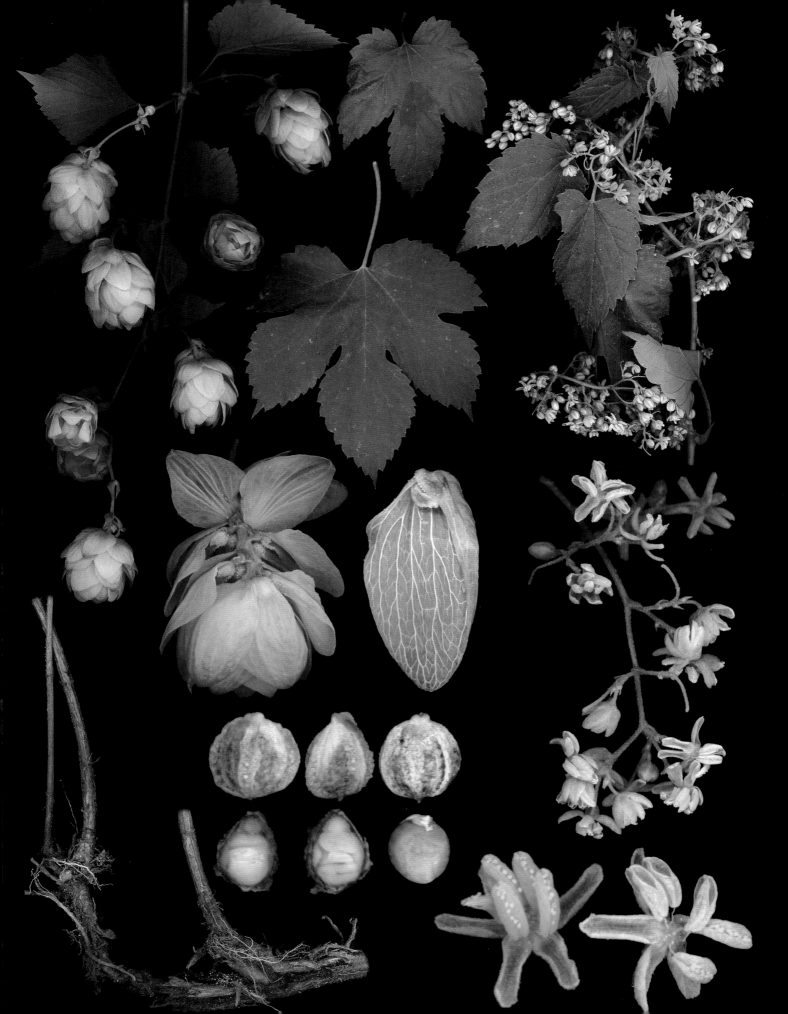

Common Hop

Humulus lupulus

FAMILY: CANNABACEAE

Active elements:

Lupulin (powder taken from the cones): flavonoids, tannins, aromatic oil rich in sesquiterpenes and bitter principles (including lupulone, humulone and valerian acid). It may also contain oestrogenic compounds.

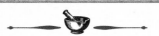

METHOD OF USE

- **INTERNAL: Infusion.** 10 to 15g (¼ to ½oz) of root per litre (quart) of water. As a tonic, it stimulates the appetite and digestion. For use as a sedative, increase the dose of cone-shaped heads up to 40g (1½oz) per litre.
Lupulin powder. 1g as a sedative, 2g as a hypnotic.
Lupulin tincture. 10g (¼oz) of lupulin crushed and dissolved (by trituration) in 90g (3¼oz) of alcohol (90% by volume) Take 2 to 4g per day, depending on the desired effect.
- **EXTERNAL: Hop pillow.** Place flower cones in a cloth bag and use as a pillow to help you fall asleep quickly.

Description

Hop creepers can climb to the top of the highest trees using the stiff downward facing hairs known as bines. Common in hedgerows and on the edges of cool, damp woodland in Europe, temperate Asia and North Africa. Hops have large, opposed, lobed leaves, similar to vine leaves. Male and female plants are separate. Male plants produce tiny flowers. In late summer, the female plants produce the cone-shaped heads known as hops, clusters of soft scales that conceal a bitter-tasting, strong-smelling powder which is lupulin.

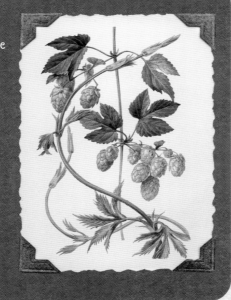

In antiquity, herbal physicians did not seem to attach much importance to Hop. However, Pliny did record its use as a delicate vegetable. In the 12th century, St. Hildegard was probably the first to attribute medicinal properties to Hop. Eminent Renaissance physicians, such as Mattioli, highlighted its aperitive, purifying, antipyretic and diuretic properties. Dodoens and Lémery, the famous botanists, advocated its use for "ailments of the liver, the spleen, to purify the blood and stimulate urination". Modern medical herbalists have acknowledged all these properties and added more.

Digestive, sedative and anaphrodisiac

- The bitter principles of the Common Hop make it a **tonic and digestive stimulant**. It is also an effective treatment for anaemia, rickets and lack of appetite.
- It reduces fever (antipyretic) and is an effective **antiparasitic**.
- Hop is also a powerful **diuretic** that eliminates uric acid.
- Its aromatic oil has **sedative** and even hypnotic properties.
- The use of Hop is advocated in cases of **insomnia and anxiety**.
- Common Hop works as a **general sedative for the genital area**, so is particularly good for period pain, as well as relieving migraines and related nervous disorders. It is also said to have an oestrogenic effect.

- The Common Hop has been recognized as having **anaphrodisiac properties (quells libido)**. Consequently, it is sometimes recommended for the treatment of certain male sexual disorders (generally those of nervous origin including premature ejaculation, excessive sensitivity in the genital region, and painful priapism caused by gonorrhoea).

OTHER USES: The Common Hop was first used to make beer around the 9th century. Its strong smell, bitter taste and sedative properties are due to its lupulin content. The young, slightly bitter, highly aromatic hop shoots can be cooked like asparagus. Whether cooked or eaten raw in salad, they are a delicious vegetable, with tonic, refreshing and diuretic properties. They were also effective in the treatment of scurvy, due to their high level of vitamin C.

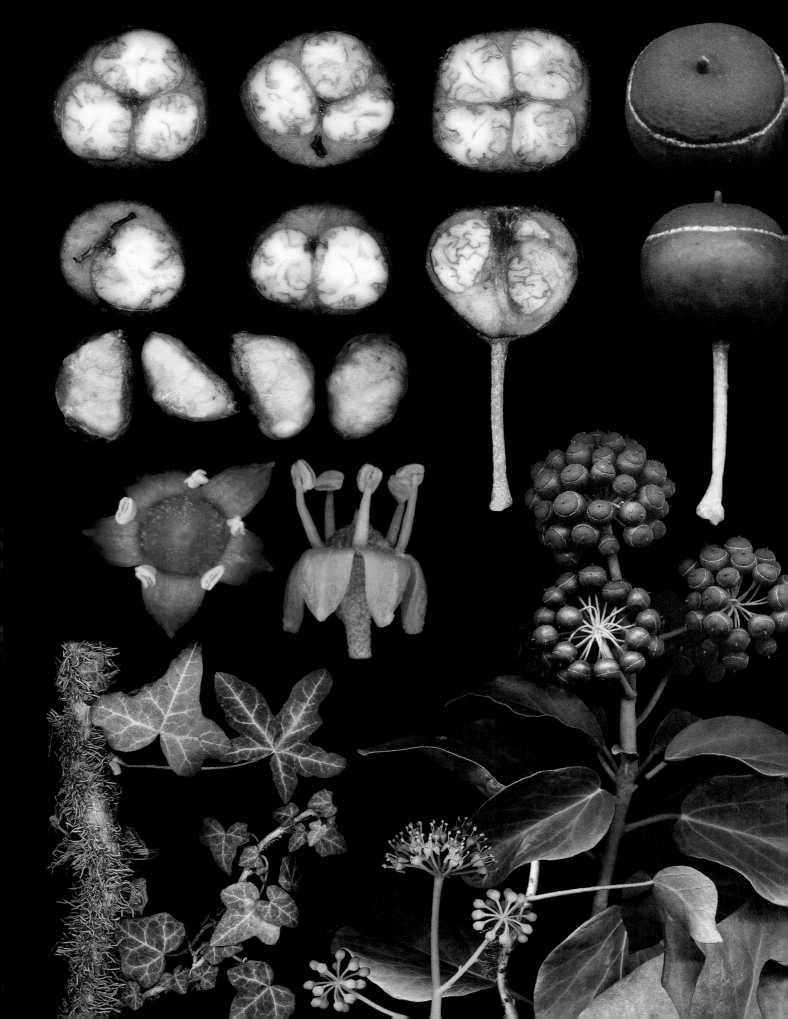

Common Ivy

Hedera helix

FAMILY: ARALIACEAE

Active elements:

Flavonoids, triterpenic saponosides (including hederin), polyynes (including falcarinol and falcarinone), sterols. An aromatic oil.

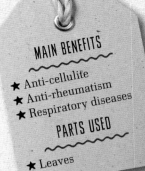

- Common Ivy is also effective against stretch marks.
- It is used to **treat cracks, chapping and insect bites**.
- It is also an excellent **remedy for rheumatic pain**, neuralgia, lower back pain and sciatica.

The ancient Egyptians considered ivy to be sacred to the god Osiris, while the Greeks and Romans dedicated it to Dionysus/Bacchus, the God of Wine, because it was alleged to protect people from drunkenness. It also symbolizes the victory of warriors. Ivy wood was well known in folk medicine as a remedy for coughs and whooping cough. Peasants used a beaker carved out of the trunk of an old ivy tree to steep wine to treat the sick.

A good anti-cellulite

- Ivy leaves are used to **soothe respiratory tract spasms** (effective in cases of chronic bronchitis, severe laryngitis, tracheitis and whooping cough) in the form of dry extract-based preparations: tablets, suppositories and alcoholic drops.
- However, its classic use is to **tackle cellulite**. Many commercial anti-cellulite creams are based on Common Ivy. It reduces skin tension, significantly improves the dimpling effect and softens rough patches.

METHOD OF USE

- **INTERNAL: Alcoholature** of leaves. Steep 10g (¼oz) of fresh leaves in 100g (3½oz) of alcohol. Administer 10 to 40 drops per day, on five occasions throughout the day. Do not exceed the stated dose. Use for respiratory ailments.
- **EXTERNAL: Decoction.** 200g (7oz) of leaves boiled for 3 hours in a litre (quart) of water. For the treatment of cellulite and pains, soak compresses in this decoction while it is hot. **Poultices** of fresh, crushed leaves, replaced every 2 hours, over aches and pains.
Rubs. Steep a large handful of fresh, chopped leaves in a litre of boiling vinegar for 6 hours, then strain. The steeped leaves are effective applied to a painful corn.
Ivy oil. Made of 10g (¼oz) of alcoholature of ivy leaves, 30g (1oz) of camomile, (1oz) base oil. Use to massage painful areas.

TOXICITY

The fruits are purgative and cause vomiting. They are a strong irritant and can trigger digestive, nervous and respiratory problems. Contact with the leaves can also cause dermatitis, probably due to the falcarinol. Ivy-based preparations can occasionally cause an allergic reaction.

Description

This climbing plant is commonly found on rocks, old walls and trees throughout Europe, Asia and North Africa. Stems, as long as 50m (164ft), creep along the ground then climb using their short, modified roots as crampons. Its tough, leathery leaves can take two forms. Those on branches without flowers are divided into dark green, marbled, triangular lobes; those on flowering branches are oval or diamond-shaped, and a lighter, glossy green. The small greenish-yellow flowers form globular umbels. The fruit are black, fleshy berries, ringed at the top.

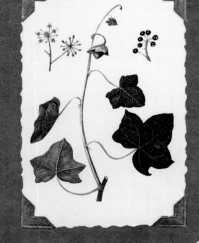

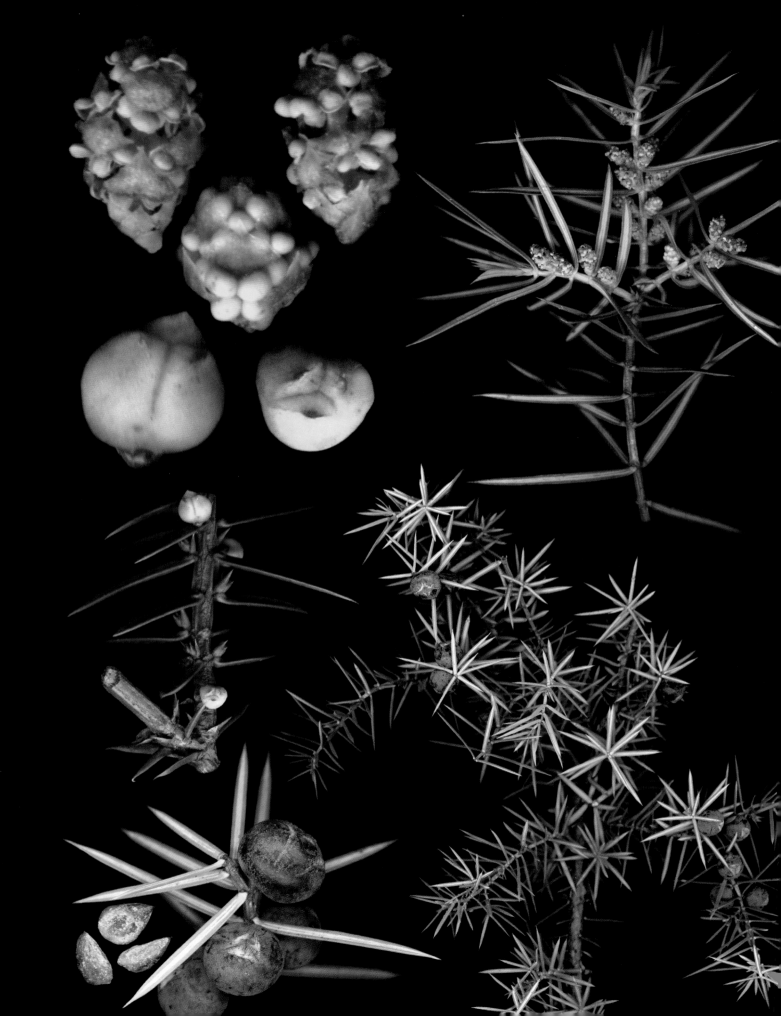

Common Juniper

Juniperus communis

FAMILY: CUPRESSACEAE

Active elements:

Cones: tannins, sugars, resin, bitter principle (juniperin), diterpenes, aromatic oil rich in carbides (pinene, myrcene, sabinene, limonene, terpineol).

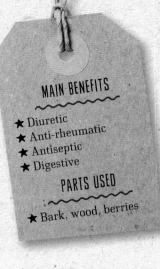

MAIN BENEFITS

★ Diuretic
★ Anti-rheumatic
★ Antiseptic
★ Digestive

PARTS USED

★ Bark, wood, berries

Mattioli, the 16th-century physician and naturalist, recommended the wood of Common Juniper in baths to treat gout. Leaves and flowering tops, and particularly their ashes, were used as purgatives. The second bark (white bark) is still used in some areas of the countryside as a remedy for furunculosis (infected hair follicles). However, it is the berries that are said to have particularly useful properties. Cato the Elder, in the 2nd century BC, advocated diuretic wine made from juniper berries. Juniper was seen as a panacea in the Middle Ages, and many of the properties it was acknowledged as having in the 18th and 19th centuries have been accepted following laboratory testing.

Pleasant smell of violets

• Juniper berries are an **effective diuretic**, which makes urine smell of violets. They are used to **treat generalized oedema**, gallstones, kidney stones and bladder inflammation, as well as **gout, arthritis and rheumatism**.
• They can be used as **antiseptics** to treat leucorrhoea and gonorrhoea.
• They are effective **as a digestive**, especially when the symptoms are flatulence and belching.

OTHER USES: Juniper berries are used to flavour a variety of dishes, especially sauerkraut. They are used as the botanicals for the production of gin, and the juniper-flavoured liqueur called *jenever* also known as "Dutch gin".

OTHER SPECIES: Cade (*Juniperus oxycedrus*), is a shrub found in Mediterranean regions. Incomplete combustion of its wood produces black, strongly smelling "cade oil" or "juniper tar oil". It is widely used in dermatology, to treat eczema, acne, psoriasis, impetigo and ringworm.

METHOD OF USE

• **INTERNAL: White bark decoction.** 20 to 30g (¾ to 1oz) per litre (quart) drunk throughout the day, to treat furunculosis (infected hair follicles).
Decoction. Steep 30 to 60g (1 to 2oz) of wood chips per litre, to induce sweating (sudorific).
Infusion of berries, 20 to 30g (¾ to 1oz) per litre, as a diuretic, tonic and stimulant of the stomach and appetite.
Diuretic **wine.** Crush 60g (2oz) of berries in a mortar. Add to a litre of wine, and bring to the boil. Leave to steep for 3 days. Bottle, and drink a glass every morning on an empty stomach.
Cure (recommended by Sebastian Kneipp, a 19th-century priest credited with being one of the forefathers of the hydrotherapy movement). Start with 4 berries per day, then increase by 1 berry per day up to a dose of 15 berries per day. Then go back down to 1 berry.
• **EXTERNAL:** Juniper **bath.** Boil 2kg (4lb) of young branches with a good handful of berries in water, then add to the bath. To alleviate rheumatism, gout and skin rashes.

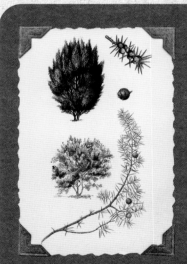

Description

Shrub reaching heights of 3 to 6m (9¾ to 19½ft), common on dry hillsides, moorland and in light woodland. Native throughout the northern hemisphere, up to 3,000m (9,800ft), where a dwarf, creeping form is often found. The trunk, with peeling, often reddish bark, bears sharp, bluish-green, needles, whorled in threes, each with a broad white band running lengthwise. Juniper "berries" are actually miniature fleshy cones, similar to pine cones, and known botanically as "galbuli". They take 2 years to mature, gradually becoming a characteristic dark blue colour, lightened by a whitish bloom. They have a sweet, aromatic flavour that smells of resin.

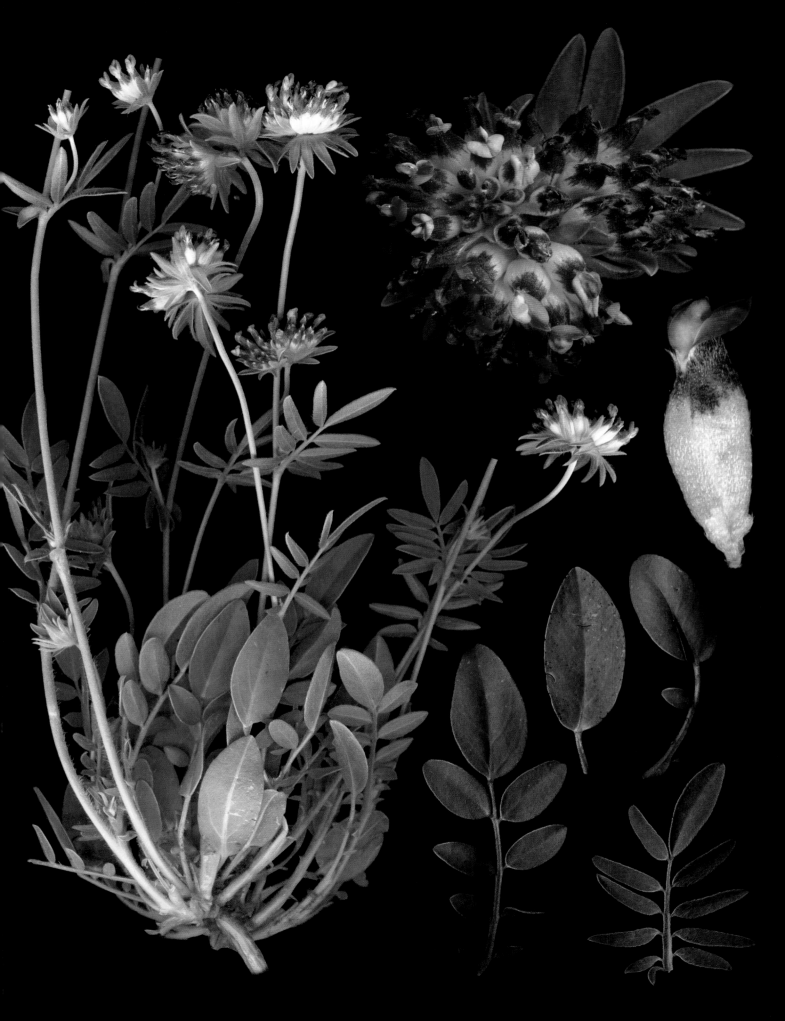

Common Kidney Vetch

Anthyllis vulneraria
FAMILY: FABACEAE

Active elements:
Tannins, saponins, mucilage,
flavonoids and organic acids.

MAIN BENEFITS

★ Cuts, burns,
inflammation of
the skin
★ Cough suppressant
★ Digestive

PARTS USED

★ Flowers, entire plant

OTHER SPECIES: There are several other species of Kidney Vetch. Although they are sometimes referred to as "vulnerary", they are never used in herbal medicine. On the whole these other species are small plants, with the exception of Jove's Beard (*Anthyllis barba-jovis*) which reaches the height of a shrub at 1 to 1½m (3¼ to 5ft), and are only found in southern European regions (by the sea or in the mountains).

This is a plant that advertises the best known of its healing properties in its name: *vulneraria* comes from the Latin *vulnus*, meaning "wound", and vulnery was once used to describe any substance that had the effect of healing wounds. It is also called "Alpine Tea" but note that this name also applies to other plants such as the Mountain Avens (*Dryas octopetala*) and Hyssop-leaved Mountain Ironwort (*Sideritis hyssopifolia*).

A popular healer

• As its Latin name implies, Common Kidney Vetch is a popular remedy recommended for the treatment of numerous skin problems. It is advocated for **healing wounds, burns and inflammations of the skin**.

• It treats ulcerations and boils and **helps tissue to heal**. It is also used to treat eczema.

• It has disinfectant properties and can be used to treat inflammation of the gums and the mucous membranes of the mouth and pharynx.

METHOD OF USE

• **INTERNAL: Infusion.** 10 to 20g (¼ to ¾oz) of entire dried plant per litre (quart) of water or 1 teaspoonful per cup. Drink 2 or 3 cups per day to aid digestion. Sweeten with honey for coughs.

• **EXTERNAL: Decoction.** 40 to 50g (1½ to 1¾oz) of dried plant per litre of water. Use as a wash, then a compress left in place for about 20 minutes on cuts and wounds, irritation and inflammation of the skin.
Poultice. Crush the fresh whole plant and apply to intact skin in case of skin irritation or sunburn.

Description

A herbaceous plant growing to a height of 10 to 30cm (4 to 12in), commonly found in dry meadows, wasteland and slopes from the seaside to 3,000m (9,800ft) above sea level. Found in Europe, North Africa, western Asia and North America. The lower leaves are often undivided, those on the stem have uneven leaflets, the last of which is much larger than the others. The flowers, with a yellow butterfly-like corolla, bloom from May to August. The flowers are grouped into one or two dense flower heads at the end of each stem. The woolly calyx bulges into a bladder, especially after flowering. The Common Kidney Vetch is highly variable in morphology and habitat, and is subdivided into numerous subspecies and varieties.

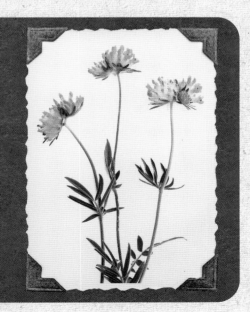

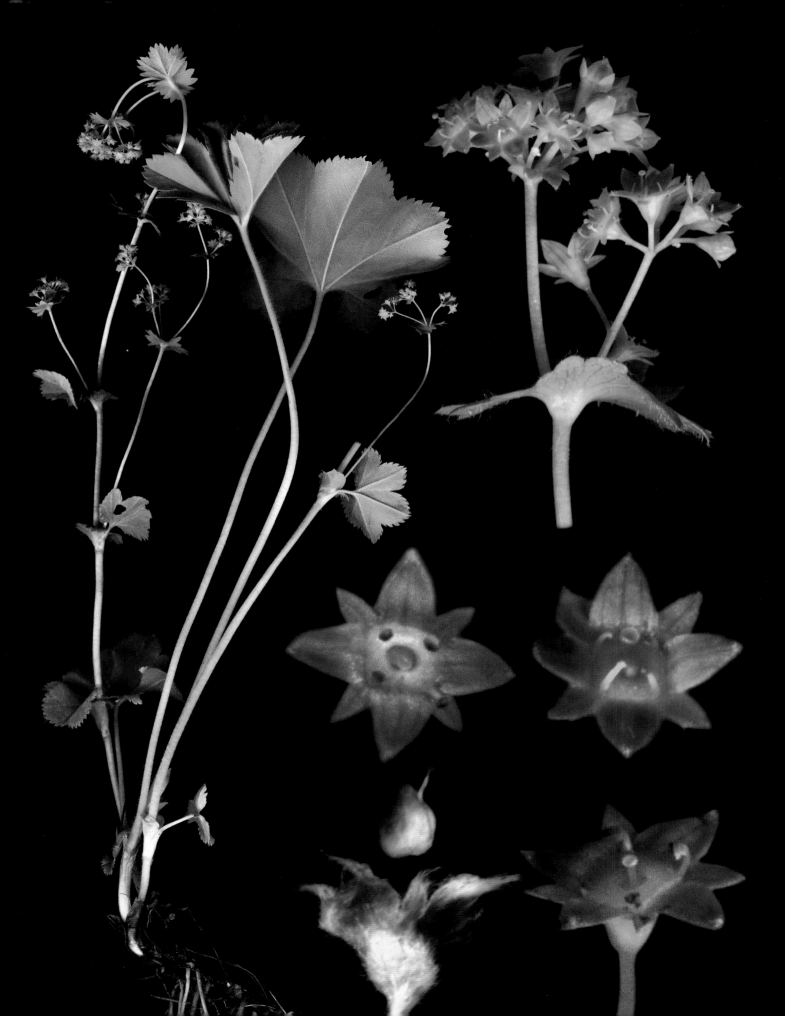

Common Lady's-mantle

Alchemilla vulgaris

FAMILY: ROSACEAE

Active elements:

Tannins, flavonoids, triterpenes, salicylic acid.

I n the 16th century, Andrés de Laguna, one of the great Spanish physicians of his age, recommended Lady's-mantle for the treatment of fractures in young children. Popular tradition granted it the status of a miracle cure for ladies who wished to regain their virginity. For the Swiss priest and herbalist, Johann Künzle, in the early 20th century, it was a panacea for the female body: he used it successfully against leucorrhoea (white discharge), uterine pain, period pain and problems related to childbirth.

A drop of holy water

• Lady's-mantle is effective in **relieving menstrual disorders**: it promotes and regulates menstruation and reduces period pain.
• It is rich in tannins giving it **astringent properties**. It has traditionally been used to treat mild diarrhoea, dysentery and gastroenteritis.
• It is also used to **reduce bleeding** and heal wounds.
• Applied topically, it can **relieve heavy legs**.

OTHER USES: The leaves of Lady's-mantle are edible, but the tannins they contain make them astringent.

DID YOU KNOW?

Alchemists gathered the dewy droplets found on the broad leaves, believing it to be "celestial water" or pure water that they needed for their work. It is formed of excess water secreted by the plant, as well as dew and rain. The plant's name comes from the wide, elegant form of its leaves.

TOXICITY

Lady's-mantle is not really toxic, but is not recommended for use during pregnancy.

MAIN BENEFITS

★ Menstrual problems
★ Anti-diarrhoeal
★ Astringent

PARTS USED

★ Whole plant

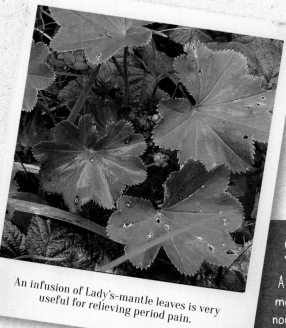

An infusion of Lady's-mantle leaves is very useful for relieving period pain.

METHOD OF USE

• **INTERNAL: Infusion.** 20 to 30g (¾ to 1oz) of plant per litre (quart) of boiling water. Infuse for 15 minutes. Drink 3 to 4 times a day just before and during menstruation for menstrual problems.
Decoction. 40g (1½ oz) of plant per litre of boiling water. Boil for 10 minutes. Use for diarrhoea.

Description

A small perennial plant around 10cm (4in) high, common in meadows, particularly at altitude. It is native throughout the northern hemisphere in numerous related forms. The rounded shape of the bluish-green leaves is particularly eye-catching. They are deeply serrated with a principal vein running from the centre. The stem bears tiny yellowish-green flowers.

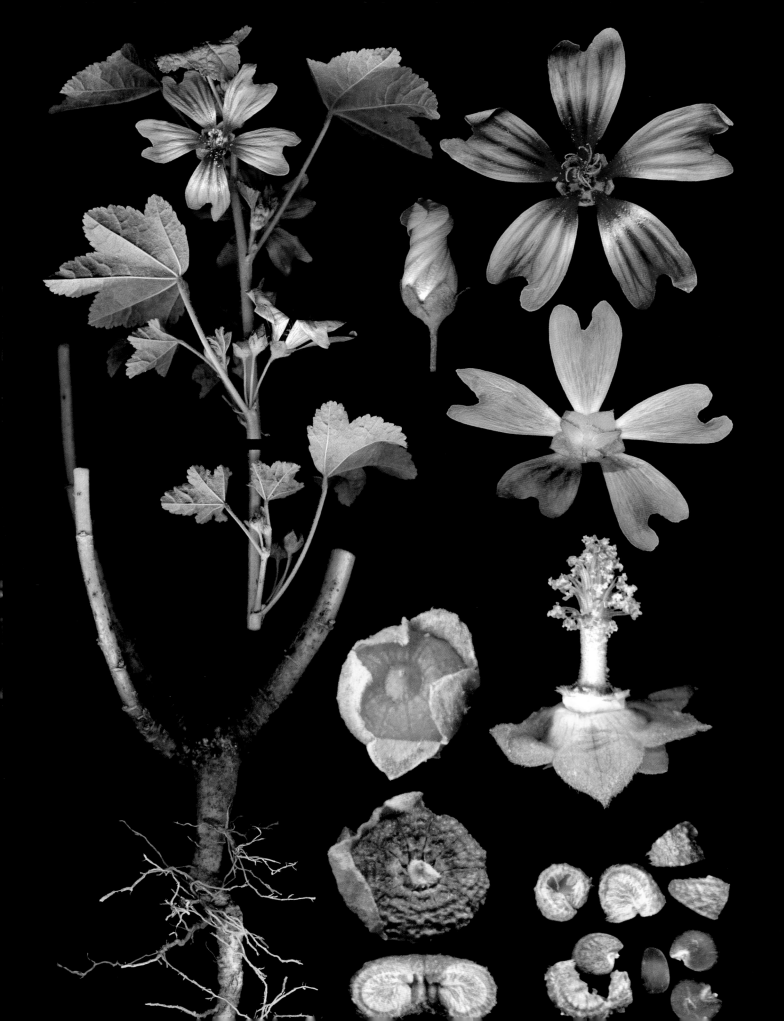

Common Mallow

Malva sylvestris

FAMILY: MALVACEAE

Active elements:
Flavonoids, mucilage. The flowers are rich in anthocyanosides.

The laxative qualities of Common Mallow have been known since ancient times. Cicero records that he underwent a copious purge in the form of a Mallow and Chard stew. Dioscorides, Celsus and Pythagoras all paid tribute to its effectiveness in treating constipation. Hippocrates advocated its use for improving digestion and Pliny claimed that a decoction of Mallow in milk would cure a cough in a few days (although warned that it could cause excessive sexual excitement). For many centuries Mallow was eaten as a vegetable. In the Middle Ages, a salad of its leaves was advocated as healthy "for what softens the belly, heals gravel and breaks down stones".

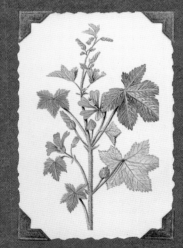

Common Mallow's flowers and leaves are emollients.

the throat. Common Mallow is one of the traditional "seven softening and bechic species" and one of the "four pectoral flowers".

• It reduces inflammation of the intestine and acts as a laxative.

• Used externally, it works wonders in treating **all kinds of irritations and inflammations**. The decoction can be used as a gargle, an enema, in sitz baths, as a douche, and in mouthwashes for mouth ulcers. It can be used as a lotion to treat rosacea and facial irritations, or as a wash or poultice, to **soften skin, soothe itching and promote healing**.

OTHER USES: The tender leaves can be used as the basis for a salad or cooked as a vegetable, but their mucilaginous texture is not to everyone's taste. It makes a delicious soup or "vegetable fondue". The flowers can be used to add a beautiful garnish to cooked dishes. The young and tender fruit is also edible, and can be added to salads after removal of the husks.

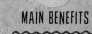

MAIN BENEFITS

★ Respiratory ailments
★ Calmative
★ Softening
★ Anti-inflammatory
★ Anti-irritations
★ Maturative on boils

PARTS USED

★ Flowers, leaves

A soothing anti-inflammatory

• Mallow leaves and flowers are emollients. They soothe irritations of the mucous membranes, and are recommended for the **treatment of bronchitis, dry coughs and inflammation of**

METHOD OF USE

• **INTERNAL:** It is generally the flowers that are used, although the leaves or a mix of flowers and leaves could be used as well.

Decoction. 15 to 20g per litre of water, drink as often as you like. To soothe coughs and irritations.

• **EXTERNAL: Concentrated decoction** of leaves. 30 to 50g (½ to ¾oz) per litre (quart) of water. Reduce by boiling. For external use, the root can also be used in a decoction with the same dose. Use to relieve inflammations.

Warm poultices of boiled leaves. Excellent for aches and pains or to maturate boils.

Description

A beautiful perennial plant commonly found on waste ground, in meadows and along paths. Its upright stem bears rounded leaves, approximately divided into five lobes. The large flowers have three whorls: an epicalyx of three free segments, the calyx with five sepals and the corolla with five pinkish-purple, heart-shaped petals. The threads of the stamens are welded between them along their entire length, forming a tube from which emerge the many styles. The small circular fruits, composed of many carpels, are sometimes called "cheeses" by children because the young fruit looks like a tiny wheel of cheese. The flowers turn blue as they dry.

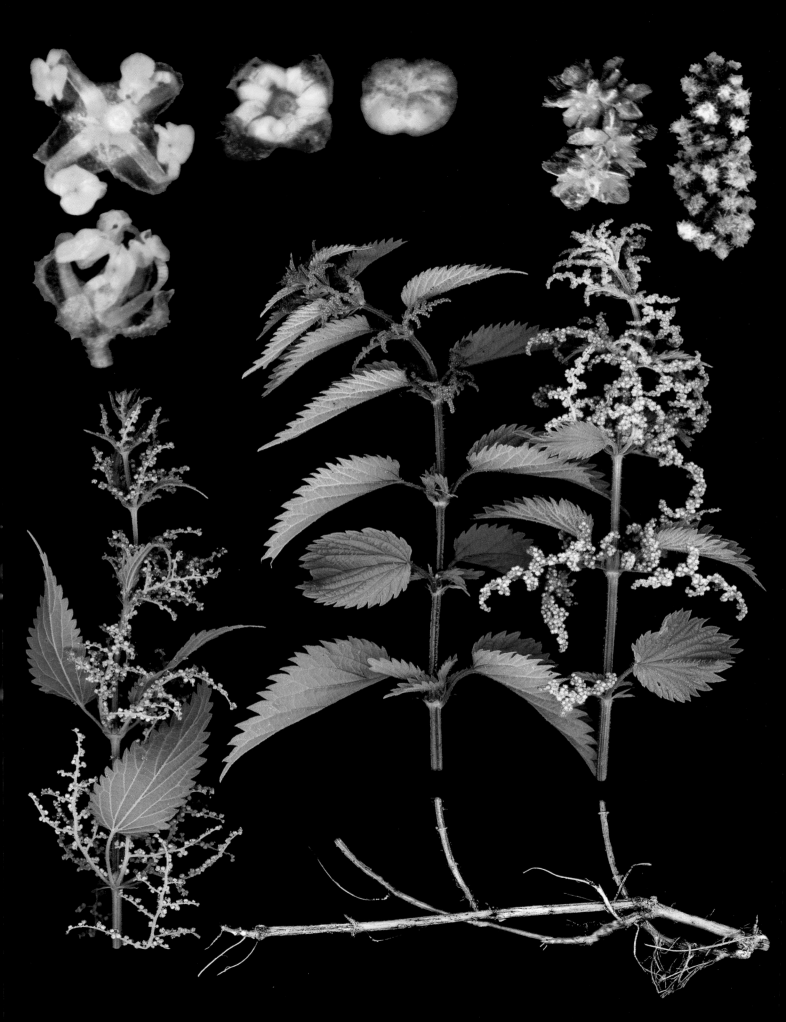

Common Nettle

Urtica dioica

FAMILY: URTICACEAE

Active elements:

Rhizome: polysaccharides, tannins, lectin, phenolic compounds, lignans, sterols.
Leaves: complete proteins, flavonoids and vitamins, mineral salts and oligo-elements: vitamin C (seven times more than oranges), iron, calcium (almost as much as cheese), provitamin A.

Used in the past in cases of paralysis, the Common Nettle was also renowned in popular medicine as an astringent. Rubbing down or whipping with a bunch of nettles used to be advocated for rheumatic pains; this "heroic" procedure is less widely used these days!

Revitalizing and detoxifying

• Nettle rhizomes are effective in treating benign prostatic gland enlargement. They are recommended for **increasing the volume and flow rate of urine** and to reduce post-urination residue.

• The leaves are **detoxifying, diuretic and anti-inflammatory**, and are effective in treating rheumatic pains, arthritis and urinary tract inflammation.

• They are used to break down kidney stones.

• The **astringent properties** of Common Nettle are effective in treating haemorrhages of various origins: coughing up blood, heavy periods, nose bleeds.

• It is an effective purifier, used to **treat rebel skin conditions** such as eczema, psoriasis and dry patches of skin.

• Nettles are used to make scalp lotions to **stimulate hair growth**. They also **keep nails healthy and enhance the complexion**.

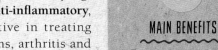

MAIN BENEFITS

★ Diuretic
★ Anti-inflammatory
★ Anti-rheumatic
★ Astringent
★ Revitalizing
★ Skin problems and hair loss

PARTS USED

★ Rhizomes, leaves, whole plant

OTHER SPECIES: The Small Nettle (*Urtica urens*), which has a more painful sting, has the same medicinal properties as the Common Nettle.

OTHER USES: Nettles can be eaten raw or cooked (soups, soufflés, quiches). For gardeners, "nettle liquid manure", made by steeping the leaves in water, is an excellent organic fertilizer and insect repellent, strengthening the natural defences of plants.

METHOD OF USE

• **INTERNAL: Rhizome decoction.** 30 to 40g (1 to 1½oz) per litre (quart) of water. Boil for 10 minutes. Drink 3 times per day for prostate troubles.
Nettle juice. 100g (3½oz) of fresh plant per day as a detoxifier.
Infusion. 30 to 60g (1 to 2oz) of leaves per litre of water Allow to infuse for 10 minutes and drink a cup before meals for rheumatic pain and arthritis.
• **EXTERNAL: Scalp lotion.** Steep 60g (2oz) of dried rhizome with 60g (2oz) of nettle in a litre of colourless spirit for one month. Administer a daily scalp rub with this lotion.

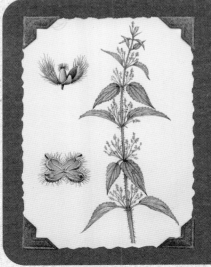

Description

A perennial that grows to 50cm to 1m (1½ to 3¼ft) with spreading rhizomes. Common in temperate regions, thriving in nitrogen-rich soils, including rubble, abandoned sites and roadsides. It is covered in many rigid hairs that break on the slightest contact, injecting a stinging, histamine-rich liquid into skin, causing an unpleasant burning sensation and raised reddish welts. The erect stems bear opposite, broad leaves, with sharply serrated margins. The greenish flowers appear in clusters in the leaf axils; plants bear only male or female flowers.

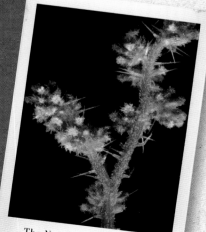

The Nettle's stinging hairs give it a bad reputation.

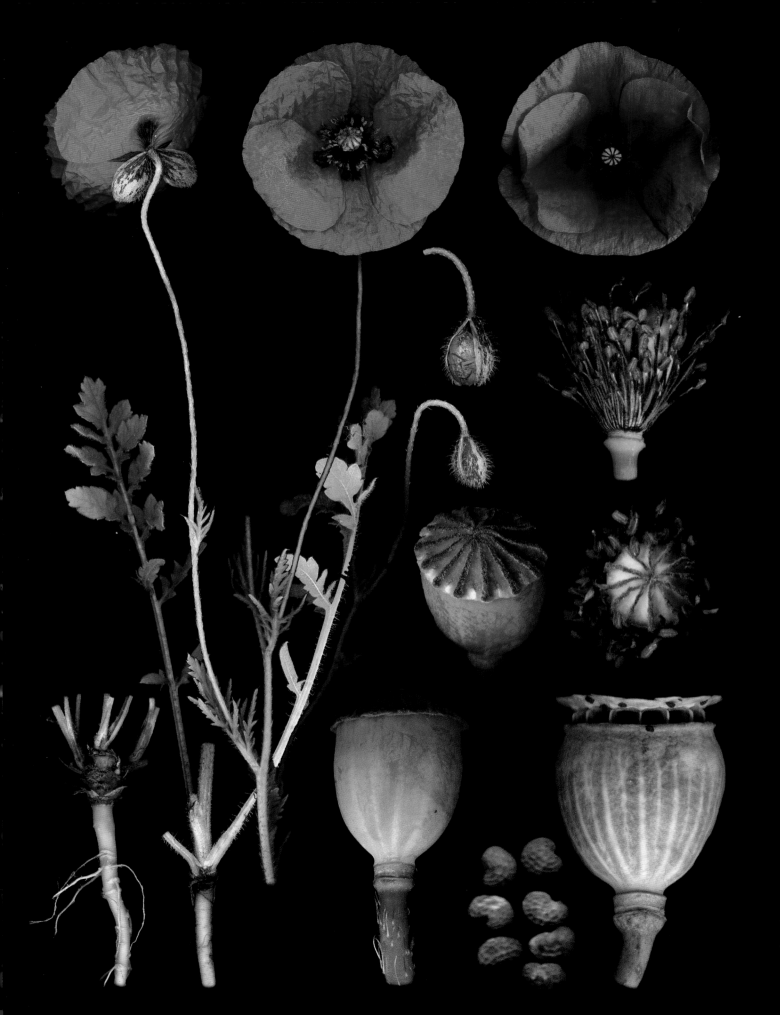

Common Poppy

Papaver rhoeas
FAMILY: PAPAVERACEAE

Active elements:
Mucilage, tannins, alkaloids (including
rhoeadine and papaverine). The Poppy's colour
is due to its anthocyanoside content.
The seeds contain a fatty oil.

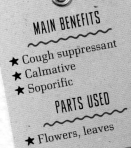

MAIN BENEFITS

★ Cough suppressant
★ Calmative
★ Soporific

PARTS USED

★ Flowers, leaves

OTHER SPECIES: Several closely related species, often confused with the Common Poppy, have the same properties. However, the Opium Poppy (*Papaver somniferum*), identifiable by its pale pink flowers, contains alkaloids that have been known to have powerful narcotic, analgesic and antispasmodic properties (in morphine and codeine) for 3,000 years. This **toxic** plant, which should only be used on medical advice, is regulated by drugs laws.

The Common Poppy has a glorious past, recommended by Dioscorides and considered a specific remedy for pleurisy during the Renaissance period. More recently, Chomel, the 19th-century French physician, prescribed it as "a more effective sudorific than goat's blood, mule droppings and other much vaunted remedies". We'll take his word for it! It was still used until recently in popular medicine as a remedy for rheumatism and colic and a recommended sudorific for whenever blood was drawn. It was also recommended for dry coughs, sore throats, pulmonary catarrh, bronchitis and whooping cough and is still prescribed for these today.

The soothing Poppy

• The soothing Poppy **relieves a cough**.
• Its **calmative and even slightly narcotic** properties make it an excellent ally in treating anxiety attacks and insomnia suffered by children or the elderly, especially when sleeplessness is due to coughing fits.
• The Common Poppy flower is sometimes used externally to **treat eye problems and dental abscesses**, and the capsule in a soothing gargle, instead of an Opium poppy capsule. The Common Poppy is one of the ingredients of the traditional "**infusion of four pectoral flowers**" (comprised, in fact, of not four, but seven flowers).

OTHER USES: Young Common Poppy leaves are traditionally eaten in a salad or boiled as a vegetable throughout the Mediterranean region. The Romans extracted a cooking oil from the tiny brown seeds.

METHOD OF USE

• **INTERNAL:** **Infusion.** 15g (½oz) of dried flowers per litre (quart) of water, which can be sweetened with the addition of honey. Drink 3 or 4 cups per day for anxiety and insomnia.
Syrup. Pour a litre of boiling water over 400g (14oz) of fresh flowers. Cover and leave to steep overnight. Strain, add 1½kg (3¼lb) of sugar and cook until it has the consistency of syrup. To relieve coughing. **Conserve.** Crush fresh flowers with double their weight in sugar to obtain a kind of paste. In dispensaries, the plant is used in a range of preparations, including Poppy lozenges.
• **EXTERNAL:** Hot, soothing **poultices** of infused flowers. Apply to swollen eyelids or to the cheek to relieve the pain of dental abscesses.

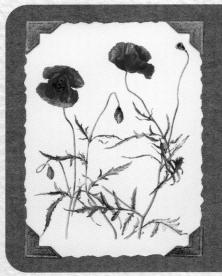

Description

An attractive annual plant, which is becoming common again after almost being eliminated by the widespread use of herbicides in agriculture. A native of the Middle East, the Common Poppy spread with the other meadow plants associated with cereal crops. Its hairy, dissected leaves form beautiful rosettes in springtime, from which a slender stem emerges to bear large, scarlet, four-petalled flowers surrounding a heart of black stamens with a globular pistil in the middle. The petals become a deep wine-red as they dry out.

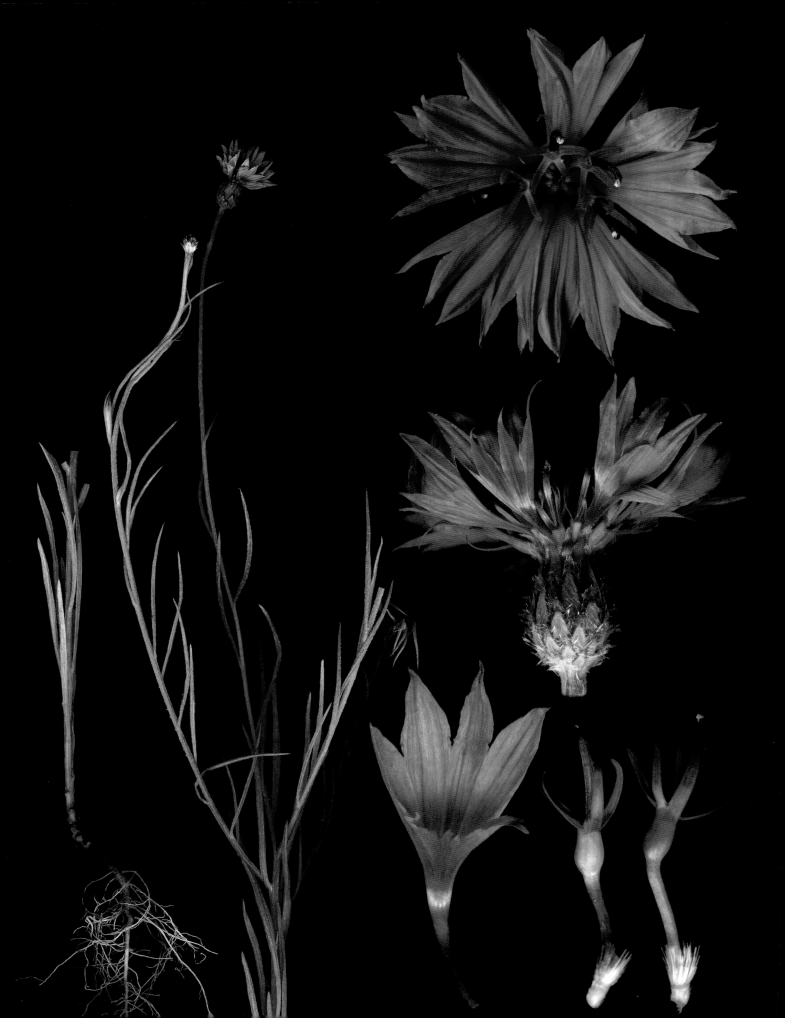

Cornflower

Cyanus segetum

FAMILY: ASTERACEAE

Active elements:
Anthocyanosides (responsible for the colour of the petals), flavonoids, acetylenic components, polyines.

I n the 12th century, Hildegard of Bingen, was one of the first to mention the properties of the Cornflower. According to the "doctrine of signatures", which stated that herbs resembling parts of the body can be used to treat ailments of those body parts, the colour of this flower evoked that of bright, healthy eyes, which made it appropriate for treating eye problems. Mattioli, the eminent 16th-century physician and naturalist, advocated Cornflowers for this purpose. Cornflowers were used in diuretic and anti-rheumatic treatments. It was not long ago that a traditional drink was still made in the north of France, using Cornflowers steeped in beer, to treat arthritis.

For the eyes and skin

• Cornflowers are mainly used as to **soothe inflammatory eye diseases**. However, their reputation for healing conjunctivitis, irritation and redness of the eyelids and styes, has not been proven in recent studies.

• Cornflowers are also slightly **diuretic and have a tonic effect**.

• Used externally, the Cornflower's **softening, astringent and anti-inflammatory properties** mean that an infusion or hydrolate of flowers is beneficial for the skin. They cause capillaries to contract and so are effective in reducing rosacea.

DID YOU KNOW? Cornflower often used to grow as a weed in cornfields, hence its name. It is not related to corn or any other grains.

METHOD OF USE

• **EXTERNAL: Infusion.** 2 teaspoonsful of cornflowers per cup of boiling water. Leave to steep, then bathe the eyelids liberally. The same infusion, with a drop or two of rosewater, applied in the form of a poultice for 10 minutes will make for sparkling eyes and rested eyelids.
Cornflower water tightens the pores of oily skin and refreshes sensitive skins. It provides good after-sun care when sprayed on to the parts of the body that have been exposed to the sun. Applied to the scalp, it acts as tonic and brings life to dull hair, while preventing the appearance of dandruff.

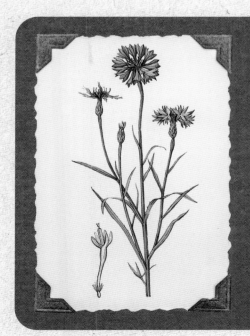

Description

In the past, Cornflowers were a common sight at harvest time. However, extensive use of modern pesticides means it has been ruthlessly eliminated, to the extent that it is no longer common, and could even be classified as rare in some areas. An annual growing up to 60cm (2ft) high, it has very fine, downy leaves and elegant, strikingly blue flower heads whose outer, tube-like florets are much longer than the inner.

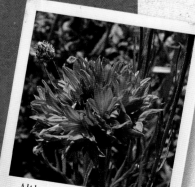

Although once common, the Cornflower is becoming rarer.

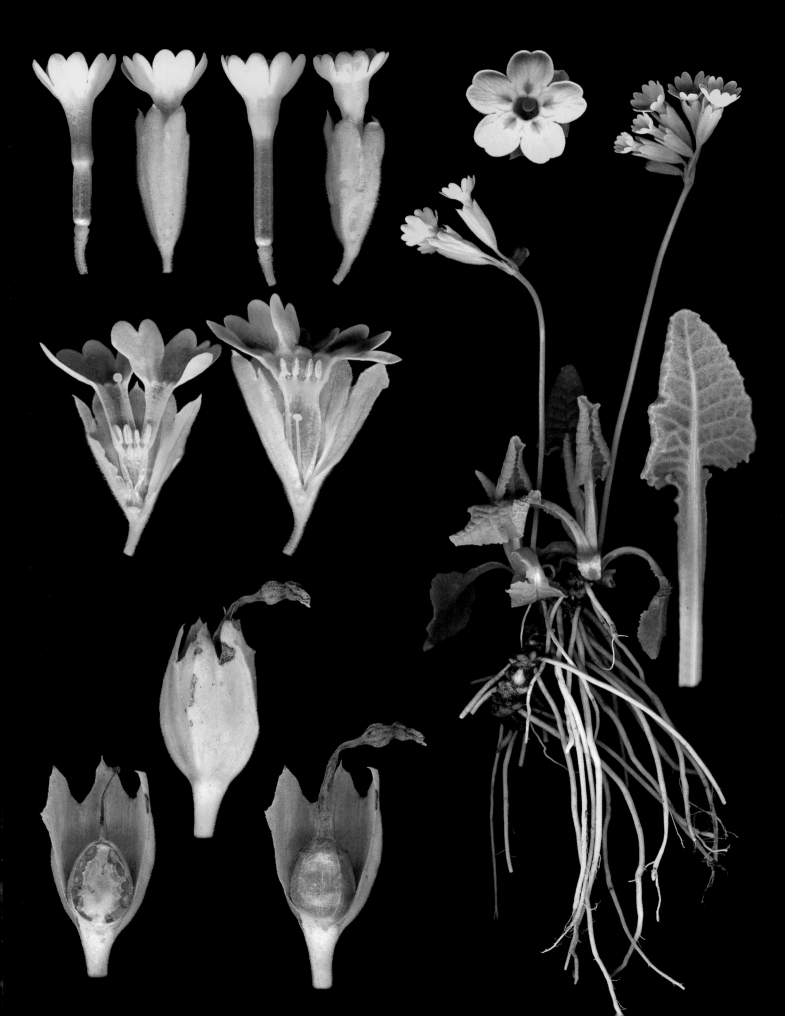

Cowslip

Primula veris
FAMILY: PRIMULACEAE

Active elements:
Flavonoids (including gossypetin),
triterpenic saponosides, phenolic heterosides.
Roots: essential oil.

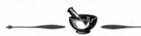

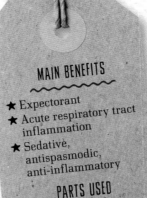

According to ancient medical tradition, the Cowslip has long been considered a remedy for paralysis. According to Chomel, the 19th-century French physician to Louis XV, this "paralysis herb" was particularly effective in curing "paralysis of the tongue and stuttering". For Linnaeus, the Swedish botanist and physician, the "flowers are sedative, soothe pain and induce sleep", properties that were later used to alleviate hysteria, apoplexy, headaches, dizziness, insomnia and stomach cramps.

METHOD OF USE

• **INTERNAL: Infusion of flowers.** Used to treat migraines, insomnia, coughs, aches and pains. A beautiful golden yellow, it exudes a pleasant fragrance and tastes delicious (Cowslip flowers infused in wine adds a delicious bouquet where it does not exist). Infuse 4 to 6g of flowers per cup of boiling water. Leave to steep for 10 minutes and drink 3 cups per day, including one just before bed. **Root decoction.** Prepare 30g (1oz) of root per litre (quart) of water. Boil for 5 minutes and leave to steep for 10 minutes. Drink 3 cups per day, between meals. Use to promote expectoration.

• **EXTERNAL: Strong root decoction.** Use 100g (3½oz) per litre of water, and boil for 20 minutes. Use in compresses to relieve bruising.
   Juice of the crushed plant on gout-related pain in joints or venomous animal bites and stings.

Free the airways

• The saponosides contained in the root increase and thin salivary and bronchial secretions. As a result, they **promote expectoration**. Recommended for bronchitis, pneumonia; chronic, productive coughs; and whooping cough. Advocated for treating acute inflammation of the respiratory tract. Sometimes used to treat rheumatism.

• The leaves have **similar properties**, but are less potent.

• The flowers are **antispasmodic, sedative and anti-inflammatory**. They are used to treat infant insomnia, asthma and allergies.

• Used topically, Cowslip works to **soothe and heal skin problems** (bruising, sunburn or spots) or in mouthwash for mouth hygiene.

OTHER USES: Cowslip flowers and very young leaves are edible. The flowers add a nice touch of colour to salads and desserts.

TOXICITY
Cowslip roots consumed to excess can lead to nausea, vomiting and diarrhoea.

Description

A perennial commonly found in fields and meadows, hedgerows and on the edge of woodland throughout Europe and Asia. Its light-green, crinkly oval leaves, in dense rosettes, create a carpet across the ground. A single stem grows to a height of about 20cm (8in) from the centre of each rosette of leaves, crowned in early spring with an umbel of golden yellow flowers, each with five orange marks at the base of the petals. The flowers are lightly fragranced. The roots give off an obvious smell of aniseed when crushed.

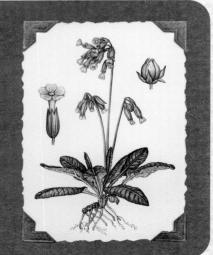

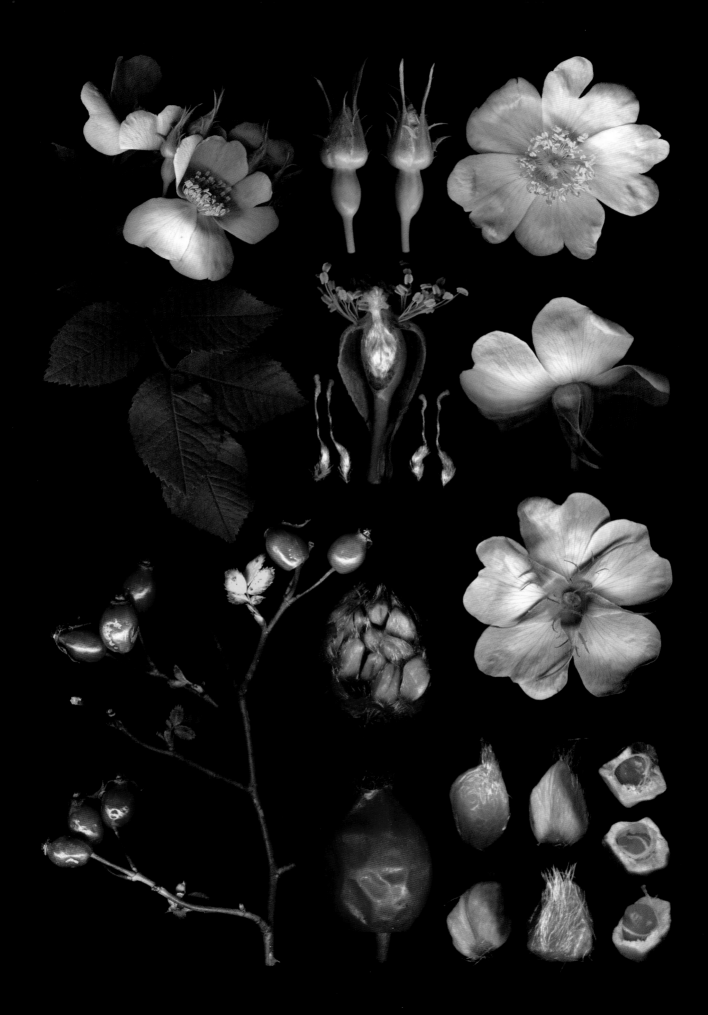

Dog Rose

Rosa canina

FAMILY: ROSACEAE

Active elements:
Leaves and flowers: tannins.
Rose hips: sugars, pectin, tannins, sorbitol, organic acids (in particular malic and citric), carotenoids, high levels of vitamin C (between 1 and 1.7%).

MAIN BENEFITS

★ Infectious diseases
★ Lack of tone
★ Laxative (flowers) or anti-diarrhoeal (rose hips, leaves)
★ Anti-rheumatic

PARTS USED

★ Rose hips, leaves, flowers

The Persians held both the modest Dog Rose hips and flowers in high regard: the former with its powers to dissolve calculi (stones) and reduce heavy menstrual flow; and the latter, mixed with sugar cane, with the power to cure consumption (pulmonary tuberculosis), and even bring people back from the dead. In the 17th century, the famous French medical writer and healer Marie Fouquet, made reference to "rose hip opiate" which "tightened the stomach" to alleviate diarrhoea. A traditional popular remedy for rabies called for the person bitten by a rabid dog to eat an omelette containing 60g (2oz) of grated Dog Rose root on an empty stomach; this may be the source of the plant's name.

A remarkable source of vitamin C

• Rose hips are highly regarded for their power to **prevent and alleviate flu and other infectious diseases**. The vitamin C content is truly remarkable: there is almost as much vitamin C in the little rose hip as in a large lemon. Rose hips are, therefore, **particularly recommended for people lacking vitamin C**—a fairly common occurrence in modern life, especially among smokers, who expend huge amounts of this indispensable substance.

• Rose hips have astringent properties which makes them an effective **remedy for enteritis and diarrhoea**. The decoction is both an efficient anti-diarrhoeal and an anthelmintic that rids the body of roundworm.

• A clinical study has shown that rose hip powder can provide significant relief from the pains of osteoarthritis. This is due to its **anti-inflammatory effect**.

• The flowers have a **slight laxative effect** while the tannin-rich leaves can be used as an astringent to treat diarrhoea.

OTHER USES: Puréed rose-hip pulp is used to make syrups, jams and desserts. In Sweden, this purée is the basis for *nyponsoppa*, the national soup, which is also available in packet form in supermarkets. While it is most commonly used in sweet rather than savoury cooking, it actually works well with dishes such as pasta or on top of pizza.

OTHER SPECIES: There are over 100 species of wild rose worldwide. Their properties vary widely from one species to another.

METHOD OF USE

• **INTERNAL:** Decoction. 30g (1oz) of hips per litre (quart) of water (5 to 10g per cup). Boil for 2 minutes. Drink 3 or 4 cups per day for vitamin C. **Infusion of flowers.** Very pleasant tasting. Made with a tablespoonful per cup, infused for 10 minutes. Use as a laxative.

Description

A bush growing to a height of 2 to 3m (6½ to 9¾ft), commonly found in hedgerows and on the edge of woodland. Found in Europe, western Asia and North Africa. Its long, upright, gently curving stems, covered with sharp thorns, bear compound leaves of serrated, oval leaflets, and beautiful, fragile flowers with five light-pink, or sometimes white, petals. They mature into the small red "pears" known as "rose hips" in autumn. The seeds inside are covered with irritating hairs which have been used by generations of naughty children to make "itching powder".

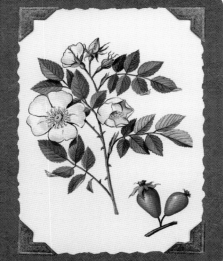

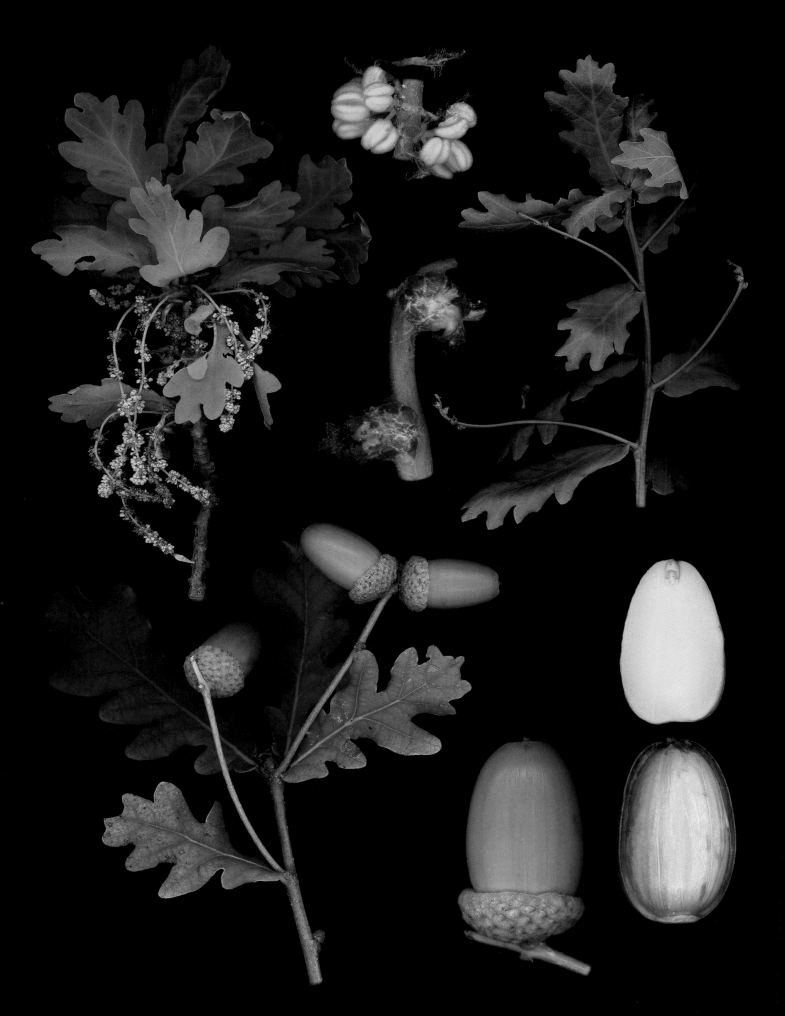

English Oak

Quercus robur

FAMILY: FAGACEAE

Active elements:

Large quantities of gallotannins, catechic tannins and ellagitannins.

As the sacred tree of the Druids and home of Mistletoe, Oak was subject to great veneration. It also had a therapeutic role: its bark is highly astringent and was used to reduce fevers and to tone the digestive system. Acorns were used to treat rickets, inflamed lymph nodes of the neck, and colic. Like the Gauls of continental Europe, the physicians of the Middle Ages and Renaissance continued to advocate Oak for the same uses.

Tannin-related properties

• **Highly astringent due to its high tannin content**, the bark can be used externally to treat leucorrhoea, anal fissures, haemorrhoids and as a gargle for sore throats.

• It soothes mouth ulcers and gingivitis and is generally useful in **treating skin problems**: itching, small sores, infections. It alleviates **excessive sweating of the feet**.

• The leaves, which contain less tannin than the bark, can be used internally **to combat diarrhoea and dysentery**.

It is best to stick to external use (see Toxicity).

OTHER USES: Acorns were once widely cooked and consumed in Europe. Powdered acorns have often been used as an alternative to coffee. It is gentle on the stomach. Pulverized Oak bark contains "tan" which gave rise to the word "tannin" and "to tan" as it was used to prepare hides during the leather-making process.

TOXICITY

Internal use of the bark or galls may lead to constipation if used wrongly or for too long. Best avoided.

MAIN BENEFITS

★ Astringent
★ Anti-diarrhoeal

PARTS USED

★ Leaves, fruit (acorns), bark

METHOD OF USE

• **INTERNAL: Decoction of leaves** (not as bitter as the bark decoction). 20g (¾oz) of leaves per litre (quart) of water. Use for diarrhoea.
Wine. Leave 30g (1oz) of fresh, washed bark to steep for 12 hours in a litre of good red wine. Strain, add sugar and drink a glass or two at mealtimes (to treat haemorrhoids, follow an 8-day course).
Acorn powder. Shell the acorns and leave the nut inside to dry. Pulverize and then leave to dry again in a thin layer. Take a teaspoonful in the morning on an empty stomach and one in the evening at bedtime, by way of a tonic.
• **EXTERNAL: Prolonged decoction.** 100g (3½oz) of bark in a litre of water. Strain and use this decoction as a douche (to treat vaginal discharge, leucorrhoea); or for soaking compresses, to be replaced 3 times a day (haemorrhoids, fissures, sores, chilblains); or add honey to use as a gargle against chronic sore throats and gum inflammation.

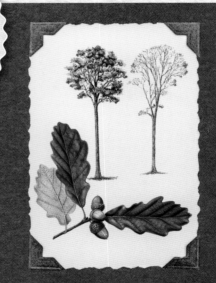

Description

This beautiful tall tree, growing to heights of up to 35m (115ft) is common throughout Europe, and as far afield as western Asia and North Africa. It is easily identifiable by its distinctive, lobed leaves which are a beautiful dark green. It flowers April–May; its male flowers forming hanging catkins while the female flowers cluster on the young branches. Its fruit (acorn) grows on the end of a long stalk, a characteristic which distinguishes it from the fruit of the Sessile Oak (*Q. petraea*). Oak apples or galls often grow on Oak leaves; they are the result of an injection of chemicals by the gall wasp.

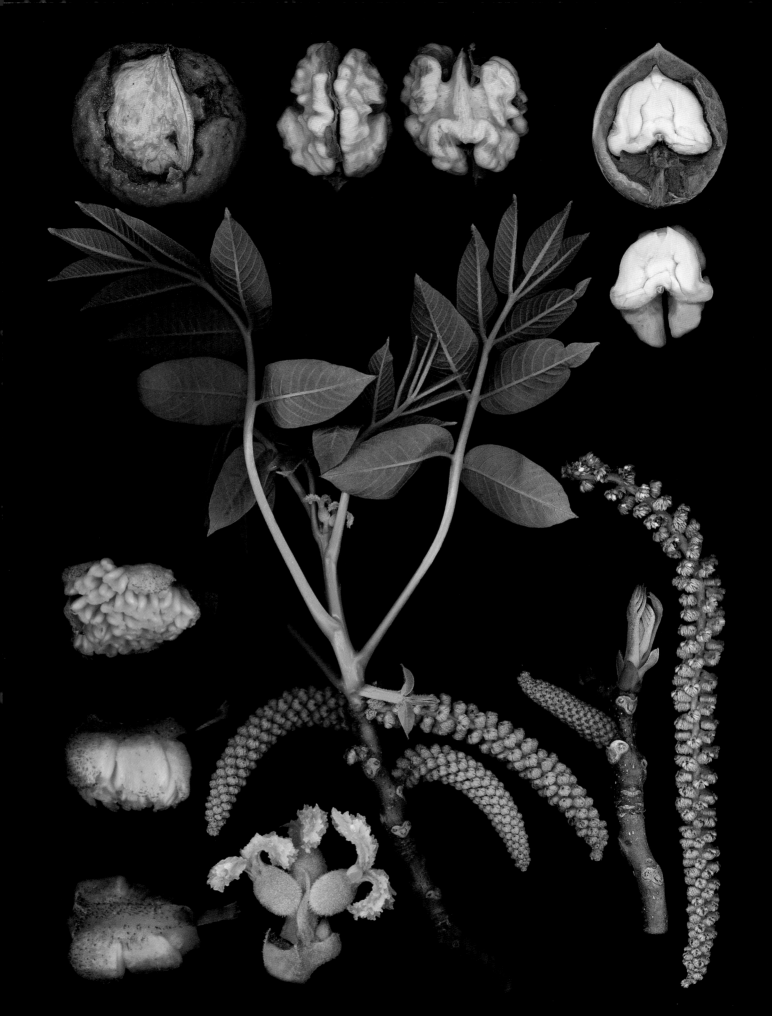

English Walnut

Juglans regia

FAMILY: JUGLANDACEAE

Active elements:

Leaves: naphtoquinones (in particular juglone), tannins, flavonoids, vitamin C, aromatic oil.
Nuts: fatty oil rich in polyunsaturated fatty acids (principally linoleic, oleic and linolenic acids).
Husks: naphtoquinones.

MAIN BENEFITS

★ Digestive tonic and anti-diarrhoeal
★ Alleviates heavy legs
★ Excessive sweating
★ Skin problems
★ Skincare.

PARTS USED

★ Leaves, nuts, nut oil

METHOD OF USE

• **INTERNAL: Infusion.** 20g (¾oz) of leaves per litre (quart) of water. Drink 3 or 4 cups per day to treat diarrhoea and gastric problems.
Depurative **syrup,** excellent for the stomach. Tightly pack the fresh leaves into a suitable container and steep for 15 days in the same volume of a colourless spirit. Filter and add 180g (6¼oz) of sugar syrup for every 100g (3½oz) of the alcoholature.
Nut wine. Steep 30 roughly chopped, newly formed green walnuts in 3 litres of red wine and a litre of colourless spirit, with cinnamon, nutmeg and cloves. Filter and add 300g (10½oz) of sugar. Leave to mature. An excellent tonic aperitif.
• **EXTERNAL: Decoction.** 50g (1¾oz) of leaves per litre of water. Use in lotions, compresses, vaginal douches and enemas for skin problems.

Walnut leaves have been used since time immemorial for their tonic, stimulant, stomachic and depurative properties. Their action on the digestive tract and muscle tone is evident. They stimulate the liver and circulation, and also purify the blood. Their antibiotic properties have been long recognized by country folk who used them to treat patients suffering from anthrax exposure. Walnut leaf is also said to be an effective treatment for diabetes, as it reduces blood sugar, and decreases the thirst and frequent need to urinate suffered by diabetics. A Walnut leaf decoction was traditionally used externally, to treat leucorrhoea (vaginal discharge), eczema, cradle cap, ulcers, irritation of the eyelids, dandruff and hair loss. The nut husk, which is tonic, stomachic and depurative like the leaves, is also an efficient anthelmintic. Walnut oil was used in the past to treat tapeworm, renal colic and bladder stones.

Your skin's best friend

• The astringent leaves are used to **treat mild diarrhoea** and gastrointestinal inflammation.
• They are also recommended for the **relief of the symptoms of heavy legs** and of haemorrhoids.
• Used externally, they can help to **soothe skin inflammations** (including nappy rash), irritation and itching.
• They are also used as a balm for **chaps, cracks, stings, sunburn** and mild burns. They are specifically renowned as anti-dandruff treatment.
• For beauty care: a bath of walnut leaves makes the skin elastic and **soft to the touch**.

• Lotion of leaves also helps dry out excessively sweaty feet and hands.

OTHER USES: It goes without saying that walnuts are a delicious, oleaginous fruit. Walnut oil (which turns rancid very quickly) is used in the manufacture of paint and soap. It was used in the past to tan hides; nowadays, the tannin-rich husk is mostly used to stain wood very dark brown.

Description

The majestic English Walnut tree, which can grow to a height of 18m (59ft), probably originated from southeastern Europe and western Asia. It is commonly cultivated in all temperate countries for its nuts and the oil that can be extracted from them. The Walnut tree is easy to identify by its smooth, light-coloured bark and large leaves made up of between five and nine elongated leaflets. It has two kinds of flowers: the females, in terminal clusters, and the males, in drooping catkins. Its fruit is enclosed in a green husk.

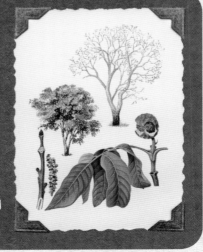

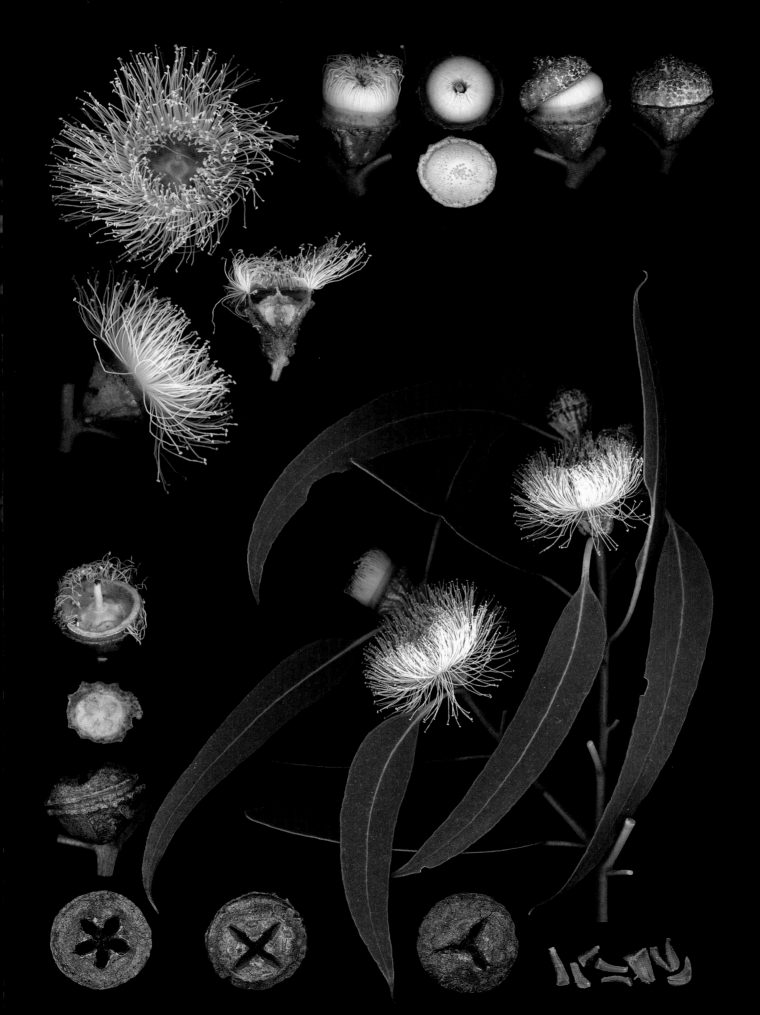

Eucalyptus

Eucalyptus sp.

FAMILY: MYRTACEAE

Active elements:

Polyphenols, triterpenes, aromatic oil rich in cineole (or eucalyptol) and other terpenes, variable depending on species: alpha-pinene and globulol (*Eucalyptus globulus*), alpha-terpineol and citrals (*E. radiata*), citronella (*E. citronnata*).

Aboriginal Australians used Eucalyptus to treat infections and fevers. It was introduced into France in 1856. In days gone by it was highly advocated as an antipyretic (fever reducer). Jules Verne went so far as to comment that the simple presence of Eucalyptus in a region, "was enough to neutralize malarial miasma". In Spain, it was also used to treat pulmonary tuberculosis. Such were its disinfectant properties it was also recommended for purulent disorders of the urethra and vagina, white discharge, and even gonorrhoea. It was also found to have significant hypoglycaemic properties; its use can cause urine sugar levels to drop significantly.

Decongestant of the nose and bronchial tubes

• Eucalyptus is first and foremost a **powerful remedy for respiratory tract ailments**. It is an excellent bronchial tube antiseptic, and is also used to make many of the targeted syrups and suppositories sold in pharmacies. Its use is advocated for acute or chronic bronchitis and all respiratory ailments in general (painful throat, mucous membranes of the nose), colds, flu and sore throats.

• It is both **aperitive and digestive**, and it is widely used when the digestive system is upset as a result of respiratory problems.

• The essential oil of the leaves of the Lemon Eucalyptus, diluted in sweet almond oil and rubbed on the body, **relieves rheumatism and neuralgia** as well as respiratory illnesses.

• The **antiseptic properties** of Eucalyptus vapours mean people suffering from colds find inhaling it helps to clear their noses.

METHOD OF USE

• **INTERNAL:** Infusion. 20 to 30g (¾ to 1oz) of leaves per litre (quart) of boiling water. Leave to steep for 20 minutes. Drink 4 or 5 cups per day for respiratory ailments.
Syrup. Prepare the infusion as above, but using 20g (¾oz) of Eucalyptus per 300g (10½oz) of water. Strain, add 300g (10½oz) of sugar and simmer until it has the consistency of syrup.

• **EXTERNAL:** Gargle with a strong infusion for sore throats. Inhale the vapours of the same infusion to stave off a cold or disinfect the respiratory tract.

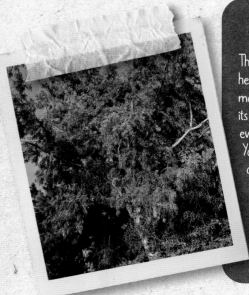

Description

This large tree is native to Australia, and can reach heights of up to 35m (115ft). It is acclimatized in most hot and dry regions of the world. The bark of its whitish trunk peels off into long strips. Its tough, evergreen leaves are a beautiful, glaucous green. Young leaves are short and broad; adult leaves are curved in the shape of a scythe. The flowers have numerous fluffy stamens enclosed in a cap, which bloom from the leaf axils. The fruits are cone-shaped capsules with a lid-like valve at the end. All the green parts of the plant give off a powerful, balsamic aroma.

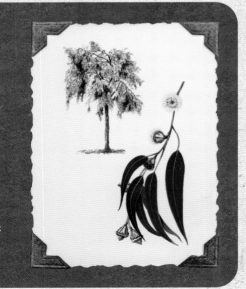

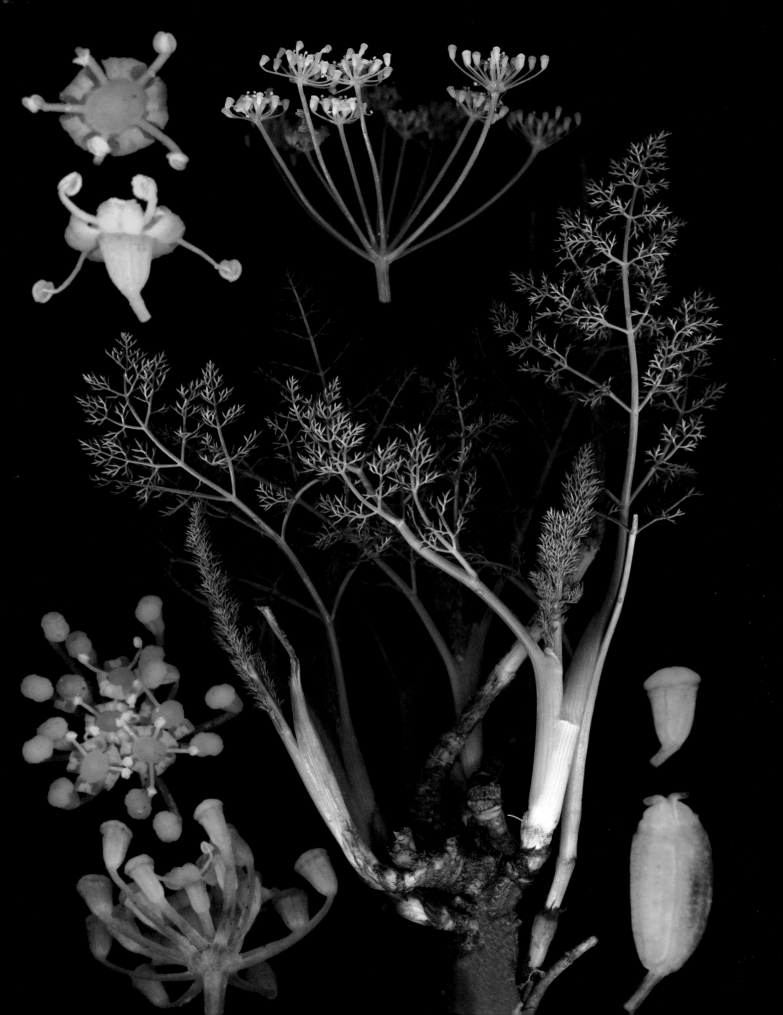

Fennel

Fœniculum vulgare

FAMILY: APIACEAE

Active elements:

An aromatic essence rich in anethole, methyl chavicol or estragole and fenchone. Flavonoids, sterols and furanocoumarins, in particular imperatorin and bergapten.

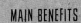
DID YOU KNOW? The cultivar of Fennel eaten in salad is the Florence Fennel. Florence Fennel originated in Italy, where it was first recorded in the 16th century. Its tightly interlocked swollen leaf bases or "bulbs" and edible leaves have a delicate aniseed taste.

Fennel was used by the Assyrians and the Babylonians to relieve stomach pains. It was later found to have diuretic properties and was advocated for the treatment of bladder stones and pains. The medieval medical school, Schola Medica Salernitana, vouched for its powerful ability to relieve flatulence.

Excellent digestive and galactogenic properties

• Fennel is **digestive, carminative and galactogenic** (it stimulates the production of breast milk); it is one of the traditional "four hot seeds" along with Aniseed, Coriander and Caraway. It stimulates contractions and activates the secretions from digestive tube glands, and is effective in treating flatulence.

• Popular medicine advocates the use of Fennel seeds to **stimulate the production of milk in breast-feeding mothers**.

• The leaves can be used in a poultice to **treat engorged breasts**.

• The root can be taken as a **diuretic**. It tackles water retention, whatever the cause and location: swollen ankles, feet and legs, swollen stomach, puffy eyelids.

• The root is also said to **stimulate appetite**.

OTHER USES: The young shoots make a delicious addition to a salad. Mature leaves can be eaten as an aromatic vegetable. The stems can also be eaten when young and tender. The flowers have an aromatic, hot, sugary taste. They contribute a fragrant flavour to dishes and make delicious infusions that have digestive properties. Fennel seeds make a tasty condiment. They are often served at the end of a meal in Indian restaurants, to freshen breath and aid digestion.

METHOD OF USE

• **INTERNAL:** Widely used in Provence to flavour fish, olives and snails. Finely chopped seeds are added to dishes that are more difficult to digest and the tasty leaves aid the process.

Decoction. 20 to 30g (¾ to 1oz) of root per litre (quart) of water, as a diuretic or to stimulate appetite.

Infusion. 15 to 30g (½ to 1oz) of seeds per litre of boiling water. Drink a cup after each meal. For a stimulating wine, steep 30 to 50g (1 to 1¾oz) of seeds per litre of wine. After 15 days, a glass drunk during a meal will aid digestion and stimulate lactation.

• **EXTERNAL:** To treat engorged breasts, apply a poultice of crushed leaves, or compresses soaked in a concentrated decoction of leaves.

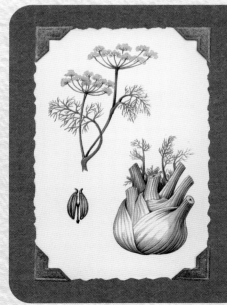

Description

A large perennial plant, growing to a height of 1 to 2m (3¼ to 6½ft), common in dry areas and on roadsides. It is found throughout the Mediterranean basin and is often cultivated as a crop. The tall straight stems grow from the sheaths of the broad bulb-like base and bear dark green, filiform leaves. The small yellow flowers form terminal, compound umbels. The yellow-green fruit has five marked ribs. When brushed, the plant gives off a mild, aromatic scent.

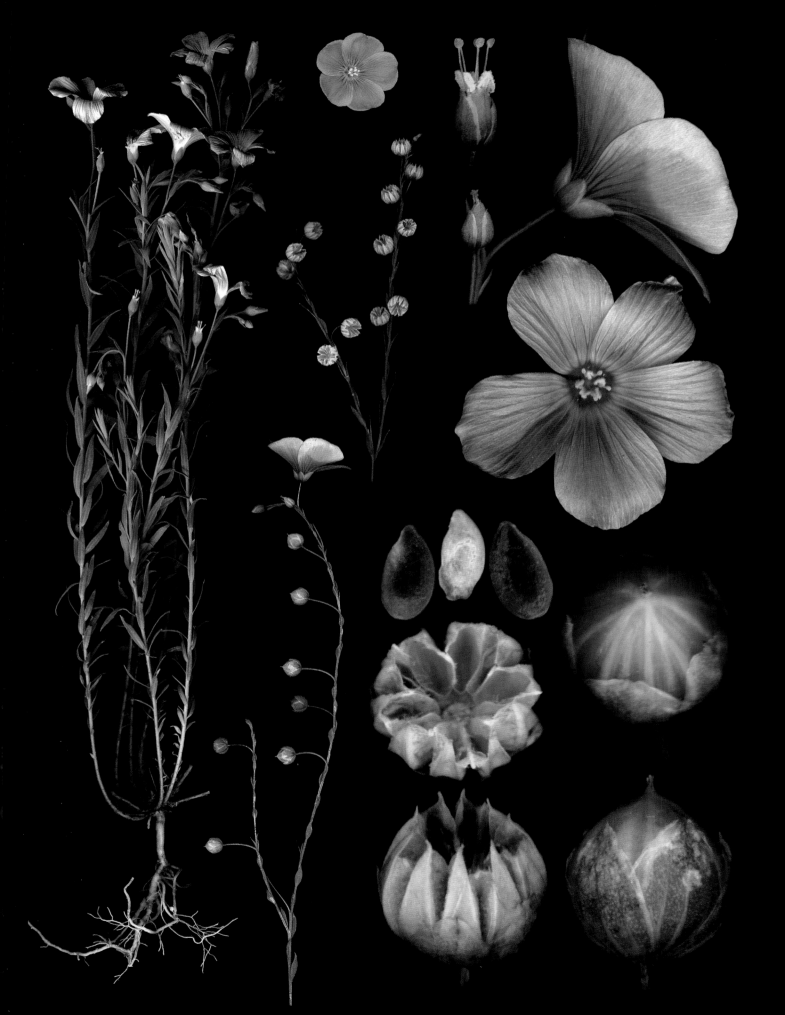

Flax

Linum usitatissimum

FAMILY: LINACEAE

Active elements:

Seeds: 40% oil rich in essential fatty acids (linolenic acid [omega-3] and linoleic acid [omega-6]), almost 25% proteins, approximately 10% mucilage, traces of cyanogenic heterosides.

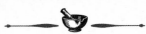

METHOD OF USE

- **INTERNAL:** As a laxative, 2 tablespoonful per day of seeds soaked in a glass of water, to be taken between meals.
Infusion. 20g (¾oz) per litre (quart) of water, for inflammation of the urinary tract.
Maceration (same uses). Steep seeds in an equal amount of hot water over night. Drink 3 or 4 cups per day of these preparations.
- **EXTERNAL: Decoction.** 50g (1¾oz) of seeds in a litre of water as an enema to treat constipation or as a lotion for skin irritation.
Flax flour poultice. Should be made with newly ground flour and soft water. Applied warm and held in place with a flannel to retain its warmth as long as possible. Also used in pulmonary illnesses, to soften the skin in the case of boils or abscesses or to treat swelling resulting from a strain.

PRECAUTIONS FOR USE

Note that Flax seeds should not be eaten where there is intestinal obstruction or narrowing of the oesophagus or digestive tract. Flax seed should be taken separately from other medications (by at least 30 minutes to 1 hour). If taking Flax seeds, it is essential to drink 1½ to 2 litres of water per day.

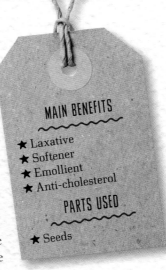

There is evidence that Flax was spun as early as the Stone Age, and right across the civilizations of the ancient world, from Egypt to Mesopotamia. In Theophrastus's *Historia Plantarum*, he recorded the use of its seeds as a cough remedy. Dioscorides advocated its properties as an anti-inflammatory. In the 16th century, the use of linseed oil made from Flax supplanted the use of the seed. During the Empire, a remedy for gout was so popular that a fortune was paid for its formula (Flax flower with the addition of hot water and a decoction of Sarsaparilla). Later, some herbal therapists recommended Flax seed for inflammation of the urinary tract or ulcers of the digestion system.

A gentle but effective laxative

- Flax seeds are **mainly used as a laxative** in the treatment of chronic constipation. On contact with liquids, their mucilage swells, forming a gelatinous mass that increases the volume of stools and promotes their expulsion.
- The seeds **soothe irritations of the digestive system**, and a Flax seed infusion calms inflammation of the urinary tract.
- In the form of flour, the seeds are used to prepare **emollient and maturative** poultices.
- Linseed oil is particularly rich in omega-3 fatty acids, similar to those found in fish oils, and is said to be **beneficial against endometrial and breast cancer**.
- Studies have shown that crushed whole Flax seeds **lower blood cholesterol levels**, thus playing a role in the prevention of heart disease. They are also beneficial in treating high blood pressure, hyperactivity and relieving menopausal disorders.

Description

An annual plant that is probably native to Asia Minor. It is cultivated for its fibres, particularly in northern France, and occasionally grows wild. Its flowers are a distinctive pale azure blue. They produce small capsules filled with light brown, oblong, flattened, shiny seeds. The seeds are used for their medicinal properties, while the stems produce the fine, luxurious cloth that is linen.

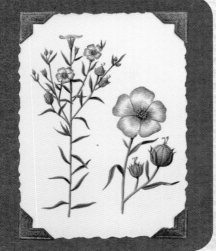

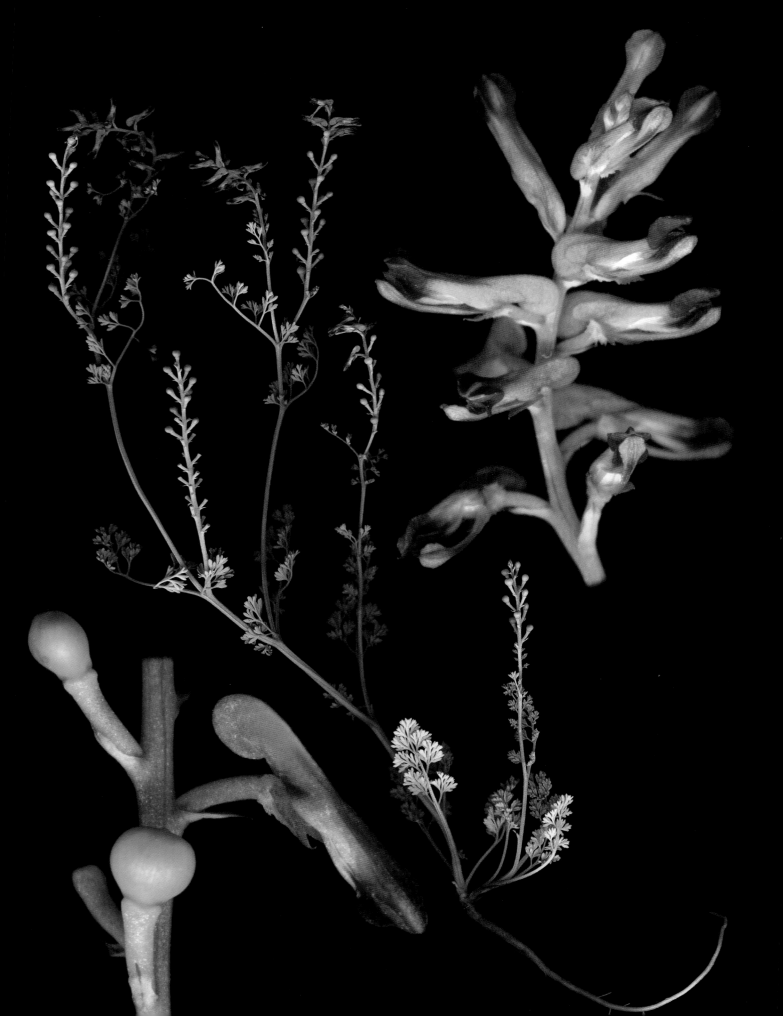

Fumitory

Fumaria officinalis
FAMILY: PAPAVERACEAE

Active elements:
Alkaloids (including protopine), organic acids (including fumaric acid).

Olivier de Serres, the French author and scientist, noted in his famous book *Le Théâtre d'agriculture* (1600), that Fumitory, "makes you laugh, cleanses the humours and is good against calculi".

A tonic in the short-term, calmative in the long-term

TOXICITY
Large doses of Fumitory are said to be toxic.

• The whole plant has **purifying** properties. It works wonders for **skin diseases** (eczema, psoriasis), and the treatment of sores and itching, as well as facilitating skin healing.

• As a treatment, it is an aperitive and tonic for the first 8 to 10 days, then the effect becomes **soothing and slightly sleep-inducing**. As a result, it can be used for 20-day treatments.

• It is also excellent **biliary tract medication**, regulating bile secretion and detoxifying the body. Fumitory is advocated for the relief of constipation and painful biliary spasms.

MAIN BENEFITS
★ Purifying
★ Skin problems
★ Aperitive and tonic
★ Soothing and soporific

PARTS USED
★ Whole plant

• It is also used to **alleviate suffering due to gallstones** and to migraines of hepatic origin.

DID YOU KNOW? In the past the Fumitory plant was thought to grow, not from a seed, but from fumes from the earth. It is to this belief that it owes its alternative name, "earth smoke".

METHOD OF USE

• **INTERNAL: Infusion.** 30 to 40g (1 to 1½oz) of the whole plant per litre (quart) of boiling water. Drink 2 or 3 cups per day, before meals. Very bitter. Use as a purifier, aperitive and to regulate bile secretion.

Wine. Make a decoction with 30 to 60g (1 to 2oz) of plant per litre of white wine (do not use iron utensils, or red wine; iron salts and tannin are incompatible with Fumitory). Take a small teaspoonful before each meal.

Syrup. Crush the fresh Fumitory. Weigh the juice obtained and add its weight in sugar. Cook to the consistency of syrup. Take 2 or 3 tablespoonsful per day. The wine and syrup are used for the same ailments as the infusion, but taste nicer.

Description

A small annual plant that is very common in cultivated lands and ploughed fields. It is native to Europe, temperate Asia and North Africa. Its glaucous leaves are small but deeply incised. The small flowers grow in pink clusters, turning purple at the apex, and bloom from May to September. Only the roots of the plant cannot be used.

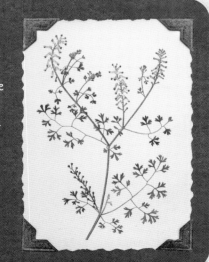

Fumitory is an excellent purifying plant.

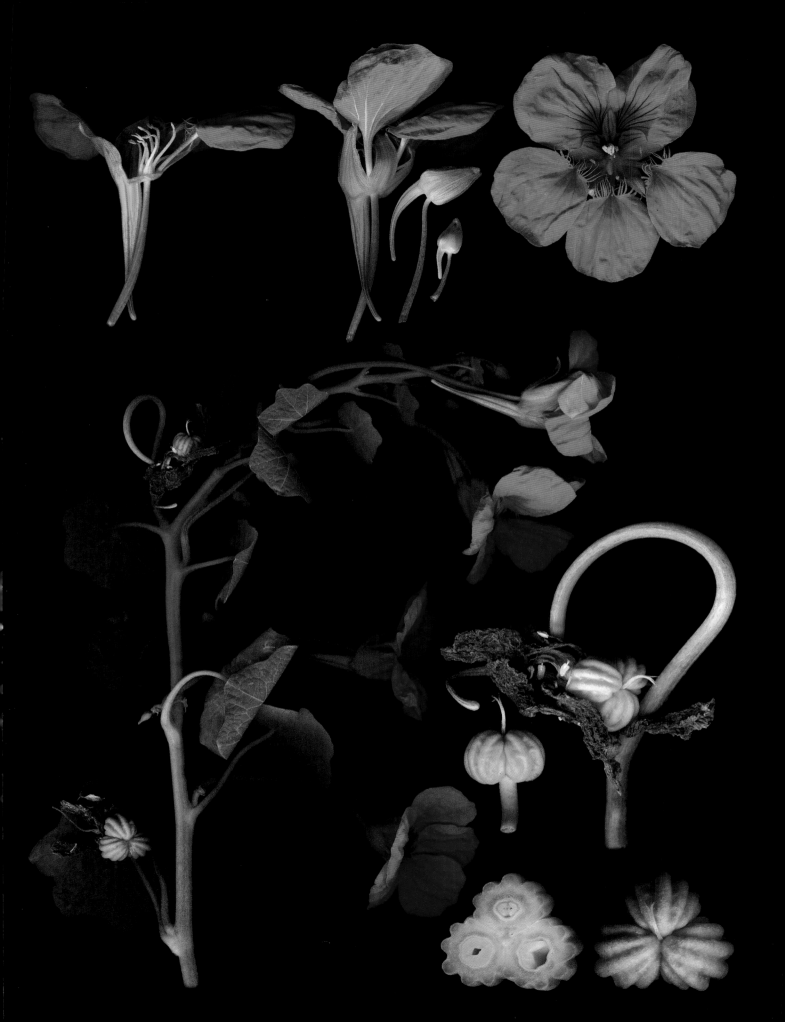

Garden Nasturtium

───── ◆ ─────

Tropaeolum majus

FAMILY: TROPAEOLACEAE

Active elements:

Plant: flavonoids and a sulphur heteroside (glucotropaeolin), which is released by hydrolysis from benzyl isothiocyanate. Seeds: rich in erucic acid.

The "blood flower of Peru" was introduced into Europe in the early 17th century and was reputed to trigger menstrual flow. Its antiscorbutic properties were also vaunted, and it was much sought after in times when scurvy on sailing ships was common: 100g (3½oz) of fresh leaves contain 285mg of vitamin C, five times that of an orange. It appeared to be forgotten for some time and then came back into fashion in 1805, as Cartheuser, the German physician and naturalist, had attributed it with being diuretic, laxative, pectoral and anthelmintic. Leclerc, the French physician and renowned medical herbalist, highlighted the Garden Nasturtium's expectorant properties, namely its ability to thin bronchial secretions.

For the body and head

• Garden Nasturtium is credited with having **antibiotic properties** useful for treating bronchitis, respiratory inflammations and urinary infections.

• Its high vitamin C content strengthens the immune system, and it is recommended for **boosting resistance to infections**.

• Used externally, the plant is antiseptic and works **to relieve itching**, superficial burns, sunburn and nappy rash. It is also advocated for **muscle pains**.

• It can be used as a **hair lotion** for scalp problems. It is said to slow down hair loss and is used in anti-dandruff shampoos.

OTHER USES: Garden Nasturtium flowers can be used to decorate salads, to which they add a touch of spice not dissimilar to watercress. The leaves can be eaten raw or cooked in the same way as watercress. Buds and the young fruit can be used instead of capers.

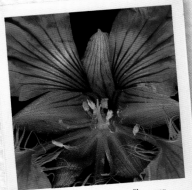

Garden Nasturtium flowers can be added to salads.

METHOD OF USE

• **INTERNAL: Decoction.** 15 to 30g (½ to 1oz) of leaves per litre (quart) of boiling water. Use to strengthen the body against infection.
Alcoholature. Macerate fresh leaves pressed into the same volume of colourless spirit for 15 days. Filter, then store in a bottle and take a teaspoonful 3 times a day. The advantage of the alcoholature is that the treatment is available all year round.

• **EXTERNAL: Decoction.** Made with a handful of flowers, leaves and fruit. As a gargle and mouthwash to prevent receding gums.
Scalp lotion. Mash 100g (3½oz) of fresh leaves, flowers and seeds of Garden Nasturtium with an equal quantity of fresh Deadnettle leaves and fresh Boxwood leaves. Steep for 15 days in half a litre of alcohol (90% by vol.). Strain and perfume with Geranium oil. Use as a daily scalp rub, applied with a rough brush.

Description

Perennial growing in warm climates, a native of the Andes. The Garden Nasturtium, with its brilliant yellow, red and purple colours, is one of the mostly widely grown ornamental garden plants. Its fleshy stems can reach lengths of 2m (6½ft). Its tender green leaves grow from long cylindrical petioles attached to the centre of the leaf blade, which is a five-cornered disc shape. The large, irregular flowers produce three-segmented fruit which has a cork-like texture when mature.

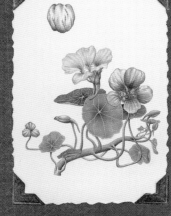

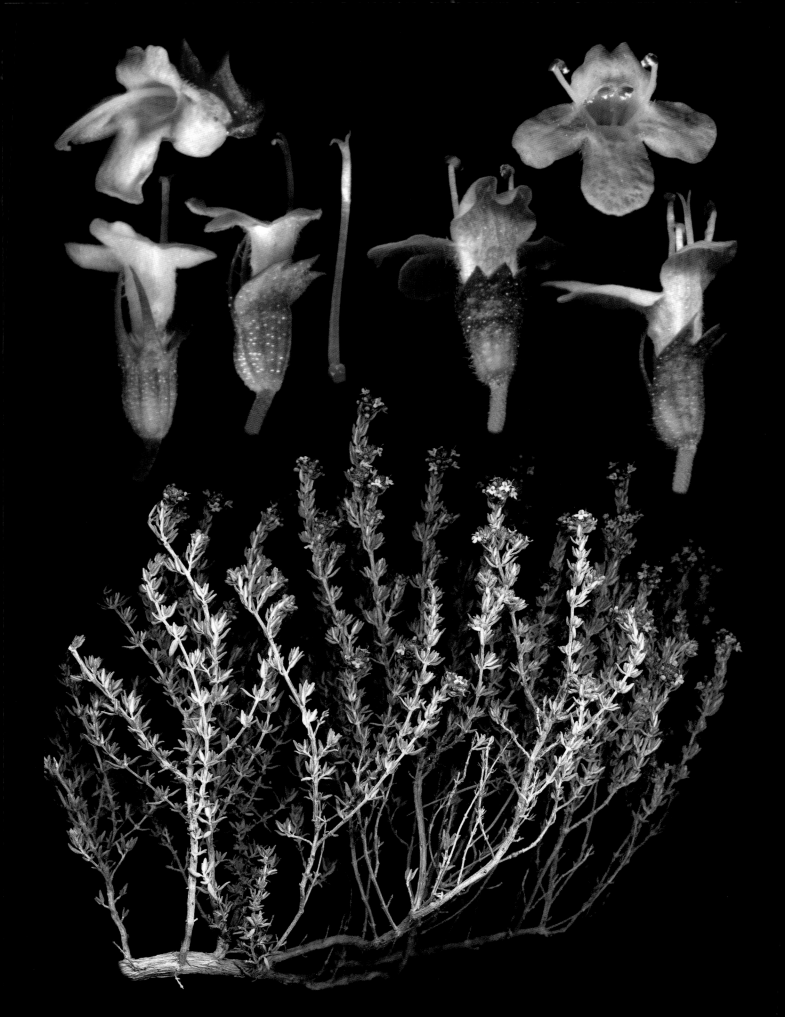

Garden Thyme

Thymus vulgaris
FAMILY: LAMIACEAE

Active elements:
Aromatic oil of variable composition depending on chemotype (dominated by thymol, linalool and geraniol).

The Egyptians used Thyme mixed with other ingredients to embalm their dead. The Greeks used it in cooking, but also to perfume their baths, and they anointed their bodies with Thyme oil. Albert the Great advocated its use in the treatment of leprosy, paralysis and lice.

Digestive, detoxifying and tonic

• Thyme is aperitive, tonic and antispasmodic, so **facilitates digestion**. It calms nervous contractions of the stomach, expels gas and prevents fermentation.

TOXICITY
Thymes rich in thymol, and especially their essential oils, should be used with caution as they are caustic. Overdoses may lead to nervous complaints.

• It is an **excellent antiseptic**, used against respiratory infections.
• It activates the detoxification process, **promoting perspiration and diuresis,** and facilitates the elimination of toxins from the body (flu, rheumatism, over-eating).
• Thyme also **stimulates the intellect**, and its infusion is recommended after a meal to tackle drowsiness.
• It is effective at relieving **rheumatic pains**, such as gout and arthritis. It can be used in a fortifying bath, ideal for sickly children.
• Garden Thyme is an excellent **scalp tonic**, preventing hair loss, thickening hair and triggering regrowth.
• It works as a toothpaste, **strengthening gums**, disinfecting the breath and preventing plaque.
• It **purifies the air** when used in a diffusion.

OTHER USES: Garden Thyme is used as a condiment on its own, or as one of the dried herbs in *Herbes de Provence*, in particular on meat. It is used in marinades, especially for well-hung game, flavouring and disinfecting.

MAIN BENEFITS
★ Digestion
★ Antiseptic
★ Detoxifying
★ Stimulant
★ Anti-rheumatic
★ Anti-hairloss
★ Effective toothpaste

PARTS USED
★ Whole plant

METHOD OF USE

• **INTERNAL: Infusion.** 20 to 30g (¾ to 1oz) of plant per litre (quart) of boiling water. Drink 3 or 4 cups per day to treat colds and poor digestion. At a higher dose of 50g (1¾oz) the infusion becomes more of a stimulant.
Cough syrup. Dissolve 175g (6oz) of honey in 100g (3½oz) warm Thyme infusion.
• **EXTERNAL:** Fresh Thyme is used for aches and pains. Heat in a dry frying pan on the hob. When nice and hot, apply between two layers of muslin to the painful area.
Thyme bath. Add a decoction of ½kg (1lb) of Thyme boiled in a few litres of water to bath water. Tonic, reinvigorating, analgesic.
Scalp lotion. Using a concentrated decoction, of 100g (3½oz) per litre of water, reduced to half by boiling. Rub the scalp with this lotion and use it to rinse hair after shampooing. Tonic. This can also be applied in washes or compresses to wounds.
Toothpaste. Clean teeth several times a week with crushed dried Thyme applied to a toothbrush.

Description

A sub-shrub growing to 10 to 30cm (4 to 12in), common in arid and rocky areas of the Mediterranean basin, from Spain to Italy. This Thyme is commonly cultivated in gardens. It is a favourite ingredient of the *bouquet garni* that is so dear to home cooks. Most people would recognize its tiny, narrow, greyish-green leaves and pale pink flowers. Like its cousin, Wild Thyme (described later), different thyme plants can exude a wide range of smells.

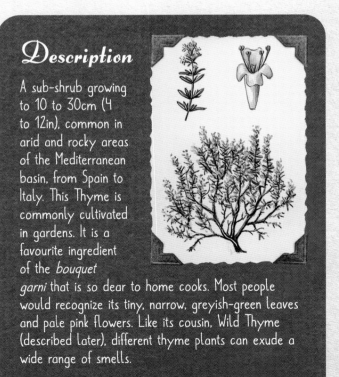

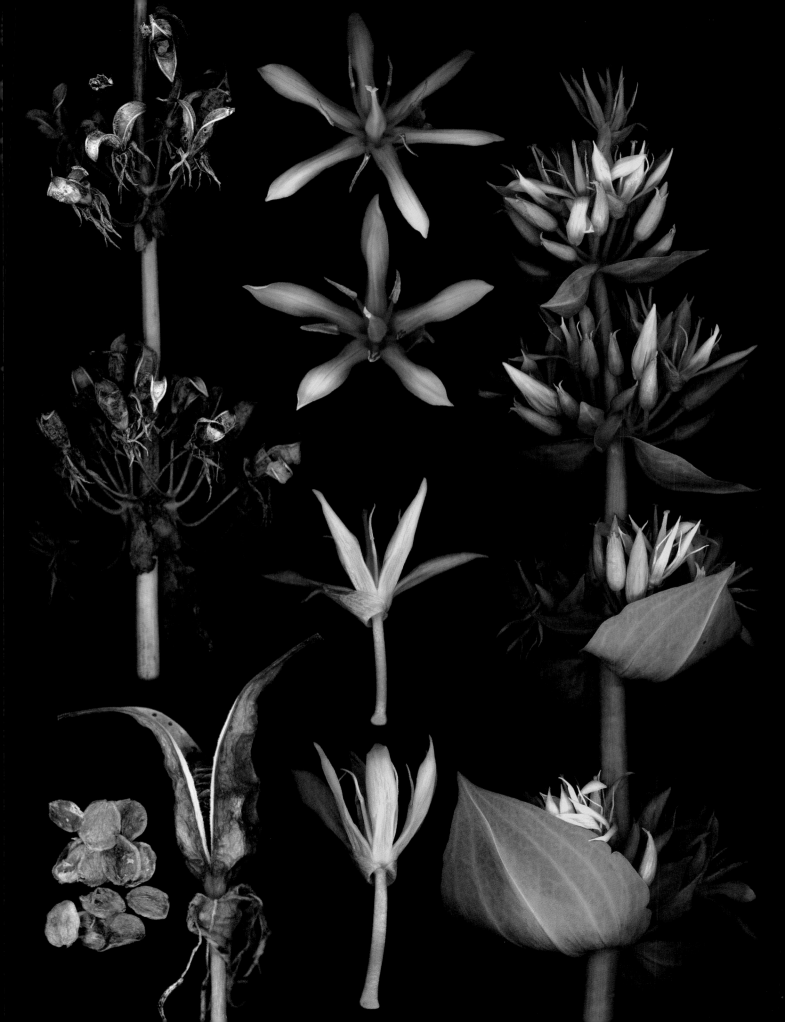

Gentian

Gentiana lutea

FAMILY: GENTIANACEAE

Active elements:

Bitter principles, including gentiopicroside and amarogentine), oligosaccharides, pectin, phytosterols, phenol acids, xanthones (yellow colourings, including gentisin).

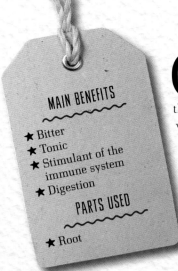

MAIN BENEFITS

★ Bitter
★ Tonic
★ Stimulant of the immune system
★ Digestion

PARTS USED

★ Root

Gentian owes its name to Gentius, the king of Illyria, who is said to have been the first to discover its properties. After the Romans invaded Gaul, they extolled the virtues of this attractive plant. Olivier de Serres, the French Renaissance author and soil scientist, advocated its powers as a tonic and anthelmintic, and also noted that it "helps with childbirth". Gentian was used to treat fevers of all kinds, as well as malaria. A mixture of equal parts Gentian, Camomile and Oak bark is known as "French febrifuge".

The most perfect of bitters

• Gentian is the most perfect of bitters. It stimulates salivary and gastric secretions. It is advocated for the treatment of gastric pains and loss of appetite. It **never irritates the stomach**.

• It is a general tonic and a stimulant that contributes to building the body's defences by increasing the number of white blood cells.

• A slice of the root, fresh or dried, **sucked at the end of an overly large meal** can help stave off any ill effects.

• In popular medicine it is sometimes used to **treat pinworm**.

OTHER USES: In Auvergne, France, the Gentian root is used to make a bitter liqueur. In the Jura and Savoie regions of France they distil the fermented rhizomes in a clear alcohol to produce a spirit with a powerful taste of earth and flowers. Both versions have aperitive and digestive qualities.

DID YOU KNOW? The gentiopicrin from the gentiopicroside is so bitter that it can be detected by the taste buds even at a dilution of one millionth in water.

METHOD OF USE

• **INTERNAL: Maceration.** Pour a cup of boiling water over 3g of dried root. Leave steeping for 4 hours. Drink a cup before each meal as a tonic; after a meal as a digestive. **Powdered root** (1 to 4g per day), mixed with a little honey can be used instead of the infusion which is very bitter. **Wine** (most common method of administration). Steep 40g (1½oz) of root in a litre (quart) of white wine for 10 days. Drink a small cup before meals.

• **EXTERNAL: Strong decoction.** Use 40g (1½oz) of root per litre of water then leave to steep. For the treatment of pinworm; also as an enema.

Description

A perennial growing to over 1m (3¼ft) in height, common in sub-Alpine pastures. It is native to central and southern Europe and western Asia. Its stems bear broad, bluish green, opposed leaves, which are rubbery to the touch. In summer, the big, bright-yellow flowers, comprised of five long, straight petals in a star-shape bloom, appear in dense clusters in the leaf axils and at the top of the stem. The large root (up to 1m (3¼ft) in length and several centimetres thick), brown on the outside, yellow inside, is fleshy and wrinkled.

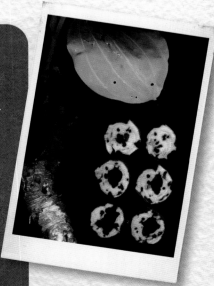

The Gentian root is a remarkable tonic.

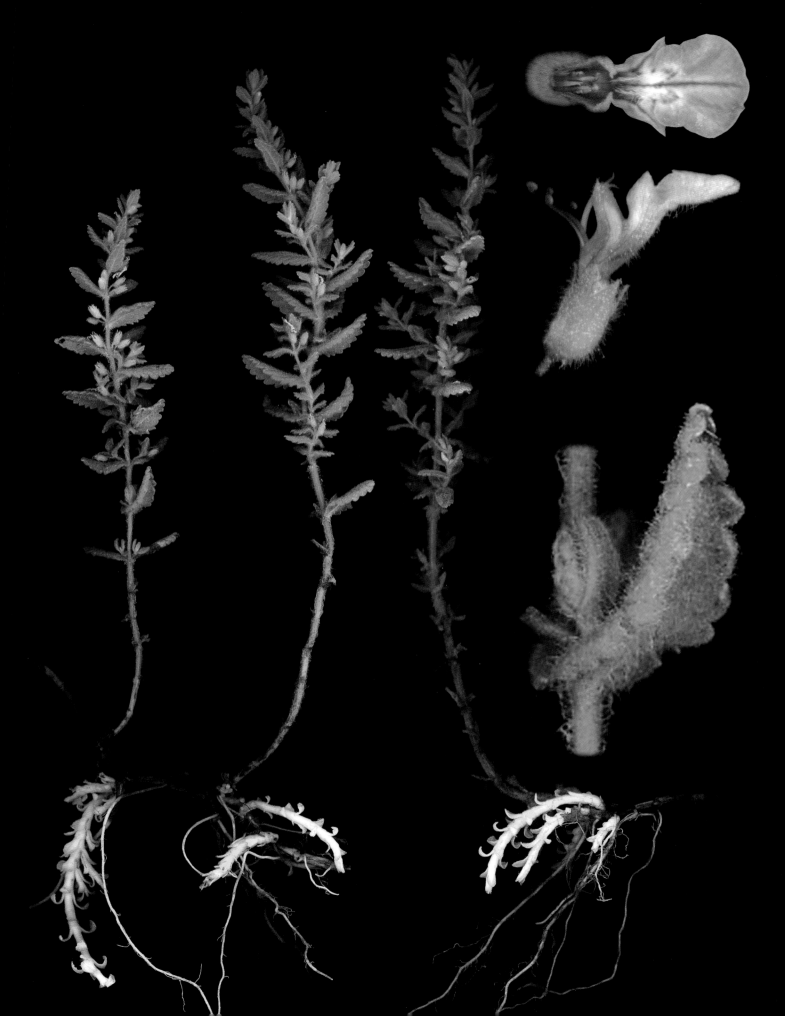

Germander

Teucrium chamaedrys

FAMILY: LAMIACEAE

Active elements:

Triterpenes, flavonoids, aromatic oil rich in caryophyllene, iridoids, lactonic diterpenes (including teucrins).

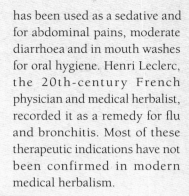

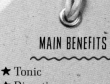

MAIN BENEFITS

★ Tonic
★ Digestive
★ Antipyretic

PARTS USED

★ Leaves, flowers

The Germander was already a renowned febrifuge or antipyretic in ancient Egyptian times. From Dioscorides until at least the 18th century it was advocated to promote menstrual flow and treat snake bites. Pliny added that it was effective against coughs and Apuleius recommended it as a treatment for gout. Traditionally, Germander has been used as a sedative and for abdominal pains, moderate diarrhoea and in mouth washes for oral hygiene. Henri Leclerc, the 20th-century French physician and medical herbalist, recorded it as a remedy for flu and bronchitis. Most of these therapeutic indications have not been confirmed in modern medical herbalism.

A bitter liqueur

• Like all bitter, aromatic plants, Germander is a **tonic** and **stimulates both appetite and digestion**. It combats a sluggish stomach, liver and the whole digestive tract. Germander is also used in the preparation of various aperitifs and digestive liqueurs such as vermouth and chartreuse.

• Germander also has **antipyretic** properties (it reduces fever).

• It is **antiseptic** and is also recommended for the treatment of chronic bronchitis, rheumatism and gout.

• Used externally, it is a vulnerary: it **relieves inflammation inside the mouth (gingivitis and ulcers)** and speeds up the healing of wounds.

OTHER SPECIES: Water Germander (*Teucrium scordium*), when crushed, gives off a smell of garlic that the common Germander does not have. It is used for the same purposes, but is additionally used externally in lotions for treating skin ulcers and, in the past, gangrene.

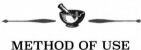

METHOD OF USE

• **INTERNAL: Infusion.** 30 to 40g (1 to 1½oz) of flowering tops or leaves and flowers in a litre (quart) of water or wine. Drink 3 or 4 small glasses (100g (3½oz)) per day as a tonic, aperitive and digestive.

• **EXTERNAL: Decoction.** 50g (1¾oz) of flowering tops or leaves and flowers in a litre of water. Boil for 10 minutes. Use to relieve gingivitis and mouth ulcers.

TOXICITY

Some cases of acute hepatitis linked to long-term consumption of Germander-based medications were recorded in France and Canada in the 1990s, probably attributable to the teucrin content. The sale of the plant and preparations containing it has been prohibited since then.

Description

A small perennial growing to 15 to 30cm (6 to 12in), commonly found in dry places, especially on limestone. Found in central and southern Europe, western Asia and North Africa. Its woody stems first creep along the ground before becoming upright. They have small, opposite leaves which are glossy on top and pale green and slightly hairy on the underside, with serrated edges like those of the oak. Its red, irregular flowers have just one enlarged, lower lip. The plant exudes a faint aromatic odour and has a bitter, astringent flavour.

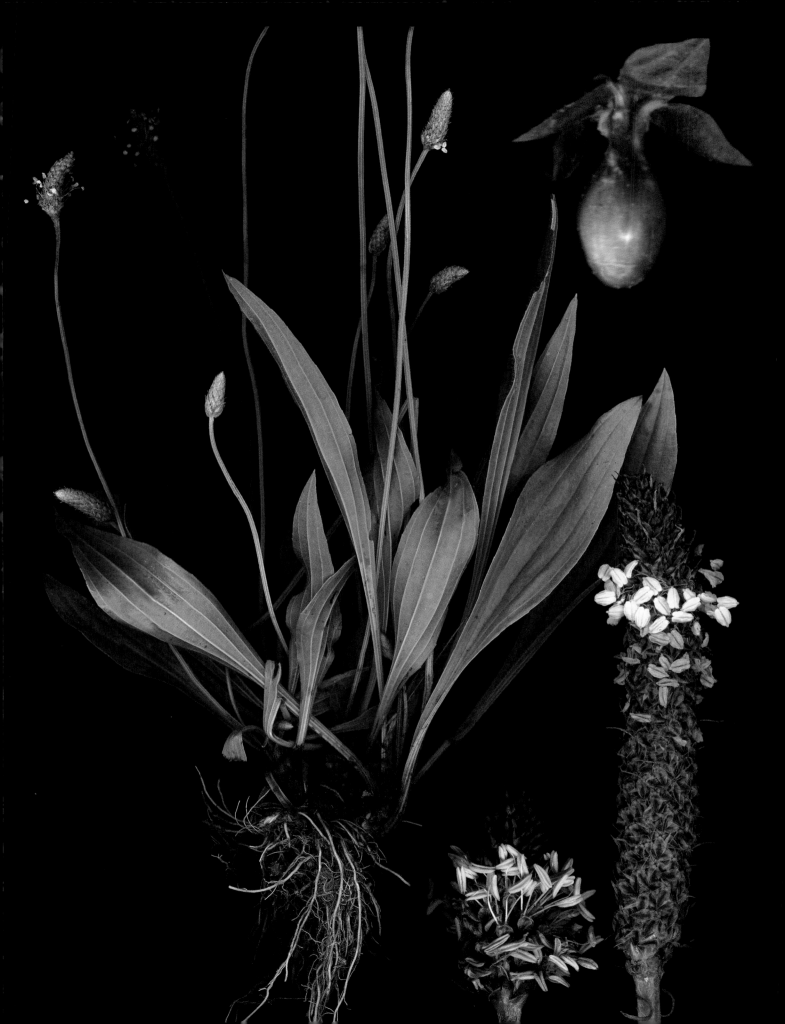

Glandular Plantain

Plantago afra
FAMILY: PLANTAGINACEAE

Active elements:
Psyllium (seeds): lots of mucilage and fibres,
carbohydrates, unsaturated fatty acids,
sterols, iridoids, alkaloids (traces).

Plantain seeds have been used as laxatives since ancient times. Egyptian physicians advocated them for this purpose as well as for inflammation of the urinary tract.

Useful mucilages

• Plantain seeds are used as a mechanical laxative to **treat constipation**, where there is no accompanying inflammatory illness, diabetes or risk of intestinal obstruction. Their mucilage inflates within the intestine, softening and increasing the volume of stools. Their softening properties also make them useful in the case of **intestinal irritation or colitis**. By softening stools, mucilages have the knock-on effect of **relieving haemorrhoids**.
• The seeds can be used to **regulate bowel function**, in the case of diarrhoea. Mucilage eliminates toxins present in the large intestine.
• Plantain **alleviates inflammation of the oral mucosa** as well as respiratory disorders.
• It **soothes irritations of the skin** and eyes (in the form of eyedrops) as well as boils. It is effective, to a degree, in bringing down blood cholesterol.

OTHER SPECIES: Sand Plantain (*Plantago arenaria*) from which we get black psyllium seeds, is as highly regarded as Glandular Plantain. Bond Plantain (*P. ovata*), sometimes known as Ispaghul or Desert Indian wheat in reference to its geographical origin, has the same laxative properties.
As long ago as the 1st century AD, Dioscorides recommended the Great Plantain or Broad-leafed Plantain (*P. major*) and Ribwort Plantain (*P. lanceolata*), for the treatment of dermatitis. This is due to their soothing action on skin and mucosa. They also counter the irritation of sore throats and act as anti-inflammatories to relieve eye irritations (in the form of eye drops or a compress). Their crushed leaves calm insect bites and Nettle stings, disinfect cuts and grazes and promote the healing process. The husks of the various Plantain seeds including this one, also known as 'psyllium', can be used to treat diarrhoea as well as acting as a gentle laxative. Psyllium is also effective in eliminating uric acid from the kidneys.

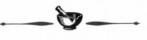

METHOD OF USE

• **INTERNAL.** 3 to 10g (¼oz) of seeds in 5 to 10cl of water, Take 3 times a day (namely 10 to 30g (¼ to 1oz) per day) for constipation.
For diarrhoea, increase the daily dose to 40g (1½oz) per day. Use a dosage of 10 to 20g (¼ to ¾oz) per day to reduce cholesterol and blood sugar.
Ensure you consume sufficient fluids.

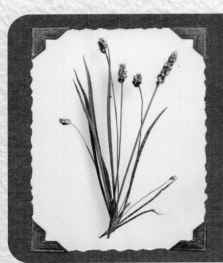

Description

A perennial growing to 10 to 50cm (4in to 1½ft), generally found on stony or sandy ground in southern France and right across the Mediterranean region (Spain and Italy), as well as in Switzerland and Austria. Its herbaceous stems bear small, opposite, linear leaves and minuscule flowers grouped in ovoid heads on long axillary stalks. Each flower produces a small capsule containing two long seeds.

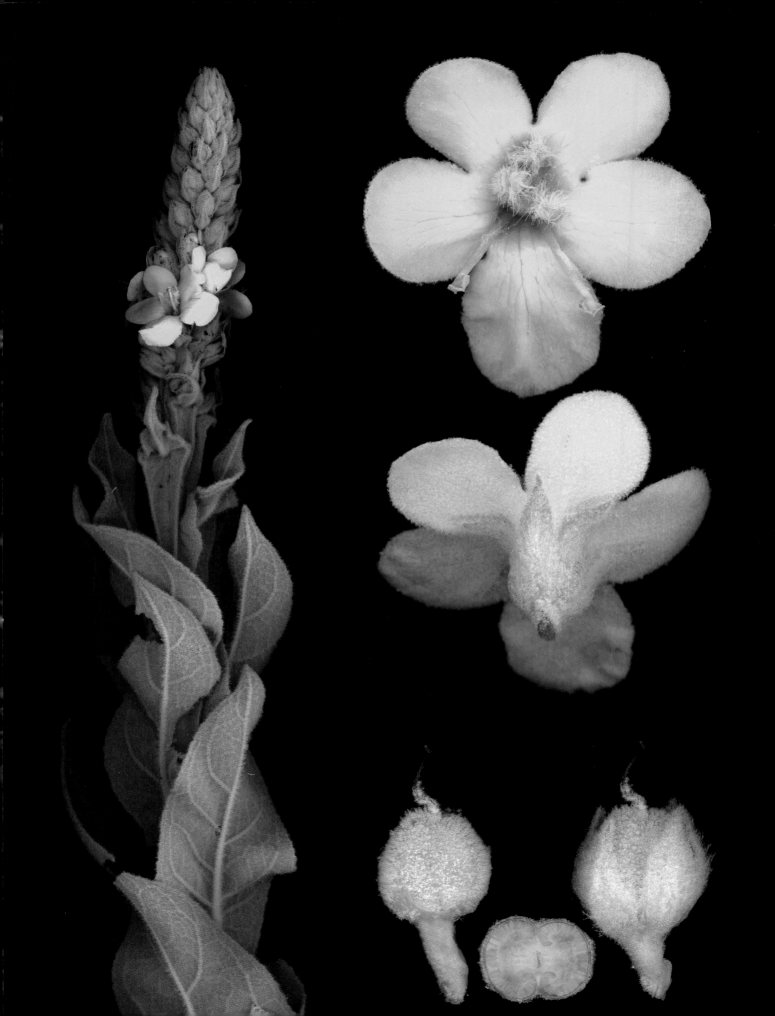

Great Mullein

Verbascum thapsus

FAMILY: SCROPHULARIACEAE

Active elements:

Mucilage, flavonoids, saponosides, iridoids, heterosidic lignans, aromatic oil.

• Their soothing powers are due to their mucilage content, which means they can also be used **to treat internal inflammation, and difficult or painful digestion**.

• Great Mullein was also used traditionally as a **diuretic**, as well as to relieve rheumatic pains.

• The leaves are **calmative and healing on the skin**. They can be used to treat haemorrhoids and skin ailments.

• As a mouthwash, they can **play a part in oral hygiene**. They dull pain linked to inflammation of the inside of the mouth and throat.

As far back as the 1st century AD, Dioscorides recommended Great Mullein for all lung ailments, as did Pliny the Elder. They did not, however, agree as to which part of the plant should be used: the former advocated the leaves, while the latter the root. In the 12th century, Saint Hildegard of Bingen, firmly believed that its flowers were an infallible remedy for hoarseness.

A pectoral flower

• A proven cough suppressant, Great Mullein was one of the ingredients of the "infusion of four pectoral flowers". Its emollient, soothing flowers **facilitate expectoration and relieve coughs**. They work wonders for chest inflammations, blocked airways, sore throats and tracheitis. A good calmative **for asthmatics**.

• The flowers likewise have **antibacterial and antiviral** properties, and to a lesser degree, are antimycotic (fungi).

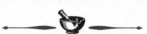

METHOD OF USE

• **INTERNAL:** Infusion. 20 to 30g (¾ to 1oz) of flowers per litre (quart) of boiling water steeped for 10 minutes. Strain through a cloth to remove the hairs of the stamen which can irritate the throat. Drink hot between meals and in the evening before going to bed. Use for inflammation of the airways and hoarseness.

• **EXTERNAL:** Decoction. 30 to 60g (1 to 2oz) per litre of water. Use either in a sitz bath or as a body wash to treat haemorrhoids and irritation of the female body parts, or as a lotion to treat dry patches of skin, burns, ulcers and chilblains.
A **poultice,** made with leaves boiled in water, can be used for boils, nail infections and abscesses.

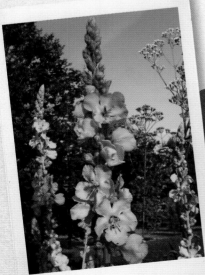

Description

A large biennial plant that can grow to 2m (6½ft) in height, common on uncultivated land, stony soil and rubble. It is found throughout Europe, Asia, North Africa and in North America where it is naturalized. Its robust, upright stem, covered in white hairs, bears large, soft, cottony, almost white leaves. Its attractive yellow flowers, which bloom in July and August, exude a light fragrance and are arranged in a large compact spike at the end of the stem.

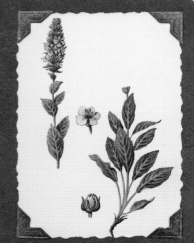

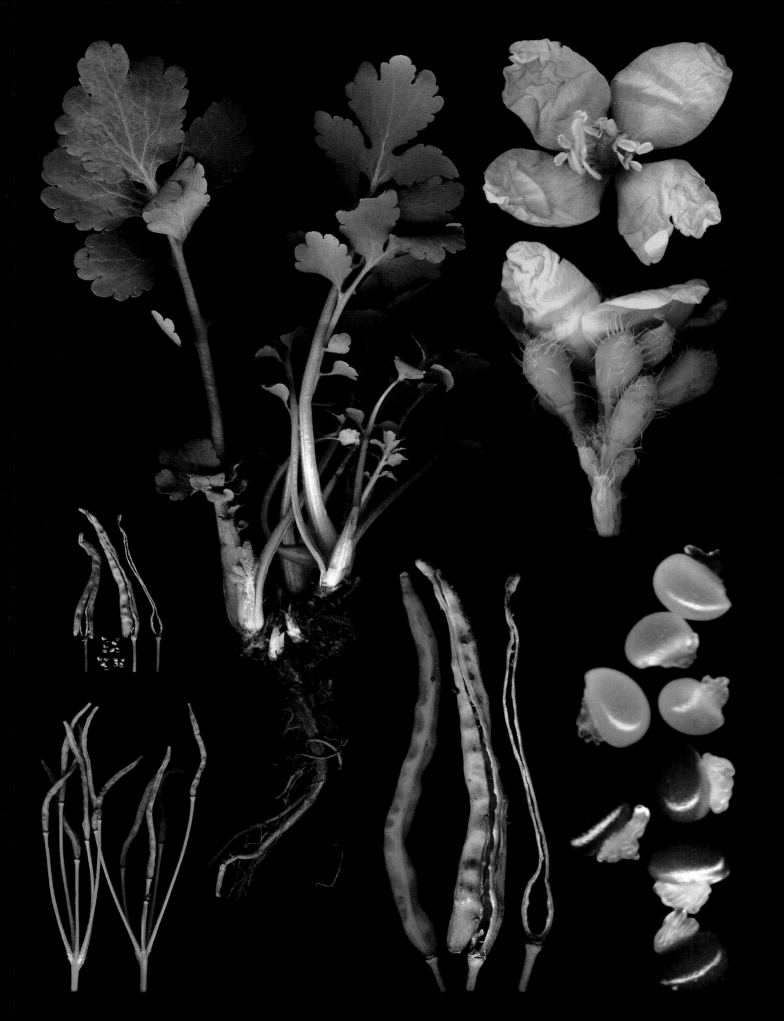

Greater Celandine

Chelidonium majus

FAMILY: PAPAVERACEAE

Active elements:
Alkaloids, including chelidonine, sanguinarine, berberine and coptisine.

Herbalists of antiquity held that swallows dropped juice from the Celandine stalk into the eyes of their fledglings to help them open. So it is sometimes known as Great Light and said to have the unproven property of improving eyesight. Deninsenko, a Russian doctor, used Celandine extract to treat cancerous tumours. In the early 20th century Henri Leclerc, the French physician, concluded that it could not cure cancer, but could slow its spread. As the plant is toxic and dangerous, he recommended it only as an extract or tincture for internal use. Jean-François Cazin, the great 19th-century French medical herbalist, used it only in dried form and in limited doses.

Goodbye warts and calluses

• Celandine is considered a **powerful choleretic**, believed to increase bile-secretion fivefold. It is also a bladder sedative and can soothe liver pains.

• It is recommended for the **treatment of abdominal spasms**, digestive cramps and bladder problems.

• It relaxes the muscles of the bronchi and intestines, has a **purifying action** and **stimulates the immune system**.

• The plant is mainly used externally; its juice is **effective against warts, corns and calluses**, which can disappear completely with repeated application.

TOXICITY
The ingestion of fresh leaves and latex occasionally causes serious digestive, nervous and cardiac problems. The use of Greater Celandine is not recommended during pregnancy.

MAIN BENEFITS
★ Stimulates bile production
★ Antispasmodic
★ Warts, corns and calluses

PARTS USED
★ Leaves, roots, sap, juice

METHOD OF USE

• **INTERNAL:** Caution strongly advised. Only use dried and never exceed the doses below:
Infusion. 15g (¼oz) of dried leaves per litre (quart) of water. Or as a decoction of 10g of dried root boiled for 10 minutes. Drink 1 or 2 cups over 24 hours, to stimulate bile secretion and treat digestive problems. **Wine.** Pour a litre of boiling white wine over 15g (¼oz) of dried root. Drink a half to one small glass (100g (3½oz)) every morning. Use to treat the same conditions.

• **EXTERNAL: Sap of fresh plant.** Obtained by snapping a stem. Apply three times a day to warts, corns or calluses. Take care not to apply to an open wound.
It is also possible to crush **the juice** from the plant and mix it with an equal quantity of glycerine in order to keep it for the full duration of the treatment.

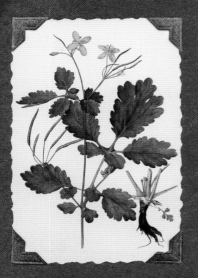

Description

A perennial plant growing to 30 to 60cm (1 to 2ft) in wasteland and at the foot of walls. It is widespread in the northern hemisphere. Its large blue-green leaves are pinnate with deeply lobed margins, forming a wide rosette. The stem bears flowers of four yellow petals that only bloom briefly. The elongated fruit are full of tiny black seeds, attached by a white, fleshy structure that attracts ants to disperse the seeds. When snapped, the stem produces a pungent yellowy-orange liquid.

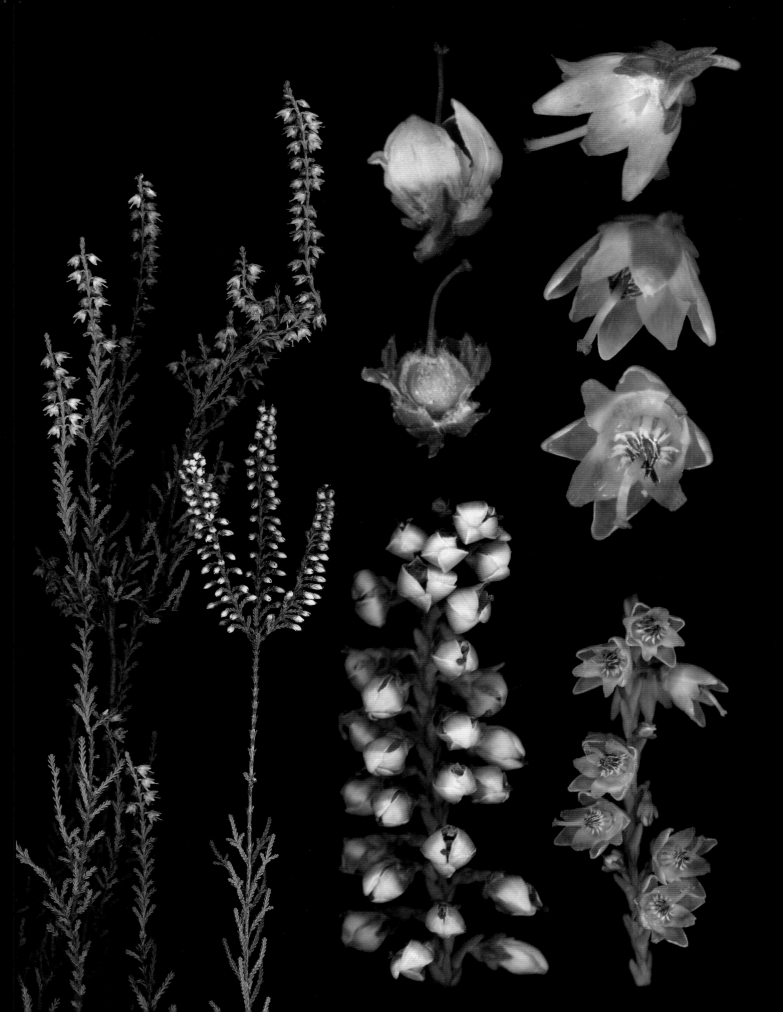

Heather

Calluna vulgaris

FAMILY: ERICACEAE

Active elements:
Tannins, flavonoids, arbutoside, ericodine.

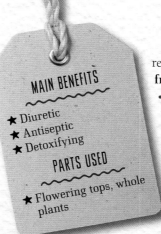

MAIN BENEFITS

★ Diuretic
★ Antiseptic
★ Detoxifying

PARTS USED

★ Flowering tops, whole plants

Dioscorides advocated the use of Heather for snake bites and the Roman physician Galen recorded its use as a sudorific (sweat inducer). During the Renaissance, Mattioli and Dom Alexandre noted that it was effective in breaking down kidney and bladder stones.

A urine disinfectant

• The flowering tops are recognized as **active and quick-acting diuretics, antiseptics and urinary tract sedatives**. Ericodine has a proven disinfectant action. Heather increases urine volume, and clears and deodorizes problematic or fetid urine. It is used to treat kidney ailments, as well as heart failure, rheumatism and gout.

• Its **purifying and detoxifying properties** help eliminate harmful waste products such as urea, uric acid and oxalic acid from the body. Heather is also **highly recommended for people with a rich diet**, or one high in meat, and therefore full of purines, which cause the body to build up waste products.

• Its high arbutoside content means it is effective in treating prostate inflammations of infectious origin. It is therefore recommended **for cystitis resulting from a prostate infection**.

• Add to a warm, full-body bath, to **relieve muscle ache**. Useful for athletes and convalescents who are weak from a long spell in bed.

OTHER USES: The Celts made a mead from a decoction of Heather flowering tops fermented with honey. A similar drink could until recently be found in the Hebrides, which used germinated barley instead of honey.

OTHER SPECIES: The real Heathers are cousins belonging to the *Erica* genus. Their medicinal properties are similar to those of the genus *Calluna*. The Bell Heather (*Erica cinerea*, see below left) is also commonly found on heathlands and in siliceous woodland. Tree Heath (*Erica arborea*) is one of the characteristic species of Mediterranean maquis shrubland.

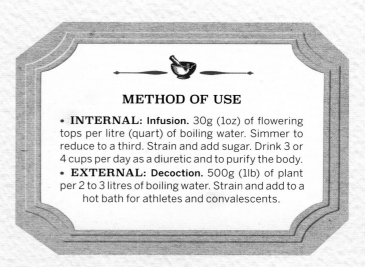

METHOD OF USE

• **INTERNAL: Infusion.** 30g (1oz) of flowering tops per litre (quart) of boiling water. Simmer to reduce to a third. Strain and add sugar. Drink 3 or 4 cups per day as a diuretic and to purify the body.

• **EXTERNAL: Decoction.** 500g (1lb) of plant per 2 to 3 litres of boiling water. Strain and add to a hot bath for athletes and convalescents.

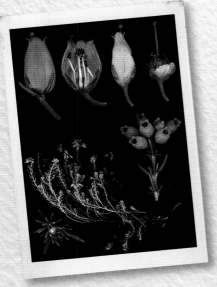

Bell Heather has the same properties as Common Heather.

Description

Common Heather (*C. vulgaris*), is a sub-shrub, growing to a height of 30 to 80cm (1 to 2½ft), very common in heathland and woodland in siliceous regions. Its numerous reddish twigs bear small, opposite leaves, close-set in four vertical rows, and bright pink flowers with four separate petals in loose terminal clusters.

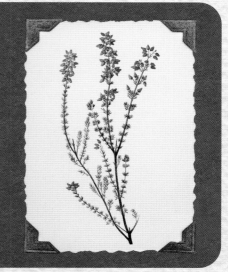

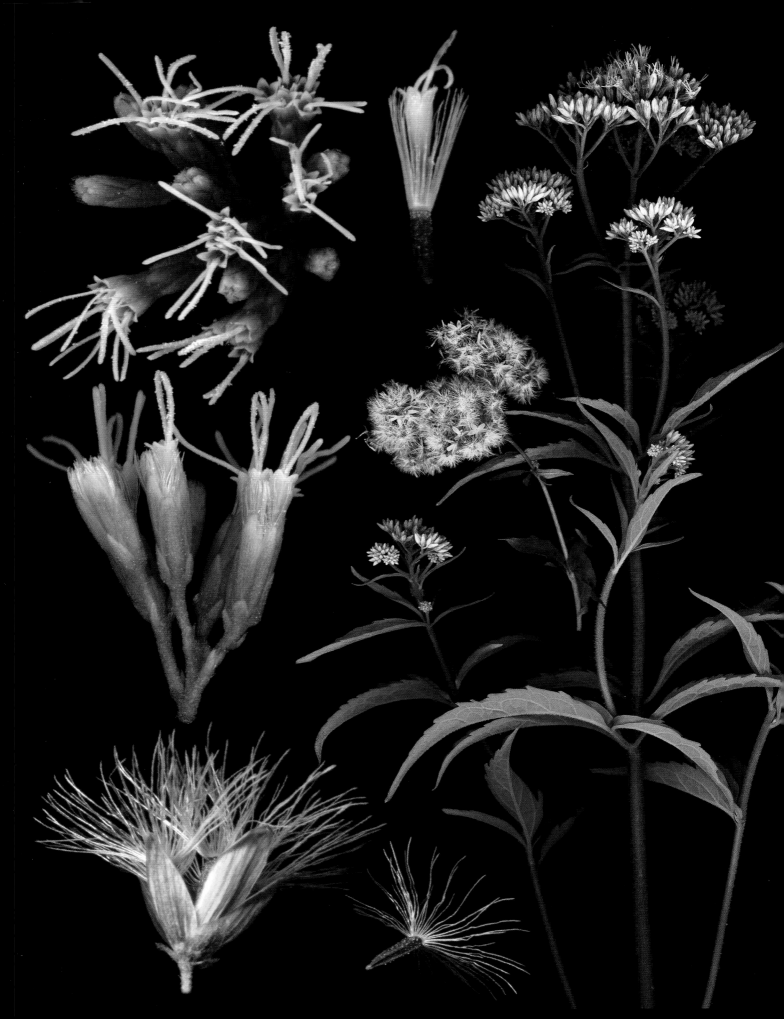

Hemp Agrimony

Eupatorium cannabinum

FAMILY: ASTERACEAE

Active elements:

Polysaccharides, flavonoids, benzofurans,
sesquiterpene lactones (including eupatoriopicrin),
an aromatic oil containing alpha-terpinene,
p-cymene and thymol, and pyrrolizidine alkaloids.

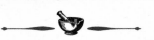

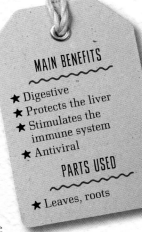

Mithridates Eupator Dionysius, King of Pontus in the 1st century BC, gave his name to the Eupatorium which he discovered. It was one of the plants in the medicinal garden of Olivier de Serres, the 16th-century French agronomist. He described it as "good for dysentery, snake bites and improving liver humour". The plant was used to treat colds and fevers, and especially advocated for liver obstructions and constipation caused by liver failure and atonic internal organs. Used externally, it was widely reputed to cure tumours of the backside or scrotum.

METHOD OF USE

- **INTERNAL: Infusion of leaves.** 30g (1oz) per litre (quart) of water taken for the liver.
Decoction. 30g (1oz) of chopped root per litre of water, boil for 2 minutes. Use to stimulate the immune system.
Maceration. 40g (1½oz) of chopped root, steeped for one night, in 1 litre of white wine or beer. For the same purposes as above.
- **EXTERNAL:** To treat tumours, use a **poultice** made of layers of leaves, or warm compresses soaked in a concentrated decoction of the root.

Stimulates bile and immunity

- *Eupatorium* has **cholagogic properties** (stimulating the discharge of bile from the digestive system) and protects the liver.
- It is considered to stimulate the immune system and **fight viral ailments**.

OTHER SPECIES: In North America, related species, particularly *Eupatorium perfoliatum*, have been used to treat colds, fevers, arthritis and rheumatism and are believed to stimulate the immune system.

TOXICITY

While the plant itself has never been known to cause any health disorders, pyrrolizidine alkaloids have induced liver tumours under experimental conditions.

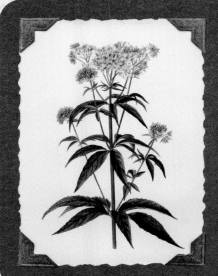

Description

A large perennial plant growing to a height of over 1m (3¼ ft), common in damp and shady places, along streams and in marshes. Native to Europe, Asia and North Africa. Its tall, upright, reddish stem bears opposite leaves, divided into three narrow, toothed leaflets. The tiny pink flowers grow in dense clusters at the top of each terminal stem. The root is grey and fibrous.

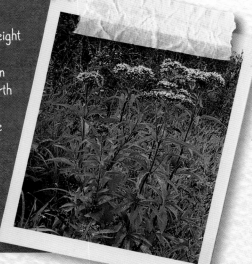

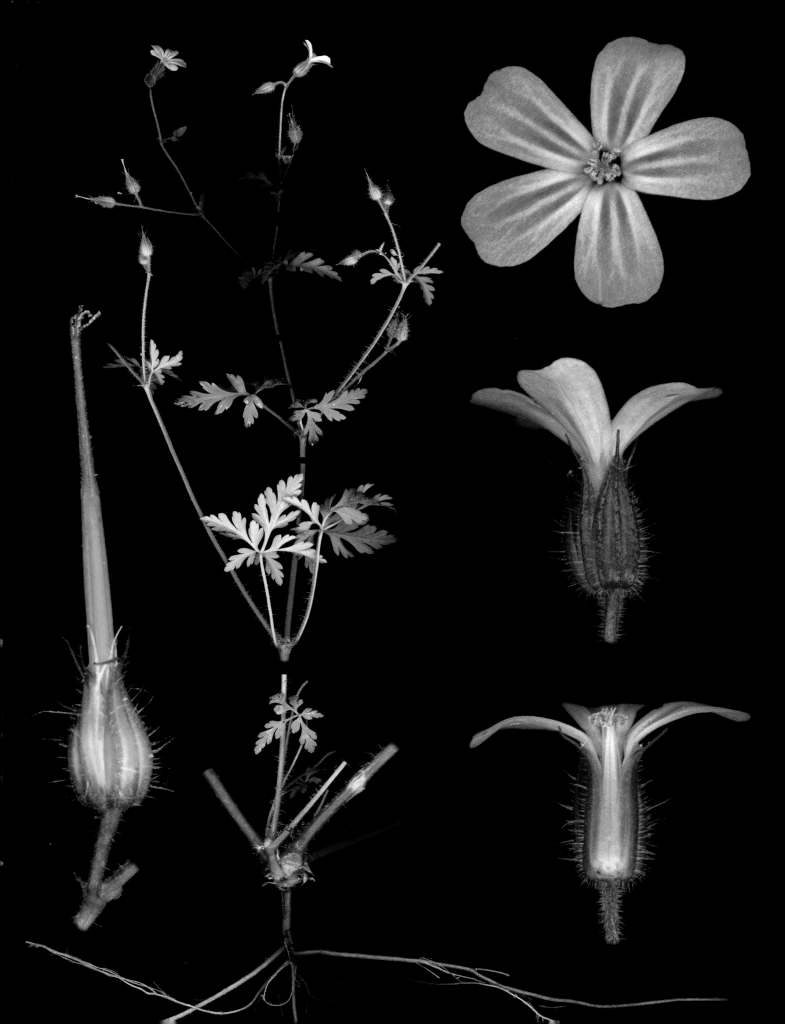

Herb Robert

Geranium robertianum

FAMILY: GERANIACEAE

Active elements:
Tannins, bitter principle, aromatic oil.

Daniel Sennert, a German physician in the early 17th century, advocated the use of Herb Robert for the treatment of cancer.

Particularly as a gargle or lotion

- Herb Robert is **astringent and antispasmodic** and so is sometimes used to treat diarrhoea and uterine haemorrhages.
- Several writers recorded its use in the **treatment of diabetes**: it reduces glucosuria (an excess of sugar in the urine).
- It is most often used externally: as a **gargle** for sore throats or swollen tonsils, as a **lotion** for eye problems, sometimes as a **poultice** on the painfully engorged breasts of nursing mothers, and to stimulate the healing of wounds.

DID YOU KNOW? The plant is not named after a hypothetical Robert, but comes from the Latin *ruber*, meaning "red", the colour the leaves of this delicate geranium turn at the end of the season. The plant's unpleasant smell has earned it the nickname Stinking Bob. The genus name, *Geranium*, comes from the Greek *geranos*, meaning "crane", as the fruits of these plants evoke the bird's long beak. The geraniums on our balconies are in fact Pelargoniums, from the Greek *pelargos*, "stork", for the same reason.

OTHER SPECIES: The Wild Geranium (*G. maculatum*) was traditionally used by American Indians to treat sore throats, mouth ulcers and inflammation of the gums. Even today, it is more widely used in herbal medicine than its European cousin. It is advocated for the treatment of colon irritation, haemorrhoids and to staunch small external haemorrhages.

MAIN BENEFITS

★ Anti-diarrhoeal
★ Anti-diabetic
★ Inflammation of the mouth and throat

PARTS USED

★ Flowering tops, dried plant

METHOD OF USE

- **INTERNAL: Infusion.** 20g (¾oz) of flowering tops or 50g (1¾oz) of dried plant per litre (quart) of boiling water. Steep for 20 minutes and drink 3 to 4 cups per day for diarrhoea or as an anti-diabetic.
- **EXTERNAL:** Gargle the same infusion (or a slightly more concentrated decoction) to soothe a sore throat.
   Apply the juice or **poultices** of the crushed plant to cuts or sores.

Description

A small plant growing to a height of around 30cm (1ft), common in shady places, hedgerows, undergrowth and along walls. Found throughout the northern hemisphere (native to Europe and Asia, acclimated in North America). Its spindly, hairy stems often have a reddish tinge. Its leaves are dissected into three or five segments, which are themselves deeply divided, and give off a smell of Indian ink when crushed. Its flowers have five, pink petals and produce a long-beaked fruit.

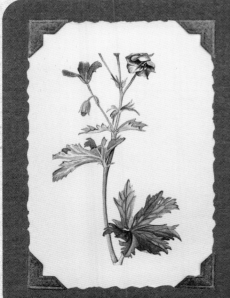

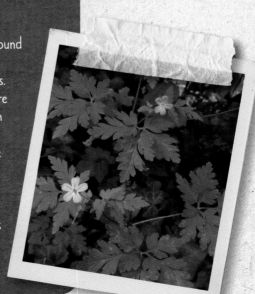

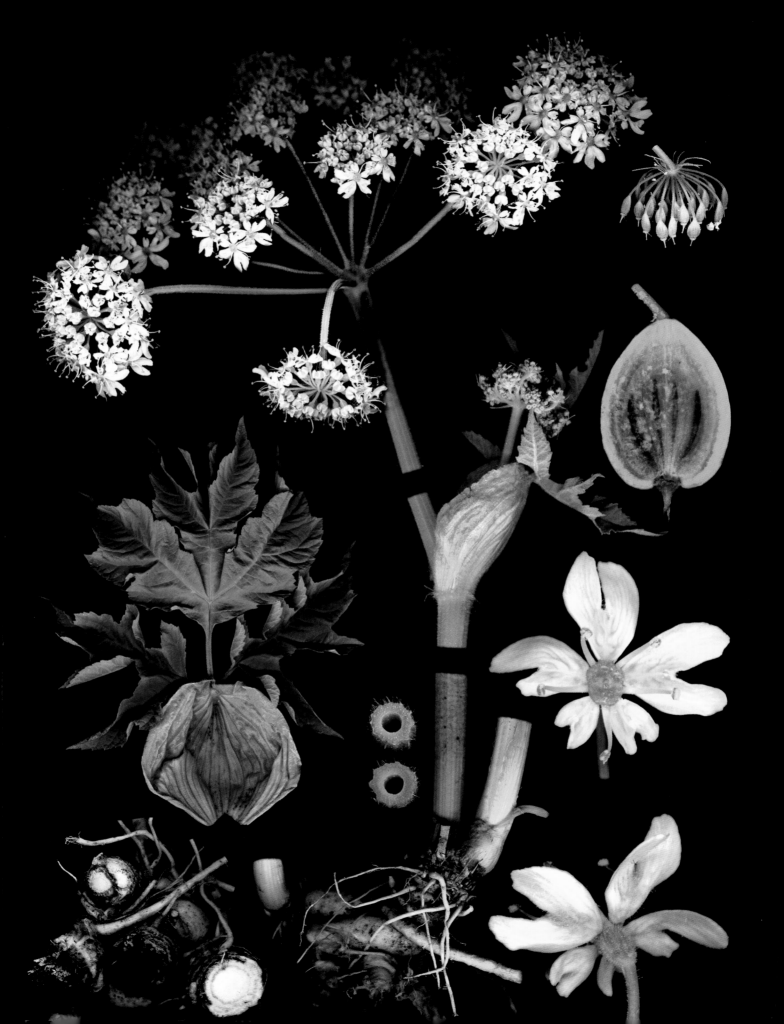

Hogweed

Heracleum sphondylium

FAMILY: APIACEAE

Active elements:
Aromatic oil, furanocoumarins (including bergapten, pimpinellin and xanthotoxin).

They are crunchy and deliciously sweet. The buds, hidden in the hollow of the enlarged petioles, resemble small broccoli and can be steamed and served with a sauce in the same manner as asparagus. The flat fruits give off a strong citrus smell when crushed. Their pungent, aromatic flavour is reminiscent of ginger. It is a strongly flavoured condiment, perfect for savoury dishes or desserts.

OTHER SPECIES: Giant Hogweed (*Heracleum mantegazzianum*) is often blamed for causing outbreaks of severe dermatitis. This imposing plant, growing up to 3m (9¾ft), is known for its photosensitizing effect. This means that juice applied to the skin may result in second-degree burns if subsequently exposed to the sun.

TOXICITY

Because of the furanocoumarins contained in Hogweed, it can sometimes cause inflammation in people with sensitive skin.

Fresh Hogweed leaves were a widely used folk remedy for abscesses, boils and bites.

Goes the whole hog

• The roots and leaves are **tonic and digestive**.
• Their **calmative** properties were used for epileptic seizures.
• Henri Leclerc, the French physician and medical herbalist, recommended Hogweed as an **aphrodisiac**, having used it for "genital asthenia" (weakness).
• Applied topically, it **cures boils**, abscesses and acne.
• In homeopathy, Hogweed (Branca Ursina) is prescribed for **headaches, ovarian pain and contact dermatitis**.

OTHER USES: The young, soft, tender leaves make a tasty salad. As they get older, they can be eaten as a vegetable. When cut, the young stems exude a smell of mandarin and coconut.

METHOD OF USE

• **INTERNAL: Infusion.** One teaspoonful of roots and leaves per cup of boiling water. Infuse for 10 minutes. Drink 3 cups per day between meals, to invigorate the body, or after a meal to stimulate digestion.
• **EXTERNAL:** Decoction. 30g (1oz) root per litre (quart) water in washes and compresses for boils, pimples, abscesses.

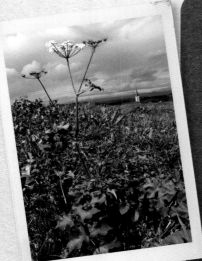

Description

A large perennial plant growing to 1m (3¼ft) or more, commonly found on roadsides and in meadows. Its huge leaves are incised and deeply lobed, forming a dense tuft at the plant's base. Leaves are also borne on its stout, hairy stem, whose thick petiole expands at its base into a large reddish sheath enclosing the young flower heads. The white flowers are clustered in large, flat umbels. The fruits are broad, winged schizocarps. The plant gives off an aromatic scent when crushed, especially the root and fruit.

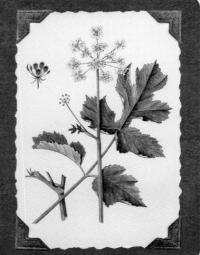

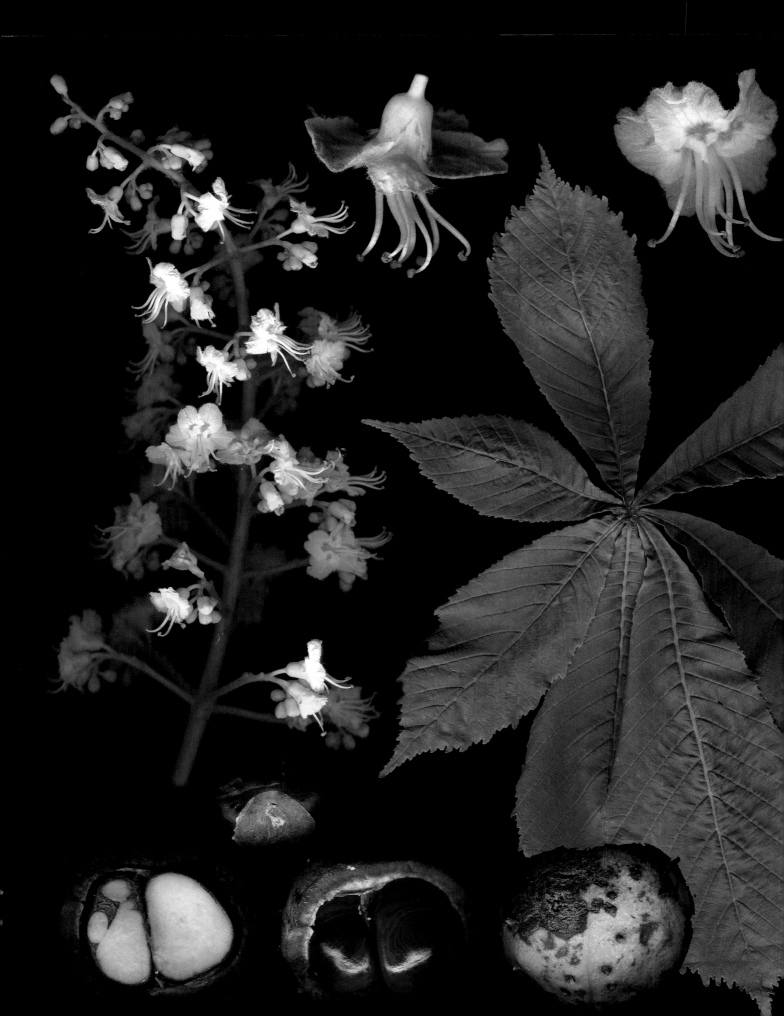

Horse-chestnut

Æsculus hippocastanum

FAMILY: SAPINDACEAE

Active elements:

Tannin, esculin (a coumarin compound).
Seeds: lots of starch, lipids, flavonoids and
triterpenic saponosides, including aescin.
Seed coat: proanthocyanidins.

• Useful for **treating congestive problems** in the pelvic region, including those that affect the prostate.
• Medicines based on Horse-chestnut are used to **treat bruising** and problems resulting from fragile skin capillaries.

OTHER USES: Horse-chestnuts are nutritious and can be eaten, although the toxic saponosides must be removed from them first. North American Indians did this by boiling the seeds of various local species of Horse-chestnut in water for a long time.

It was Clusius, gardener to Emperor Maximilian in Vienna, who planted the first Horse-chestnut tree, imported from Constantinople, in Europe. Bachilier subsequently introduced it to France in 1615. In the 17th century, many authors advocated the use of the bark and fruit of the Horse-chestnut tree as effective substitutes for *Cinchona* bark in the treatment of fevers. Under Napoleon I, at the time of the Continental Blockade, when doctors were obliged to use indigenous drugs, the Horse-chestnut tree came back into favour. Despite this, *Cinchona* remained the treatment of choice as, though more expensive, it was also safer. Latterly, the Horse-chestnut's antipyretic (fever-reducing) properties were outstripped by its universally acknowledged effectiveness in treating circulatory problems.

Heavy legs, varicose veins, haemorrhoids...

• The Horse-chestnut (seed) is recommended for the **treatment of chronic venous conditions** such as varicose veins and heavy legs.
• It **combats water retention**.
• It **relieves the pain of haemorrhoids** and acts on the varicose walls.

METHOD OF USE

• **INTERNAL:** Horse-chestnuts taste bitter and unpleasant so it is better to use capsules or tablets based on the dry extract. Use for vein problems. **Bark wine.** Steep 30 to 60g (1 to 2oz) of bark in a litre (quart) of white wine. Drink a glass before each meal. As preparations taste unpleasant, in the past people were advised to carry a conker in their pocket instead!
• **EXTERNAL: Bark decoction.** Use 50g (1¾oz) per litre as an antiseptic for bruising. This decoction is also used in lotions and washes for haemorrhoids, or in douches for congestion in the female pelvic region.

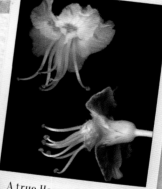

A true Horse-chestnut has white flowers (never pink).

Description

This beautiful tree, which originated in the forests of the Balkans and Turkey, is often seen majestically adorning parks, paths and school playgrounds. It has large sticky buds, beautiful palmate leaves composed of five to seven leaflets and tight clusters of white flowers with red or yellow markings. The green and spiny fruit contains large, shiny brown seeds with a lighter spot, known as horse-chestnuts or conkers.

DID YOU KNOW? The name Horse-chestnut tree comes from its traditional use in Turkey (and subsequently in Europe), for invigorating sluggish horses.

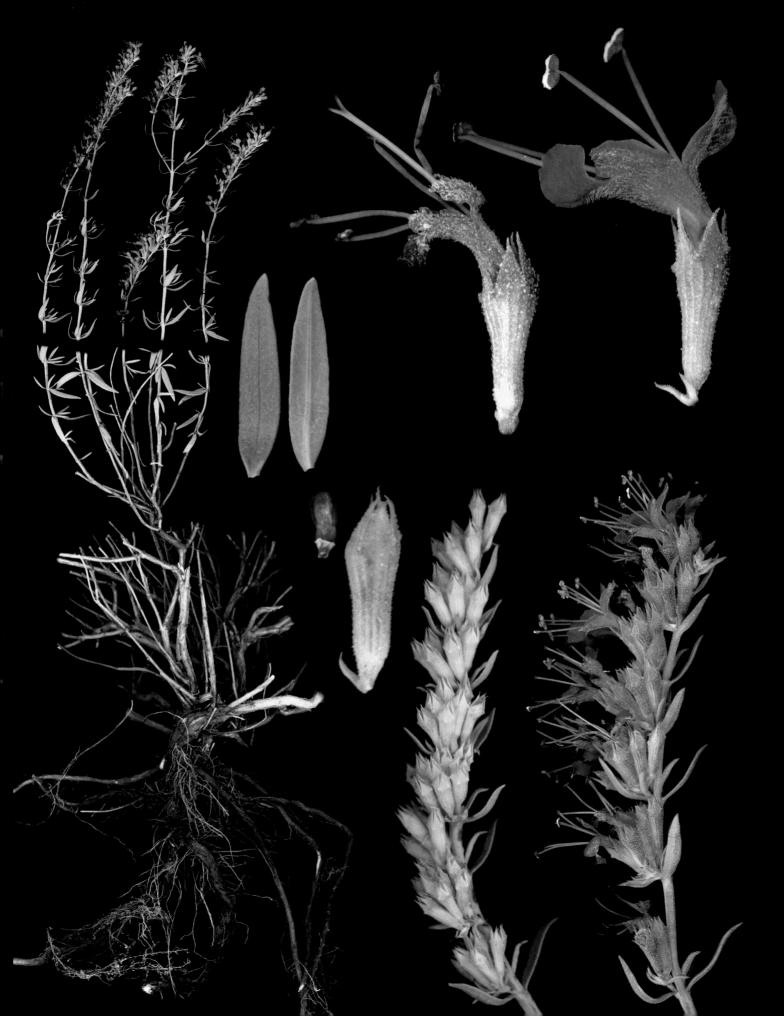

Hyssop

Hyssopus officinalis

FAMILY: LAMIACEAE

Active elements:

Flavonoids, phenolic compounds, bitter principle marrubiin and an aromatic oil rich in ketones including pinocamphone and isopinocamphone.

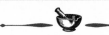

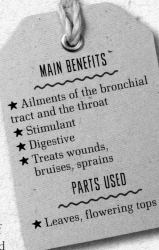

METHOD OF USE

- **INTERNAL: Infusion.** Infuse 20g (¾oz) of leaves and flowering tops per litre (quart) of boiling water. Take 2 or 3 cups per day to stimulate digestion and treat respiratory ailments.
Syrup. Prepare as a concentrated infusion, using 100g (3½oz) of plant per litre of boiling water. Leave to infuse for several minutes. Strain, add 1½kg (3¼lb) of sugar and cook until it has the consistency of syrup. Take 5 tablespoonsful per day to relieve coughing.
  - **EXTERNAL: Concentrated infusion.** Use as a **gargle** or in **hot compresses.**

"**W**ash me with Hyssop and I shall be clean," said King Solomon, who used this sacred plant with cedar wood to heal leprosy. In the Middle Ages, St. Hildegard used it, with liquorice and cinnamon, as "a powerful remedy for liver and lung ailments", and combined it with an infusion of the "four pectoral flowers", "to bring relief to nuns whose singing caused hoarseness". In turn Trotula, the "wise matron"—one of the leading figures at the famous Schola Medica Salernitana—recommended its use to purge phlegm from the lungs, especially combined with figs: "for cold cough, use the wine or Hyssop and dried figs that have been cooked".

For bronchial problems

- Hyssop is used to **treat bronchial disorders**. Its high marrubiin content makes it an excellent expectorant, while also drying out the airways, making breathing easier by acting on the nerve centres. It is advocated for the treatment of coughs and bronchial diseases with shortness of breath, and asthma.
- It is a **stimulant**, which restores energy following a cough, however people who suffer anxiety should use it in small doses.
- Hyssop also has **digestive properties**. It is a bitter which stimulates the appetite and aids digestion.
- When used externally, the plant is **restorative and heals wounds**. It is also one of the ingredients of the official "vulnerary tincture". It can be gargled for ailments of the throat and used in poultices against wounds, bruises and sprains.
- Inhaling Hyssop is said to help cold-sufferers to **clear blocked noses**.

OTHER USES: Hyssop is a great condiment to use in salads and a variety of warm dishes. It is a pleasant seasoning for grains, vegetables and meat. The plant is also used to flavour liqueurs.

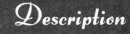

Description

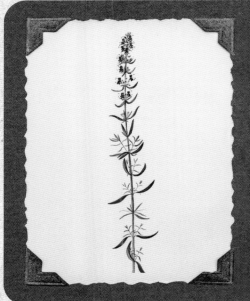

A perennial growing to a height of 20 to 60cm (8 to 24in), found in arid, stony areas, sometimes on old walls. It is native to southern Europe, western Asia and Morocco. Hyssop is grown for its medicinal properties and as a condiment. The stems are woody at the base from which a number of upright branches grow, densely covered with long, narrow, leaves in opposition, with bunches of smaller leaves in their axils. Intense purplish-blue, double-lipped flowers bloom on the long, compact terminal spikes in summer. Leaves and flowering tops give off the spicy smell of peppery honey.

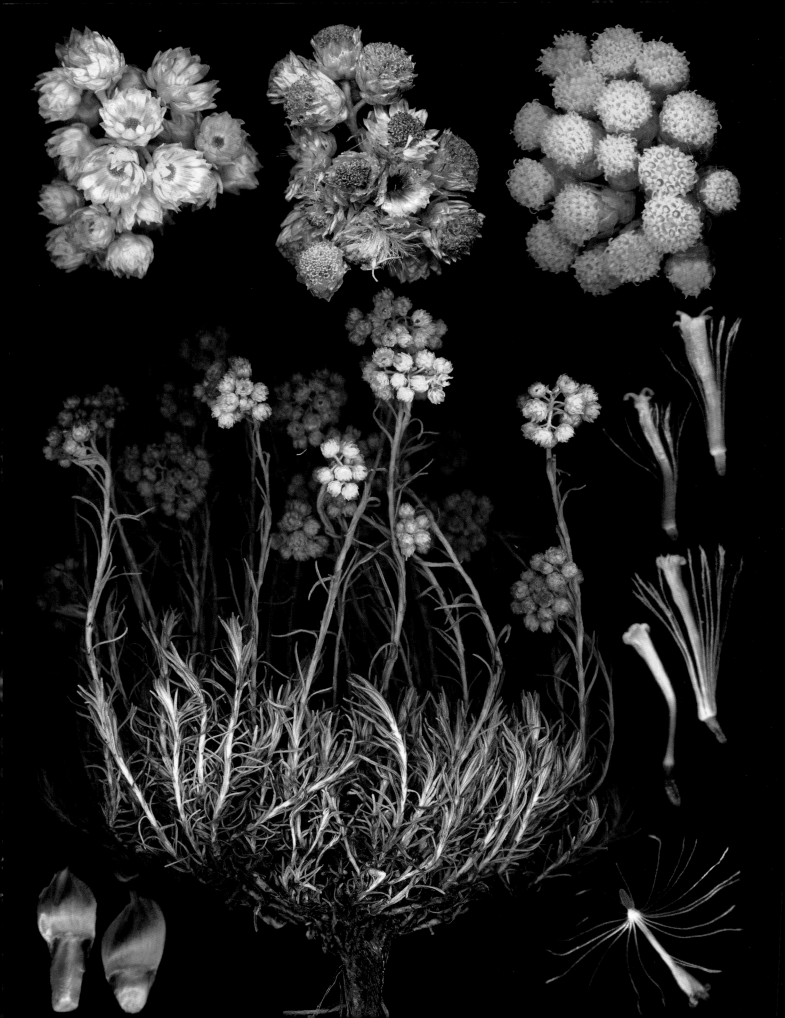

Immortelle

Helichrysum sp.

FAMILY: ASTERACEAE

Active elements:

Flavonoids, phthalides, coumarins, pyrone derivatives, phytosterols, tannins, bitter principles (including sesquiterpene lactone). Curry Plant (subspecies *Helichrysum italicum*): essential oil (including neryl acetate, diones and curcumenes).

Immortelle, a symbol of immortality, is so named because the flowers dry without withering and can keep for over a year. They crowned the head of Apollo, God of the Arts, Masculine Beauty and Healing. Their medicinal properties have, however, remained largely unknown over the centuries. Although one subspecies, the Curry Plant, was burned during the Second World War and the great flu epidemic of 1918 to purify the air in French hospitals, it was only in the second half of the century that any real interest was shown in its healing powers.

Excellent for the digestion and healing bruises

• Immortelle flowers are used to **stimulate the production and discharge of bile**. They can also protect the liver and detoxify the body.
• Its bitter properties stimulate secretions from the stomach and pancreas, and it is effective at **soothing difficult and painful digestion**. It is also a diuretic.

• Like Arnica, essential oil of Curry Plant is good for treating **bruises, swelling, knocks and bumps**.
• In skincare, it provides effective **treatment for acne**, blotchiness and varicose veins.

OTHER USES: As its name would suggest, Curry Plant can be used to give vegetable or rice dishes a slight curry flavour (remove the plant before serving). In Corsica, a torch of Immortelle (or fern) was traditionally used to burn off the bristles on a wild boar before it was spit roasted.

DID YOU KNOW? 700kg to 1 tonne (up to 19½cwt) of Curry Plant flowers are needed to obtain a litre (quart) of essential oil. That's 3½ to 5kg (up to 11lb) of flowers for a tiny 5ml bottle. It is little wonder that this essential oil is so expensive.

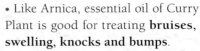

MAIN BENEFITS

★ Gall bladder and liver
★ Detoxifying
★ Digestive
★ Bumps and bruises (Curry Plant)

PARTS USED

★ Flowers, parts of the plant above the ground

TOXICITY

Do not used Immortelle if your bile ducts are obstructed. If you suffer from gallstones, medical opinion must be sought first.

METHOD OF USE

• **INTERNAL**: Infusion. 1 small teaspoonful (~1g) for 5 to 10 minutes in 150ml of simmering water. Drink 1 to 3 glasses per day.
Curry Plant essential oil. Oral administration, for adults only, requires a medical opinion.
• **EXTERNAL: Curry Plant essential oil.** For adults, topical application, 2 to 5 drops three times a day, pure or diluted in a vegetable oil.

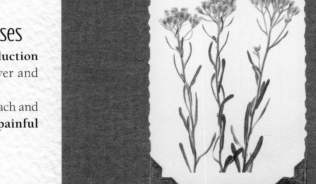

Description

Immortelle grows to a height of 20 to 50cm (8in to 1½ft) and has conglomerations of small, tightly packed, yellow flowers which are very fragrant. Various species, such as the Common Shrubby Everlasting (*H. stoechas*) and Dwarf Everlast (*H. arenarium*), are widely used in herbal medicine. The Curry Plant (*H. italicum*) provides an essential oil used in aromatherapy. Do not confuse Immortelle with Mountain Everlasting (*Antennaria dioica*), another member of Asteraceae, whose flowers are white or pink.

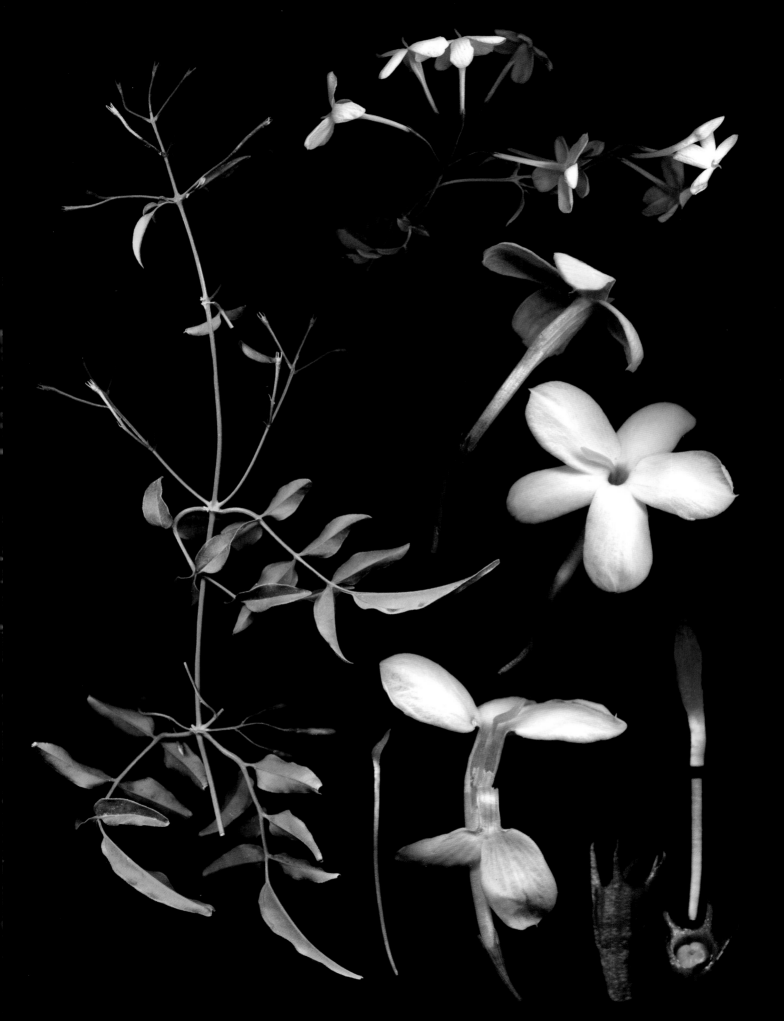

Jasmine

Jasminum officinale

FAMILY: OLEACEAE

Active elements:
Highly scented aromatic oil rich in linalyl acetate and jasmone.

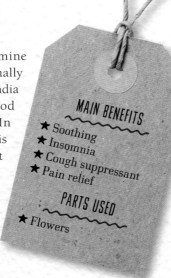

OTHER SPECIES: Arabian Jasmine (*Jasminum sambac*) is traditionally used in the Middle East and India to calm nerves, improve mood and build self-confidence. In Ayurvedic medicine, the flower is recommended for the treatment of depression, insomnia, coughs and respiratory infections, while the leaves are used to treat skin conditions, ulcers and wounds. In China, its flowers are used to perfume tea and rice.

Originally from the foothills of the Himalayas, Jasmine was introduced to Spain in the 16th century, before spreading throughout the entire Mediterranean basin. Its flowers were recommended by François-Joseph Cazin, the 19th-century French doctor and botanist, for the treatment of headaches.

TOXICITY

Note that the essential oil of Jasmine should not be used during pregnancy or breast-feeding, or on children under the age of six.

Sedative with scent

• Jasmine flowers **calm nervous tension**, induce sleep and soothe spasmodic coughs.
• A preparation of highly scented flowers steeped in oil can be used as an excellent rub for **treating the pains of nervous paralysis**.

OTHER USES: The aromatic oil extracted using the enfleurage process is highly prized in the perfume industry, but extremely costly. No less than 1,000kg (2,205lb) of flowers is required to obtain 1kg (2lb) of this absolute oil.

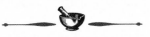

METHOD OF USE

• **INTERNAL: Infusion.** 20g (¾oz) of flowers per litre (quart) of water Drink 2 cups per day and one before going to bed. It is delicious.
• **EXTERNAL:** Tightly pack the flowers in a suitable container and add double their volume in olive oil. Leave to steep for at least one month, then use as a rub.
Essential oil. Use diluted in a vegetable oil, on the solar plexus, the back and wrists, for its calming properties.
Diffusion. For a calming atmosphere.
Haircare and skincare. A few drops in shampoo or a moisturizing cream.

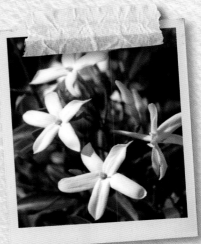

Jasmine flowers, with their strong, heady scent, are some of the most commonly used in perfumery.

Description

A perennial climbing plant that is commonly grown in countries with a mild climate, now naturalized in the hedgerows and rocky places of southern Europe. Its long, twining stems bear dark, evergreen, pinnate leaves, made up of leaflets. Its loose clusters of large, tubular white flowers, bloom from June to October and give off an incredible scent, particularly in the evening. The fruit is a round black berry.

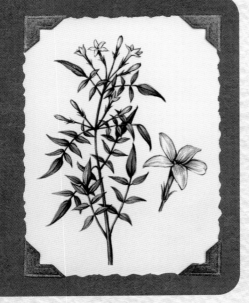

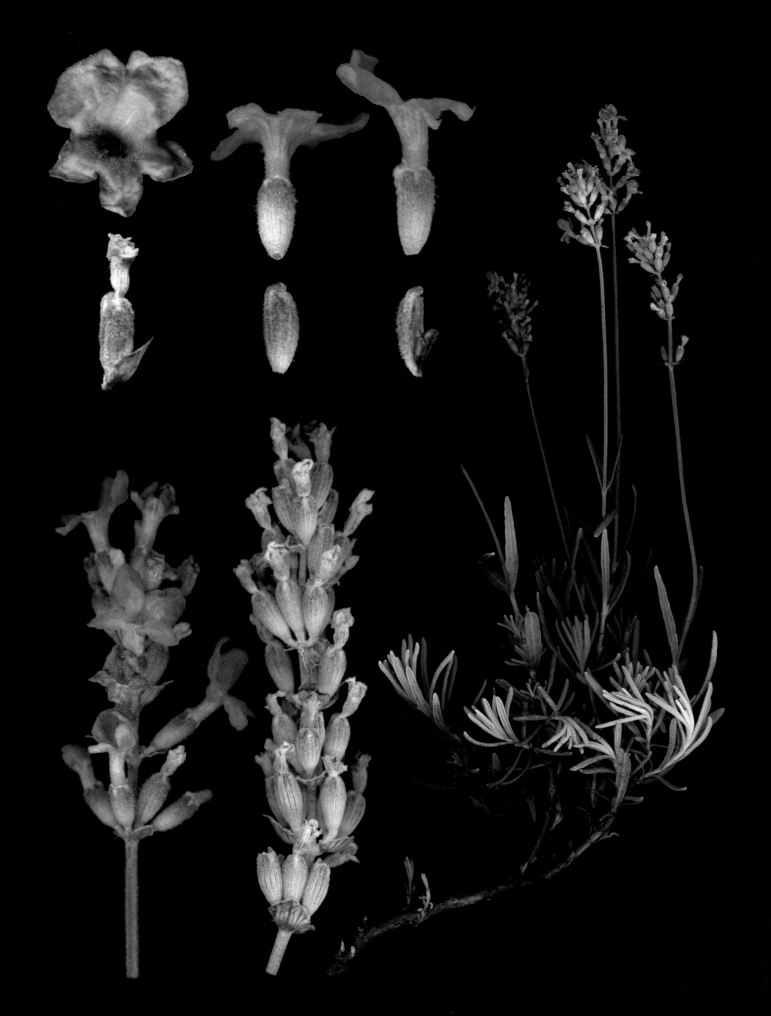

Lavender

Lavandula angustifolia

FAMILY: LAMIACEAE

Active elements:
Aromatic oil particularly rich
in linalyl acetate and linalool.

In the early 19th century, Henri Leclerc, the French physician and renowned medical herbalist, acknowledged Lavender's power to "dull painful sensitivity" and reduce fever. In high doses, Lavender is both a tonic and cordial, and its use was advocated for inflammation of the lymph nodes due to tuberculosis, anaemia related to iron deficiency and white discharge (leucorrhoea).

Calming, digestive, antiseptic and scented

• Lavender's calming properties are effective in **cases of insomnia or irritability**. It dulls headaches, migraines and vertigo.
• A scented stimulant which **facilitates digestion**, it combats colic, bloating and flatulence.
• Its **diuretic** and sudorific (sweat inducing) properties mean its use can relieve rheumatic pain.
• Lavender is **antiseptic** and has an effect on bronchial secretions.

External applications to the chest can be an excellent **treatment for lung congestion** or pneumonia.
• The essential oil distilled from the flowers is also antiseptic and antibacterial. It can be applied to **wounds, burns and insect bites** and soothes itching. When massaged on the temples, Lavender dulls headaches and can induce sleep.

OTHER USES: Widely used for its refreshing smell, Lavender is also ornamental. Its aromatic oil is a **powerful insect- and moth-repellent**. Lavender is also used to flavour cooking, particularly desserts and syrups.

OTHER SPECIES: There are numerous species and varieties of lavender, each with different properties. The essential oil of English Lavender (*Lavandula spica*), is anti-infective and fluidizing, and is helpful in the treatment of all ear, nose and throat conditions, as is that of the French Lavender (*L. stoechas*) —take care, however, as these essential oils can be neurotoxic in strong doses. The essential oil of Lavandin (*L. hybrida*) is calming, antispasmodic and wards off lice.

Description

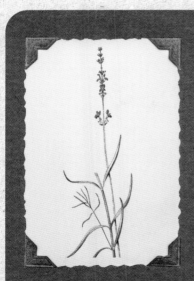

A perennial shrub growing to 40 to 80cm (16 to 31½in), widely found on limestone hillsides, at altitudes of 400 to 2,000m (1,300 to 6,500ft). Native to the western Mediterranean basin. Its simple, unbranched stems bear opposite, narrow, elongated, greyish leaves and small, purplish-blue, double-lipped flowers clustered densely around the terminal spikes. The whole plant, but particularly the flowers, gives off a delightful smell when lightly crushed.

METHOD OF USE

• **INTERNAL: Infusion.** 15 to 30g (½ to 1oz) of flower per litre (quart) of boiling water. 3 or 4 cups per day. To alleviate headaches and induce sleep.
Digestive wine. Steep 15 to 30g (½ to 1oz) of flowering tops in a litre of good red wine for a fortnight. Drink two small glasses per day.
• **EXTERNAL: Infusion.** Can be used as a vaginal douche (leucorrhoea), an inhalation (bronchial ailments) or compress (cuts and sprains).
Alcoholic tincture. Steep 100g of flowers in 500g of alcohol for one month. Multiple uses: rubs to treat headaches and bronchial problems; disinfection of cuts and wounds; dissipation of migraines; as an antispasmodic, on a sugar lump, to treat hiccups and stomach cramps; as an antiseptic toothpaste; as an aromatic water.
Lavender oil. Steep a handful of flowers in a litre of olive oil, leaving for 3 days in the sun. Use to treat aches and pains, cure wounds and dry eczema and reduce swelling after a fall. For insect bites, **crush some leaves** and apply the juice to the relevant area.
Put a **sachet of lavender** under the pillow to calm migraines and induce restorative sleep.

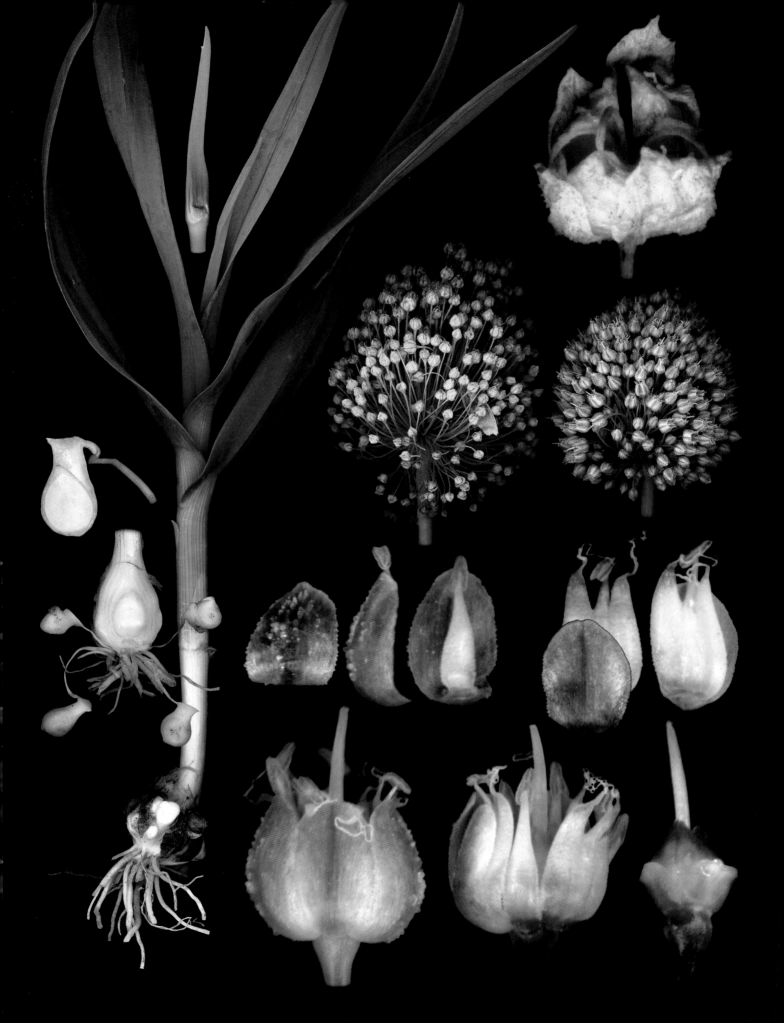

Leek

Allium porrum

FAMILY: ALLIACEAE

Active elements:
Sulphur heterosides.

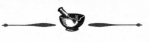

MAIN BENEFITS

★ Diuretic
★ Aids constipation
★ Respiratory diseases
★ Skincare

PARTS USED

★ White (stem), green (leaves) and seeds

for the **treatment of constipation**.

• It is effective for acute and chronic **inflammation of the respiratory tract**, and a Leek syrup works wonders for sore throats, hoarseness, coughs, and pharyngitis.

• Our grandmothers were well aware of the soothing, healing properties of Leek poultices, using them to treat **boils, ulcers, joint swelling, gout and sore throats.**

• A lotion made from the juice reduces redness and spots and **soothes insect bites.**

Leeks were held in particularly high regard by the Egyptians according to the famous Satire of Trades which recounts how King Cheops paid a skilled physician who had cured a urinary infection with 100 jars of leeks. It was highly esteemed by the Hebrews for its refreshing properties and is mentioned in the Book of Numbers. Among Greeks and Romans, it was both a valued vegetable and a genuine remedy. Hippocrates was the first to list its many virtues—it "increases diuresis, increases the milk of nursing mothers and cures consumption". The Emperor Nero ate nothing but Leeks for a few days a month as he believed this habit gave him an exceptional singing voice. As a result he was derisively nicknamed *porrophagus* ("leek-eater"). In the Middle Ages, it was likewise for this purpose that physicians generally prescribed Leeks.

The salutary Leek

• The Leek is a **popular diuretic** used in cases of urine retention. Leek broth or a decoction of seeds in white wine are both equally effective.

• It has a salutary effect on the gut, and is particularly useful

METHOD OF USE

• **INTERNAL: Leek broth** can be drunk as a herbal tea for its diuretic effects. Regular consumption is said to be a beauty aid, as it is apparently a good way to protect the skin from premature ageing.
Syrup. Obtained by mixing a strong and well-boiled decoction with an equal weight of honey. Very effective in respiratory tract inflammations.

• **EXTERNAL: As a poultice.** The poultice is prepared with boiled Leek leaves and applied hot. For the aforementioned conditions.

AN EQUALLY HELPFUL COUSIN: Garlic, the superstar of the Alliaciae family, is the Leek's cousin, and can be eaten fresh — either raw or cooked—or in the form of capsules, tablets or garlic oil. It is said to have numerous medicinal properties: it can **reduce blood pressure**; stimulate the heart and circulation; and thin the blood. It is recommended for lowering cholesterol and blood sugar, and can be used **preventatively against cardiovascular diseases**.

Its **antiseptic, antibacterial and expectorant properties** make it an excellent preventative and cure for colds, flu and other respiratory infections. The liquid pressed from it (known as allicin) has proven antibiotic action. Garlic is also an excellent anthelmintic. Chinese studies have shown a significantly lower rate of cancer among a population that has a high rate of garlic consumption (20g (¾oz) per day) in comparison with places where this condiment is only used occasionally.

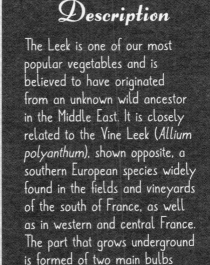

Description

The Leek is one of our most popular vegetables and is believed to have originated from an unknown wild ancestor in the Middle East. It is closely related to the Vine Leek (*Allium polyanthum*), shown opposite, a southern European species widely found in the fields and vineyards of the south of France, as well as in western and central France. The part that grows underground is formed of two main bulbs surrounded by numerous bulblets.

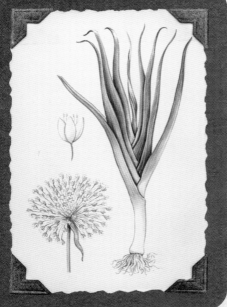

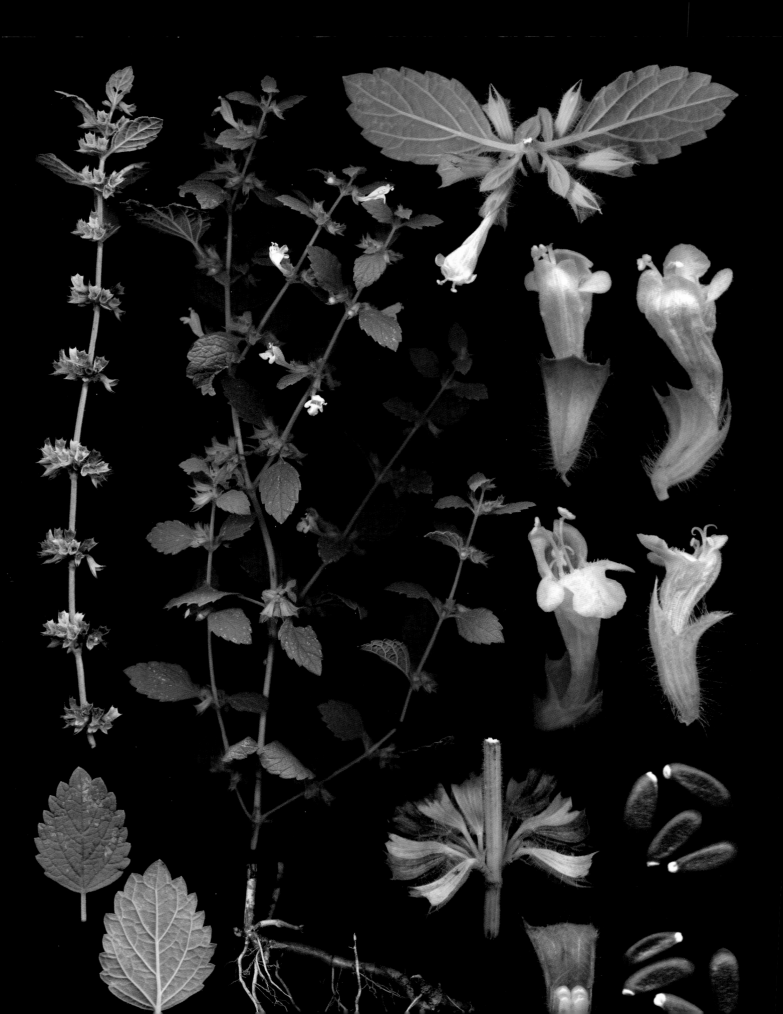

Lemon Balm

Melissa officinalis

FAMILY: LAMIACEAE

Active elements:

Triterpenes, phenolic acids, flavonoids, aromatic oil rich in citral, citronellal, caryophyllene and geranyl acetate.

Arab doctors vaunted the virtues of this highly renowned antispasmodic plant. Avicenna, the Persian polymath, attributed it with the property of rendering the heart joyous. In the 17th century, it was used by doctors to treat nervous depression—not only a 21st-century affliction. Lemon Balm is the basis of the famous "Carmelite Water" which in the 17th century became known as a miracle water, considered a panacea for a wide variety of ailments.

For all nervous complaints

• Lemon Balm is recommended for the treatment of **digestive difficulties** and disorders with palpitations, dizziness and fainting fits.

• It is advocated for the **treatment of anxiety, nervousness and mild depression**. It is effective in alleviating **sleep disorders**.

• It can also relieve the nervous tension and stress that may precede or accompany menstruation.

• By stimulating the release of bile, its flowers act on nervous disorders related to liver and gall-bladder failure.

• Lemon Balm has **antiviral** properties, probably due to the phenolic acids. The extract-based ointment effectively relieves herpes and **reduces the frequency of eruptions**. It is also effective against chickenpox and shingles.

• It is said to balance the function of the thyroid gland.

OTHER USES: Young Lemon Balm shoots can be added to salads, giving them a citrus note. Fish or vegetables steamed on a bed of Lemon Balm absorb its flavour. It can be used to flavour desserts and is a delicious addition to drinks.

DID YOU KNOW? Lemon Balm is occasionally erroneously referred to as "Lemon Grass". However, the real plant of this name is a large, strongly scented, tropical grass, *Cymbopogon citratus*, which has long, sharp leaves. Lemon Balm's scientific name, *Melissa*, means "bee" in Greek, and its nectar-rich flowers are popular with bees.

Description

A perennial, growing to 30 to 70cm (12 to 27½in), native to the Mediterranean basin. Frequently cultivated in gardens and sometimes found growing wild in hedgerows or along forest paths. Its square stems bear large, oval leaves which grow opposite each other. They are crinkled and serrated. The double-lipped white flowers, which bloom from June to September, grow in whorls around the leaf axils. Both leaves and flowers give off a strong, fresh, lemon-like scent.

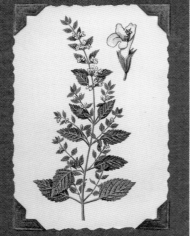

METHOD OF USE

• **INTERNAL: Infusion.** 25 to 50g (¾ to 1¾oz) of leaves and flowering tops per litre (quart) of water. Leave to infuse for 10 minutes. Drink 3 or 4 cups per day to aid digestion, calm nerves and induce sleep. It is always preferable to use the **fresh plant**, as it loses its scent when dried. Lemon Balm is very easy to grow in the garden or in a pot on a balcony. However, it is also useful to have some Lemon Balm wine or water ready prepared in case of need.
Wine. Leave 50g (1¾oz) of the fresh plant to steep for 48 hours in a litre of white wine. Take 2 tablespoonsful per day as and when needed.
Home-made Carmelite Water. Steep the following in a litre of colourless spirits for a fortnight: 50g (1¾oz) of fresh Lemon Balm, 5g of cinnamon, 15g (½oz) of fresh lemon zest, 10g (¼oz) of angelica, 15g coriander, 10g cloves, 15g nutmeg. Press through a sieve and keep bottled. One teaspoonful if feeling unwell.

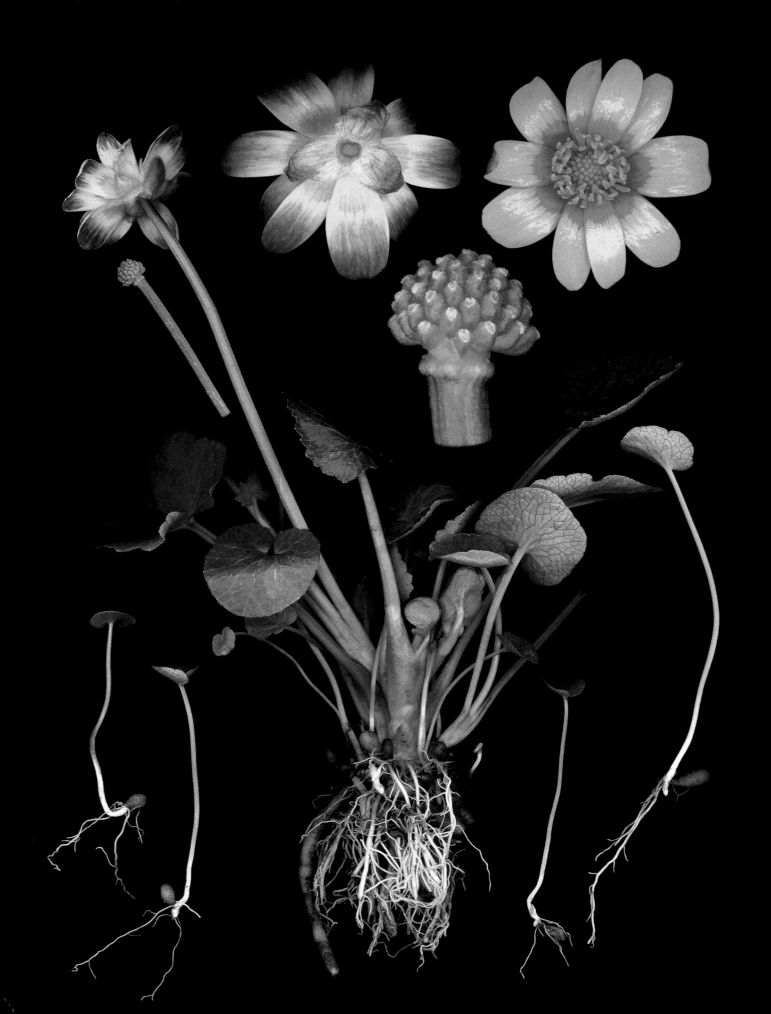

Lesser Celandine

Ranunculus ficaria
FAMILY: RANUNCULACEAE

Active elements:
Roots: starch, saponosides (heterosides). Plant: variable amounts of protoanemonin, which disappears on drying. Leaves: rich in vitamin C.

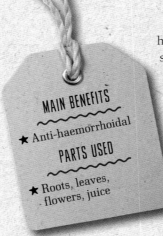

MAIN BENEFITS

★ Anti-haemorrhoidal

PARTS USED

★ Roots, leaves, flowers, juice

The small roots, in the form of tubers, bear a striking resemblance to haemorrhoids. By application of the "doctrine of signatures", they were used in the 16th century to treat piles. In this case, this dubious-sounding association has been proven to be entirely correct. Lesser Celandine, one of the plants known as Pilewort, is indeed remarkably effective against the condition. It was recorded as such, for the first time, by Rembert Dodoens, the 16th-century Flemish physician and botanist.

Remedy for haemorrhoids

• The heterosides in Lesser Celandine give it **vasoconstrictive properties** which add tone to the vein walls. The plant has remained a **specific remedy for haemorrhoids** (simple, prolapsed and inflamed haemorrhoids). It can be administered in the form of extracts, intraits, ointment, syrup, powder, infusion, decoction, balm or compress.

OTHER USES: A little gold button adorning woodland or hedgerows, the Lesser Celandine is closely related to the Meadow Buttercup, However, unlike the latter, the Lesser Celandine has a very low content of caustic substances (protoanemonin) meaning that its very young leaves, the ones right at the base of the plant, can be eaten raw. They have a high vitamin C content and can be added to a salad, but always in moderate quantities so as not to risk illness. Older leaves can be boiled then prepared in various ways.

DID YOU KNOW? The scientific species name *ficaria* comes from "fig", because of the resemblance between its bulging roots and the fig. The genus name *Ranunculus* means "little frog" because many plants in this genus grow around ponds and in other watery environments.

METHOD OF USE

• **INTERNAL:** Infusion or short decoction. 50 to 60g (1¾ to 2oz) of root per litre (quart) of water. Use to reduce haemorrhoids.
• **EXTERNAL:** Juice pressed from the fresh plant. Apply to haemorrhoids.
It can also be used in the form of an ointment.
Hot poultice. A strong decoction of boiled leaves is another option, reduced by two-thirds, mixed with flax or fenugreek flour, to make a poultice that can be applied very hot.

TOXICITY

Although the Lesser Celandine has a lower level of protoanemonin than others in the buttercup family, it can cause irritation of the skin and mucosa when used externally. With the exception of the young leaves (to be used in moderation), it should never be eaten raw, as it causes abdominal pains, vomiting and diarrhoea. Once dried, its toxicity disappears.

Description

A small perennial growing to 10 to 30cm (4 to 12in), common in cool woodland hedgerows and damp shady places. Native to Europe, western Asia and North Africa. Easily identified by its sinuous, glossy-green leaves in the form of upside-down hearts that have a rubbery texture to the touch. Its single flowers have six golden-yellow glossy petals, turning a whitish colour as they age. Underground, a short stem bears several buds and bulging roots in small tubers.

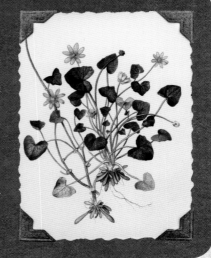

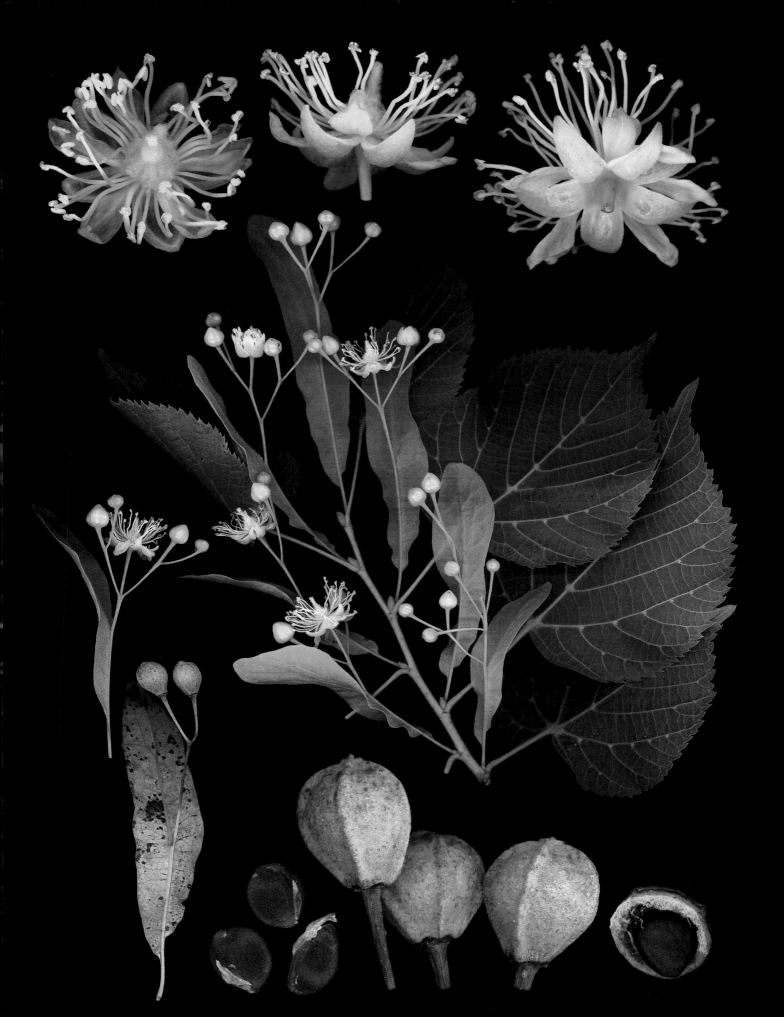

Lime (Linden)

Tilia sp.

FAMILY: TILIACEAE

Active elements:

Flowers: mucilage, tannins, phenolic acids, proanthocyanidins, flavonoids (including quercetin and kaempferol), aromatic oil. Sapwood (the recently formed wood just under the bark): phenolic acids, tannins, fraxin, esculin, amino acids.

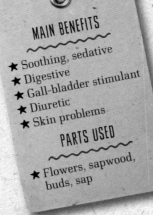

MAIN BENEFITS

★ Soothing, sedative
★ Digestive
★ Gall-bladder stimulant
★ Diuretic
★ Skin problems

PARTS USED

★ Flowers, sapwood, buds, sap

Pliny mentions the beneficial effects of Lime bark vinegar for "vices of the skin". In the Middle Ages, Saint Hildegard warded off pestilence with a ring decorated with a green stone, under which was said to be a piece of Lime wrapped in a spider's web. Numerous ancient documents related to herbal medicine record its effectiveness in treating epilepsy, paralysis, dizziness and oedema. Its importance was such that a royal decree ordered the roads to be planted with Lime trees and the product of their harvest to be reserved for the hospitals.

Calmative but fortifying

• Lime flowers are known for their **calmative, antispasmodic properties**. They act as a remarkable sedative on the nervous system, inducing **restorative sleep** even in insomniacs. However, if a dose is too high, or an infusion is left to steep for too long, it may trigger **excitant** properties which can then conversely cause insomnia.
• Lime is antispasmodic so **relieves digestive difficulties**, particularly those that are the result of excessive anxiety.
• It promotes perspiration so is an excellent remedy **for colds and flu**. It reduces nasal secretion, and relieves muscle aches and associated pains and headaches.

• Lime baths can have a **calmative** effect on over-excited children
• The decoction is recommended in lotion form to **soothe itchy skin**.
• It is also a **beauty water** that tightens the skin, and treats impurities, dry patches and spots.
• The infusion of Lime sapwood has been shown to have **remarkable cleansing powers**. It stimulates the liver and regulates bile secretion, improving slow digestion and dissolving the uric acid that causes gout and kidney stones.

OTHER USES: The leaves, when young and translucent, can be eaten in salads. Older leaves can be dried and reduced to a green powder which can be used to make pancakes, bread and cakes when mixed with flour.

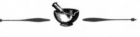

METHOD OF USE

• **INTERNAL:** Infusion of flowers. 3 to 5g per cup of boiling water (i.e. two teaspoonsful). Drink 2 to 4 cups per day as a sedative and digestif.
• **EXTERNAL:** Strong decoction. 60 to 70g (2 to 2½oz) of flowers per litre (quart) of boiling water. For lotions, compresses and beauty water.
Soothing bath. Prepare a decoction of ½kg (1lb) of flowers in a few litres of water and add to bath.

Description

These large trees are easy to identify from their broad, heart-shaped leaves with serrated margins. Their greenish-yellow flowers, hanging in clusters under long membranous bracts, exude a smell of honey in early summer. The fruit is a tiny fluffy ball containing a single seed. Three species are currently used for their medicinal properties: the large-leaved lime (*Tilia platyphyllos*), the small-leaved lime (*T. x cordata*) and the Common Lime (*T. x europea*), a hybrid of the first two. Other species may also be used, Silver Linden (*T. tomentosa*) for example. The Common Lime is often used as an ornamental tree in parks and gardens.

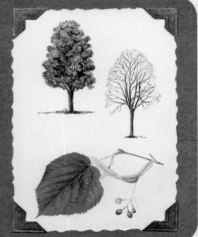

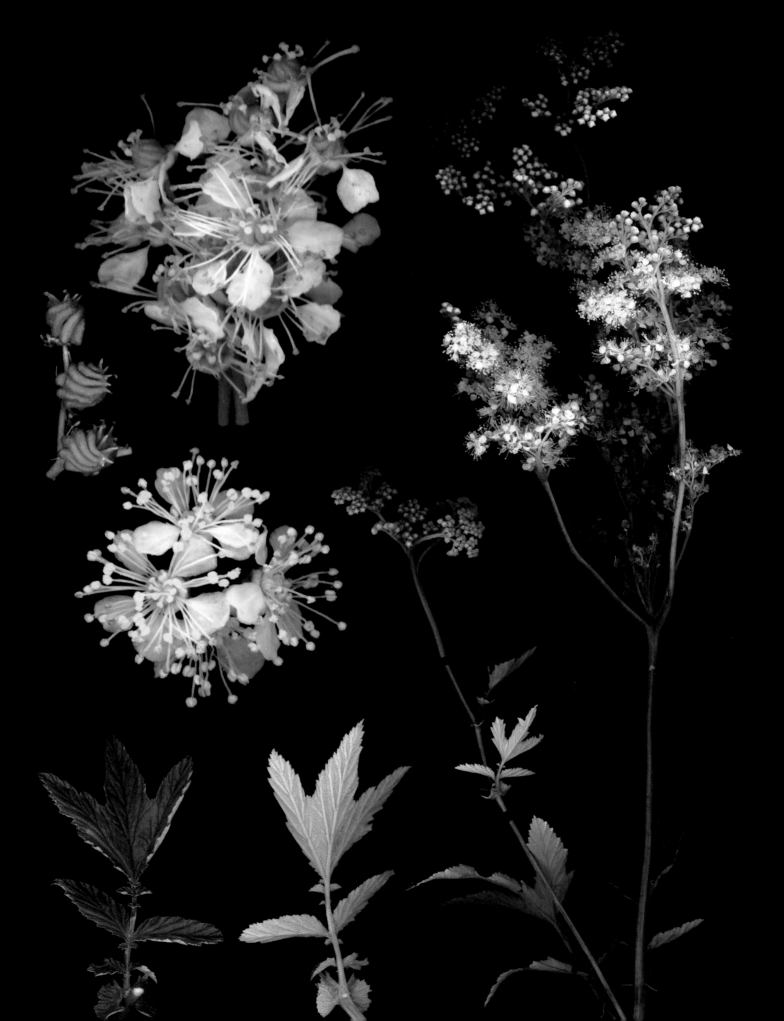

Meadowsweet

Filipendula ulmaria

FAMILY: ROSACEAE

Active elements:

Tannins, flavonic heterosides (including spiraeoside, rutin and hyperoside), heterosides of phenolic acids. Essential oil rich in methyl salicylate and salicylic aldehyde.

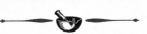

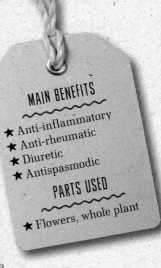

METHOD OF USE

* **INTERNAL: Infusion.** 10 to 30g (¼ to 1oz) plant per litre (quart). Drink 3 or 4 cups per day. Never boil as the salicylates will be destroyed.
Alternatively: 50g (1¾oz) of flowers per litre of hot water (fresh or dried within the last year). Infuse for 7 to 10 minutes and drink 3 to 4 cups per day for the benefits mentioned.
Alcoholature. Steep 50g of fresh flowers in 50g of alcohol (40% by volume) for 12 hours. Strain and take 1 or 2 teaspoonsful per day. Can be taken all year round.
* **EXTERNAL:** The concentrated infusion works wonders as a **compress** to treat wounds, ulcers and rheumatism pains. Hot **poultices** of infused flowers may also be applied to treat the latter.

In the Renaissance, Dodoens, a 16th-century Flemish physician and botanist, recorded Meadowsweet as a remedy for dysentery. According to the "doctrine of signatures", since the plant grew in water, it was also thought to cure ailments brought on by a damp environment. Nineteenth-century chemists studied the composition of Meadowsweet and several plants said to have similar properties. As a result, in 1829 they managed to isolate salicin from willow bark, which works wonders against fevers. In 1844, methyl salicylate was discovered in *Gaultheria*, a strong-smelling American cousin of the Bilberry. Meadowsweet owes its characteristic smell to the same chemical component. In 1897, Felix Hoffmann, the German chemist, made the less caustic compound, acetylsalicylic acid. The Bayer pharmaceutical laboratories marketed it under the name "Aspirin" (*Spiraea* being the generally accepted scientific name for Meadowsweet at that time, inspired by the spiral arrangement of the fruits).

For urinary pains, gout and rheumatism

* Meadowsweet is **anti-inflammatory and anti-rheumatic**.
* The fresh flowers (or dried within the last year) have **undeniable diuretic properties**. They efficiently eliminate uric acid and act as a sedative for urinary pains. They have antispasmodic properties and are also advocated for the **treatment of gout, rheumatic pains, cellulite and atherosclerosis**, all of which are due to a build-up of waste products in the body.
* Meadowsweet reduces gastric acidity and contributes to decreasing acidity throughout the body, which **can help with joint problems**.
* Meadowsweet's high tannin content makes it **effective in treating diarrhoea**.

Description

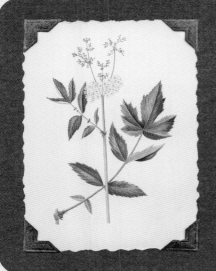

A large perennial plant, growing to over 1m (3¼ft) in height, which forms beautiful colonies in damp meadows throughout most of Europe. Its erect, reddish stems bear leaves divided into toothed leaflets, with a much larger terminal leaflet, deeply divided into three acute lobes. The creamy-white, deliciously fragrant flowers are arranged in compound clusters that flare upwards. The fruits are clustered and together take the form of small spiral green balls, very fragrant when crushed.

TOXICITY

The plant is counter-indicated in cases of hypersensitivity to salicylates.

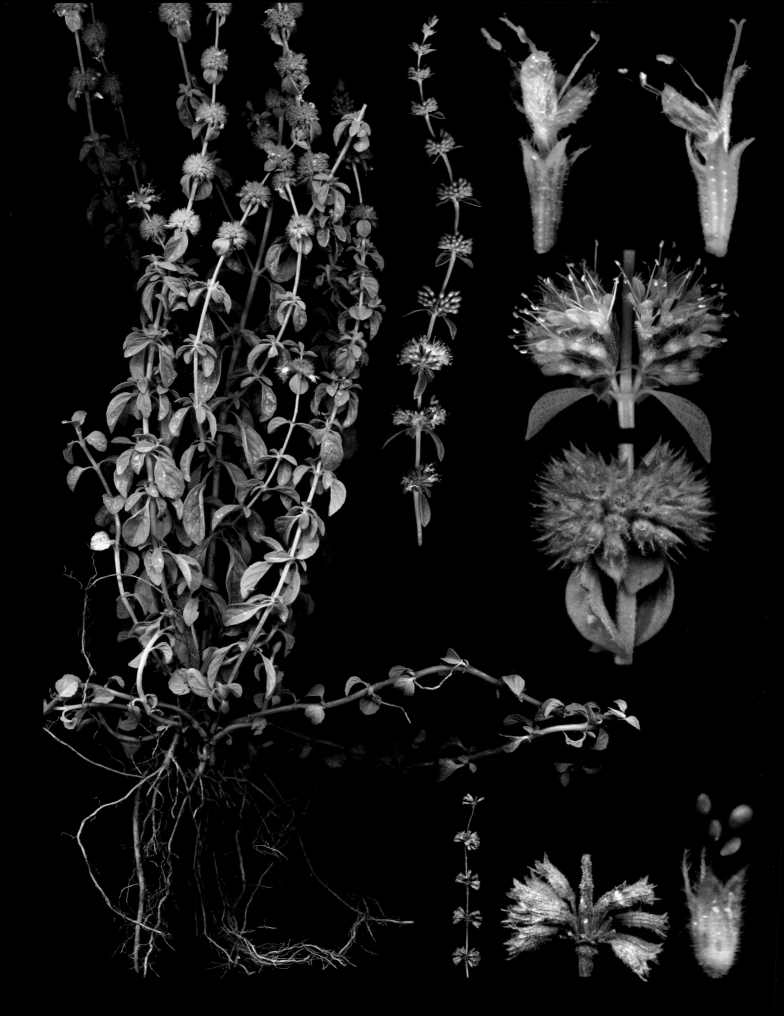

Mint

Mentha sp.

FAMILY: LAMIACEAE

Active elements:

Flavonoids, phenolic acids, triterpenes, carotenoids, aromatic oil (high in menthol, menthone and menthyl acetate).

Mint was held in high regard in antiquity. The Assyrians and the Babylonians used it to invigorate a sluggish stomach, while the Hebrews used it as a stimulant. Dioscorides found it effective in combating a weak stomach. In the 19th century, Trousseau advocated its use as a cure for vomiting, and also for stubborn, hacking coughs. In the last century, Henri Leclerc, the French physician and medical herbalist, was one of many who recommended Mint as a stimulant that was "very suitable for the games of love". The *Mentha pulegium* species of mint, commonly known as Pennyroyal, was used in the past as a flea repellent, the word *pulegium* coming from the Latin *pulex*, meaning "flea".

Effective digestive aid and breath freshener

• Peppermint (*M. piperita*) is a **remarkable stimulant of the digestive system**. It is also antiseptic, antispasmodic and analgesic and increases bile production.

• It is recommended for general **digestive problems**, stomach and intestinal pains, flatulence and bloating.

• Mint helps to **relieve migraines** and facial pain, and is indicated for the treatment of inflammation of the gums, mouth and lips.

• Peppermint and Water Mint (*M. aquatica*) are effective in freshening the mouth and **combating bad breath**.

• Pennyroyal **stimulates the nervous system**. It works as an **expectorant** which makes it useful in the treatment of asthma, hacking coughs and hoarseness.

OTHER USES: Mint is an excellent condiment that can be used in multiple ways and is the basis for Mint tea. The essential oil and menthol are widely used in pharmaceuticals, perfume, confectionery and the liqueur industry.

TOXICITY

Care should be taken with Mint essential oils. Caution should be taken with the internal use of Peppermint oil. The essential oil of Pennyroyal can cause abortions and have a harmful effect on the liver. It should be treated as toxic.

MAIN BENEFITS

★ Digestive
★ Fresh breath
★ Antispasmodic
★ Respiratory disorders
★ Tonic
★ Migraines

PARTS USED

★ Leaves, flowering tops

METHOD OF USE

• **INTERNAL: Infusion.** 20 to 30g (¾ to 1oz) of leaves and flowering tops per litre (quart) of boiling water. Drink 1 cup after each meal as a digestive and to ward off post-lunch drowsiness.

An infusion of 20g (¾oz) of mint and 20g (¾oz) of lavender flowers per litre of water is good for warding off coughs. Mint improves the taste of bland infusions and masks unpleasant ones.

Solar tea. Steep for a few hours in airtight container of water in direct sunlight. Good for False Apple-mint (*M. x rotundifolia*) and Horsemint (*M. longifolia*) which do not work well as infusions.

Fresh. Chew a leaf to refresh breath or as a digestive. Use as a rub to relieve itching and muscular pain.

• **EXTERNAL: Concentrated infusion.** 50g (1¾oz) per litre, for compresses, gargles and lotions for greasy skin and dilated pores.

Enema. 5g of Mint and 5g of Tansy, infused in half a litre of salt water. Bath. Use Mint, Rosemary and Thyme for a **scented, fortifying and anti-rheumatic bath.**

Description

Perennials growing to a height of between 20cm and 1m (8in to 3¼ft). Square stems, reddish in some species, and creeping rootstock. The leaves are serrated and the white or pink flowers are grouped in terminal spikes or whorls. Peppermint is a hybrid between Spearmint (*M. spicata*) and Water Mint (*M. aquatica*). It has a penetrating scent and an initial warm, peppery flavour, followed by a pleasant freshness.

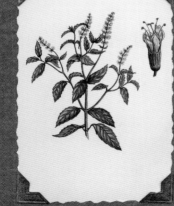

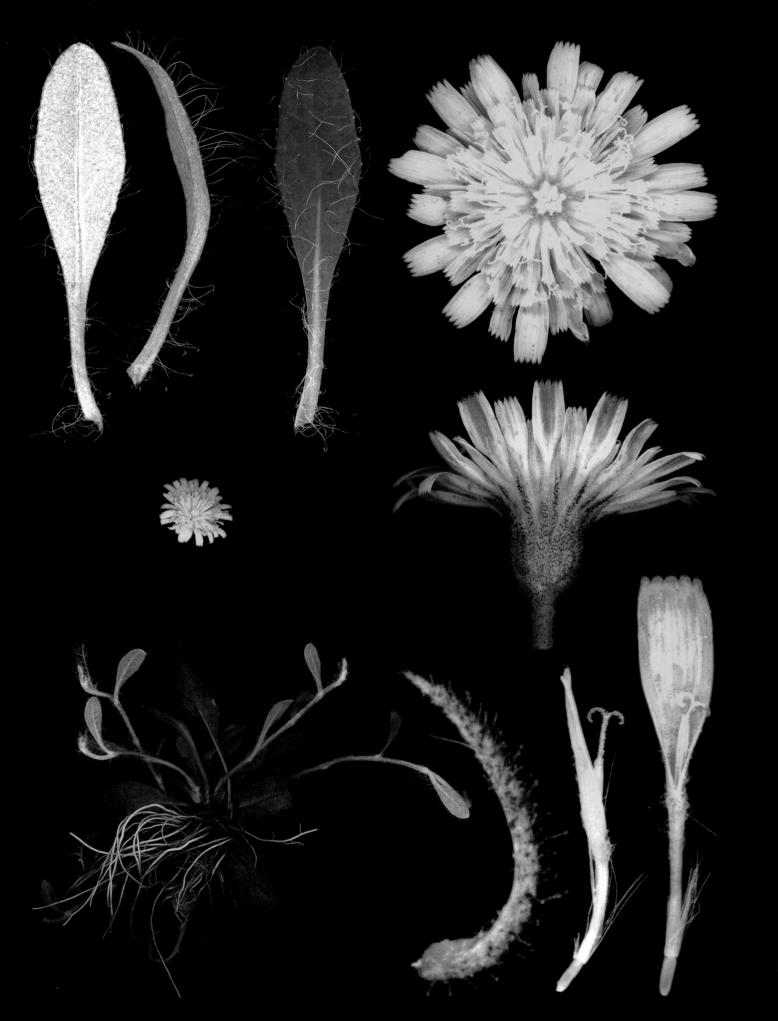

Mouse-ear-hawkweed

Hieracium pilosella
(=Pilosella officinarum)

FAMILY: ASTERACEAE

Active elements:

Flavonoids, phenol acids (including caffeic acid and chlorogenic acid), inulin (sugar) and a glucoside in the coumarin group, umbelliferone.

MAIN BENEFITS
★ Diuretic
★ Liver tonic and detox
★ Respiratory ailments
★ Healing

PARTS USED
★ Leaves

In the 12th century, St. Hildegard of Bingen, was the first to record the properties of Mouse-ear-hawkweed, as a "tonic for the heart". Popular medicine used it as an astringent, to treat nosebleeds and uterine haemorrhages and against chronic diarrhoea. Mouse-ear-hawkweed was part of the empirical pharmacopoeia of the peasants of the Landes region of France: they knew from experience that the plant flushed out toxins and used it to treat excessive levels of urea in the blood.

Farewell to toxins

• Mouse-ear-hawkweed is a confirmed **diuretic**, its high level of flavonoids making it effective in ridding the body of urea. High blood urea is often an indication of kidney disease or heart failure. The plant is also effective in reducing an excess of albumin and treating lower-limb oedema.

• The plant **promotes the production and flow of bile** which helps to detoxify the liver, and to prevent infection.

• It is used in **respiratory disorders** such as asthma, bronchitis or whooping cough.

• Externally, it can be applied to wounds to **speed up healing**.

• The umbelliferone contained in the juice of Mouse-ear-hawkweed has **antibiotic properties**, particularly against bacteria of the *Brucella* genus, which is responsible for several livestock diseases, some of which, such as Malta fever, can be transmitted to humans.

METHOD OF USE

• **INTERNAL: Infusion.** 50g (1¾oz) of leaves per litre (quart) of boiling water. Take 2 or 3 cups per day as a diuretic and to stimulate the liver.

• **EXTERNAL:** A **powder** of the dried leaves was used in the past in popular medicine to stop nosebleeds and sometimes the astringent infusion would be used for sore throats. **Crushed fresh leaves** applied to wounds hasten healing.

OTHER SPECIES: Many other European Hawkweeds have the same properties, including Meadow Hawkweed (*Hieraceum caespitosum*), identifiable by its clusters of yellow flower heads grouped at the top of the stems, and Orange Hawkweed, or Devil's Paintbrush (*H. aurantiacum*), with its yellow-orange flower heads. Several of these Hawkweeds were accidentally introduced into North America and New Zealand, and have become so invasive that their medicinal value has been overlooked.

DID YOU KNOW? The plant owes its popular name and its scientific name *Hieracium* (from the Greek *hierax*, meaning hawk) to an old belief that these birds of prey drank Hawkweed juice to enhance their eyesight.

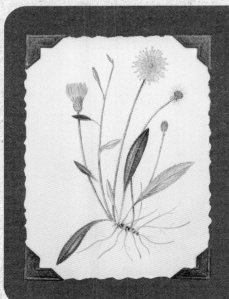

Description

A perennial plant growing to a height of 10 to 30cm (4 to 12in), with creeping shoots, common in dry places. It is found in temperate regions of the northern hemisphere. Its long leaves, covered with hairs on both sides, form a rosette. Their shape gives the plant its common name "Mouse-ear". The stem does not bear leaves, but a single flower head of pale yellow ray florets.

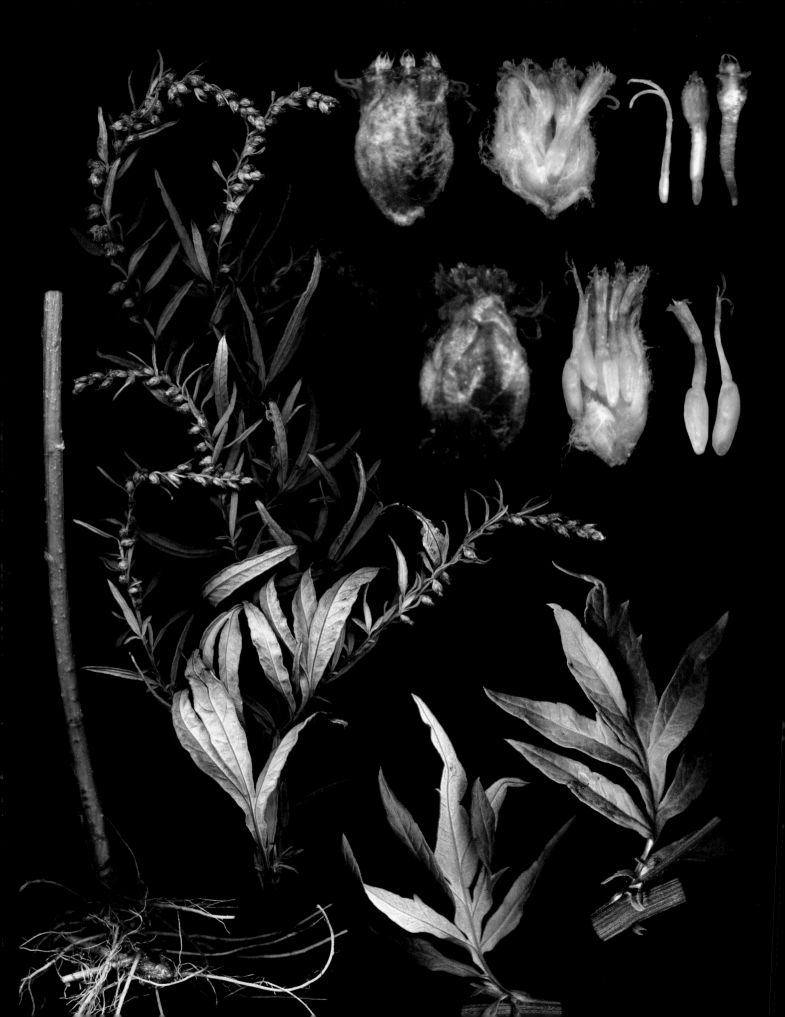

Mugwort

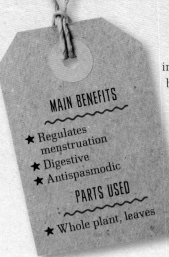

Artemisia vulgaris

FAMILY: ASTERACEAE

Active elements:
Flavonoids. Small quantities of aromatic oil containing camphor, borneol and a little thujone.

Hippocrates, Dioscorides and Pliny the Elder all referred to Mugwort's efficacy in promoting menstruation. The Ancients were said to slip it into their shoes to prevent their feet tiring during long walks. In the 17th century, the Spanish physician Diego de Torres advocated the application of a poultice of crushed Mugwort leaves to the lower abdomen to trigger contractions during childbirth. Some authors have also praised its curative properties in nervous disorders, such as hysteria, epilepsy or Sydenham's chorea (St. Vitus' Dance).

"Moxa" plant

• Mugwort is used to **regulate the frequency of menstruation or moderate its flow** as well as to reduce painful periods.
• It also has **digestive and antispasmodic qualities**.
• In traditional Japanese medicine, it is used in **moxibustion treatments**, which consist of gently burning small cones or sticks of Mugwort leaves (the "moxa") on the skin at one of the many acupuncture points along the energy meridians.

OTHER USES: Mugwort shoots and the tender ends of stems have a flavour reminiscent of artichoke, and are delicious deep-fried in batter. In Japan, the young leaves are boiled, then seasoned with roasted sesame seeds and soy sauce. They are also used to flavour and colour sticky rice balls known as "mochi". The flower heads are used to flavour creams and puddings.

DID YOU KNOW? *Artemisia* is said to have been named after Artemis, the Goddess of Hunting and protector of women. Others think it was named after Artemisia, the Queen of Caria and widow of Mausolus for whom she built the famous funerary monument. Both were experts in the field of medicinal plants, specializing particularly in gynaecology. French provincial folklore sometimes linked Mugwort to the midsummer bonfires of St. John festival. In the Moselle region, for example, Mugwort picked at the time of the solstice and thrown into the fire, was supposed to cure epilepsy and protect against against lightning and hail.

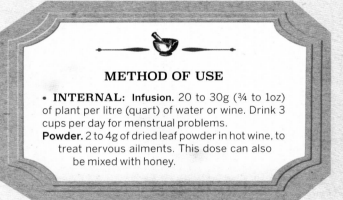

METHOD OF USE

• **INTERNAL: Infusion.** 20 to 30g (¾ to 1oz) of plant per litre (quart) of water or wine. Drink 3 cups per day for menstrual problems.
Powder. 2 to 4g of dried leaf powder in hot wine, to treat nervous ailments. This dose can also be mixed with honey.

TOXICITY

The use of Mugwort is not recommended during pregnancy. Mugwort pollen is strongly allergenic, but less so than its cousin Ragweed (*Ambrosia artemisiifolia*).

Description

A perennial growing to a height of 60cm (24in) to 1m (3¼ft), very common on wasteland, stony soils, roadsides and railway embankments. This cousin of Wormwood is widespread across most temperate regions of the northern hemisphere. When young, it grows in green tufts that turn grey as it matures. Its numerous reddish stems bear deeply divided leaves, the dark green upper surface a strong contrast with the whitish, woolly underside. They give off a sweet smell when crushed. From June to September, the tiny yellowish-green flowers grow in spikes along the stems.

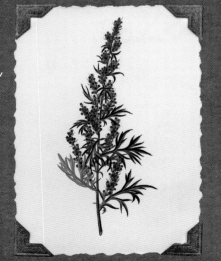

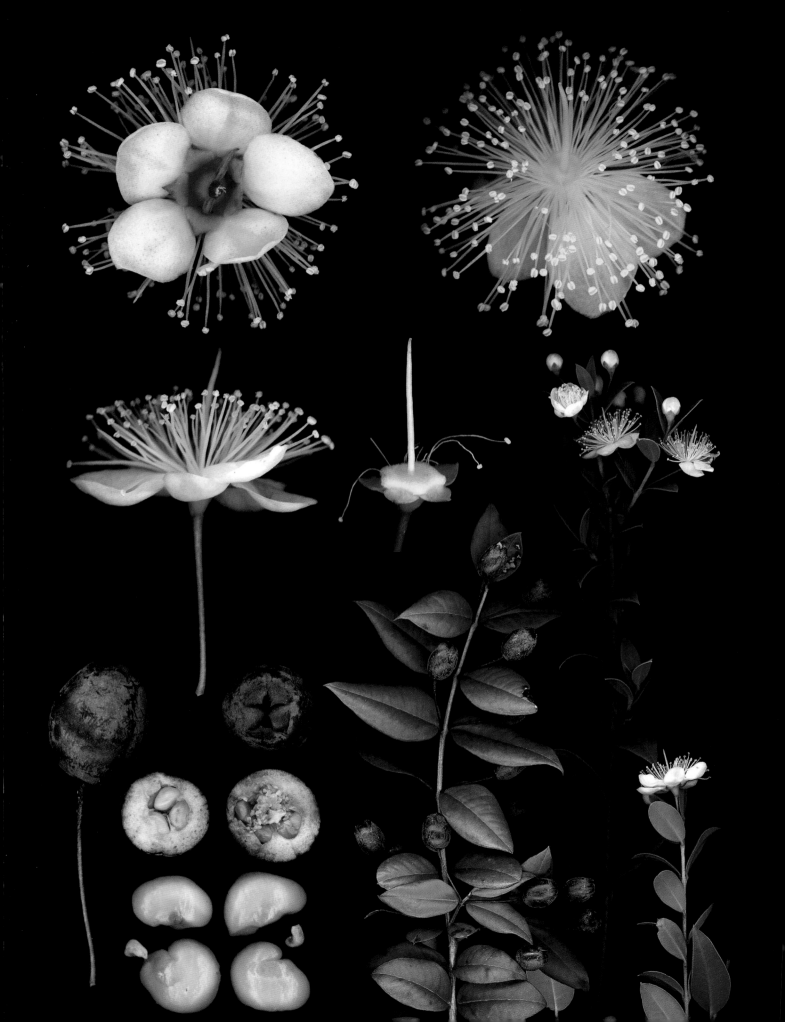

Myrtle

Myrtus communis

FAMILY: MYRTACEAE

Active elements:
Leaves: tannins, flavonoids, aromatic oil
(including myrtenyl acetate, alpha-pinene,
cineole, myrtenol and linalool.

M yrtle is mentioned in texts by ancient Arab authors as well as the Old Testament, but for the ancient Greeks it was the symbol of youth and love, dedicated to Aphrodite. Pliny recommended it to stimulate the digestive organs and as an energetic astringent, to cure diarrhoea, leucorrhoea and haemorrhages—wise advice given the high tannin content of the fruits and leaves. Its fruit-laden branches were used to make a wine known as *myrtadum*. Later, its flowers and leaves were distilled to make "Angel Water", widely renowned as a beauty aid.

Excellent antibacterial properties

• Myrtle is a **balsamic** (it soothes like a balm) and a top-class **disinfectant**. Its use is advocated for **respiratory tract ailments**, bronchitis irritated by smoking and acute catarrh.
• Used externally, it helps **heal wounds**.
• The essential oil of the leaves is a **powerful bactericide**.
• Myrtle is sometimes advocated as a **venous and lymphatic decongestant**. Good results can be achieved by massaging the legs with the essential oil.

OTHER USES: In times gone by, the dry branches and their leaves were burnt as incense. They gave off abundant clouds of strongly scented smoke as they smouldered. The fruit is used to make jam, but must be passed through a vegetable mill to ensure the numerous small pips are removed. The berries are used in the excellent, deep blackish-red liqueur of Corsica and Sardinia known as Mirto. A colourless liqueur, known as White Mirto is distilled using a variety with white berries and sometimes from young leaves. In the Mediterranean region, fresh or dried Myrtle berries are traditionally used as a spice, particularly with game.

METHOD OF USE

• **INTERNAL: Infusion.** 25g (¾oz) of leaves per litre (quart) of boiling water, drink 2 cups per day. This infusion is good for the bronchi and useful when astringent properties are required.
Syrup. Pour a litre of boiling water over 70g (2½oz) of Myrtle leaves. Leave to steep for 6 hours in a covered container. Strain, add 1.2kg (2½lb) of sugar and simmer until it has the consistency of syrup. Use for irritations of the respiratory tract.
• **EXTERNAL: Myrtle bath.** Still used in southern Europe to treat sprains, bumps and bruises following a fall.

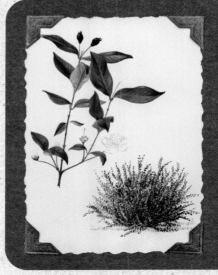

Description

A shrub growing to a height of 1 to 3m (3¼ to 9¾ft), found all around the Mediterranean, and common in the Mediterranean maquis scrubland. Its numerous branches are covered with small, pointed, glossy, light-green leaves. These give off an extraordinary smell of incense when crushed. In spring, it is covered with pretty white flowers from the centre of which numerous stamens sprout, like miniature fireworks. The fruits, in the form of small dark blue berries, survive on the branches for a long time.

TOXICITY

Great caution must be taken when using essential oil of Myrtle internally. It should not be taken by pregnant women (in particular in the first 3 months), nursing mothers and children under the age of six.

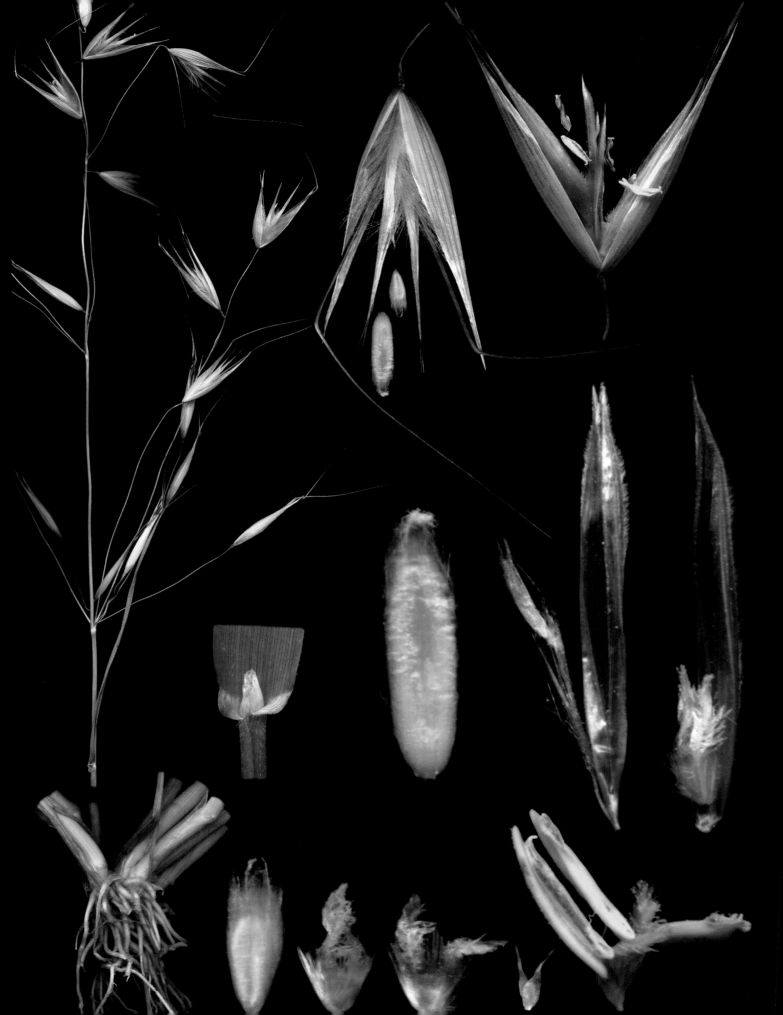

Oat

Avena sativa

FAMILY: POACEAE

Active elements:

Proteins, carbohydrates, lipids, vitamins, mineral salts, triterpenic saponosides (avenacosides), alkaloids and silicic acid.

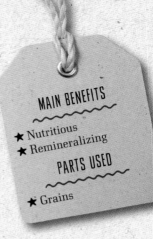

MAIN BENEFITS

★ Nutritious
★ Remineralizing

PARTS USED

★ Grains

• Bran and Oat flakes **help digestion and relieve constipation**.

• For external use, traditional medicine recommends emollient Oat baths to **soften dry, atopic, irritated, itchy skin**, as well as to relieve rheumatism and counter insomnia.

The Greeks considered Oat a weed and used it as horse fodder. The Romans seem to have been the first to use it as a cereal crop to any significant extent. It was not until the 17th century that herbalists started to use it to treat a variety of ailments, including fatigue, depression, insomnia and rheumatism.

Light and restorative

• Oats are **extremely nutritious,** and can be eaten in the form of flakes, flour or, more rarely, whole grains. Oat is light and restoratively nutritious, making it ideal for children, convalescents and the elderly.

• It has a high mineral content (silica, iron, manganese and zinc in particular), so it is perfect food for people **suffering from mineral deficiencies or recovering from illness**.

• It reduces cholesterol so is beneficial in the **prevention of cardiovascular diseases**.

METHOD OF USE

• **INTERNAL: Decoction.** 20g (¾oz) of oatmeal per litre (quart) of water. Refreshing, diuretic, slightly laxative. Also a soothing infusion for coughs.

• **EXTERNAL:** As a **poultice** to treat aches and pains (backache, rib pains). Dry roast the oats, wrap them quickly in a soft cloth and apply while still hot to the painful area. You can also boil the oats in wine and vinegar to make a poultice that can be applied as hot as possible.

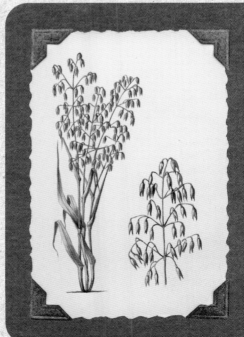

Description

Fields of Oat elegantly swaying in the summer breeze are a common sight throughout northern Europe. It is an annual cereal crop, growing to a height of approximately 1m (3¼ft), with very narrow, straight leaf-blades on swollen nodes that sheath the thin, hollow, unbranched stem. Spikelets hang down at the end of flowering.

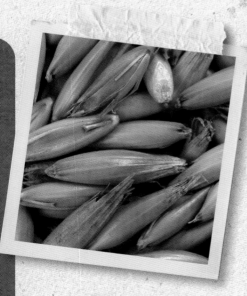

Oat grains, usually eaten as flakes or flour, are nutritious, revitalizing and lower blood cholesterol levels.

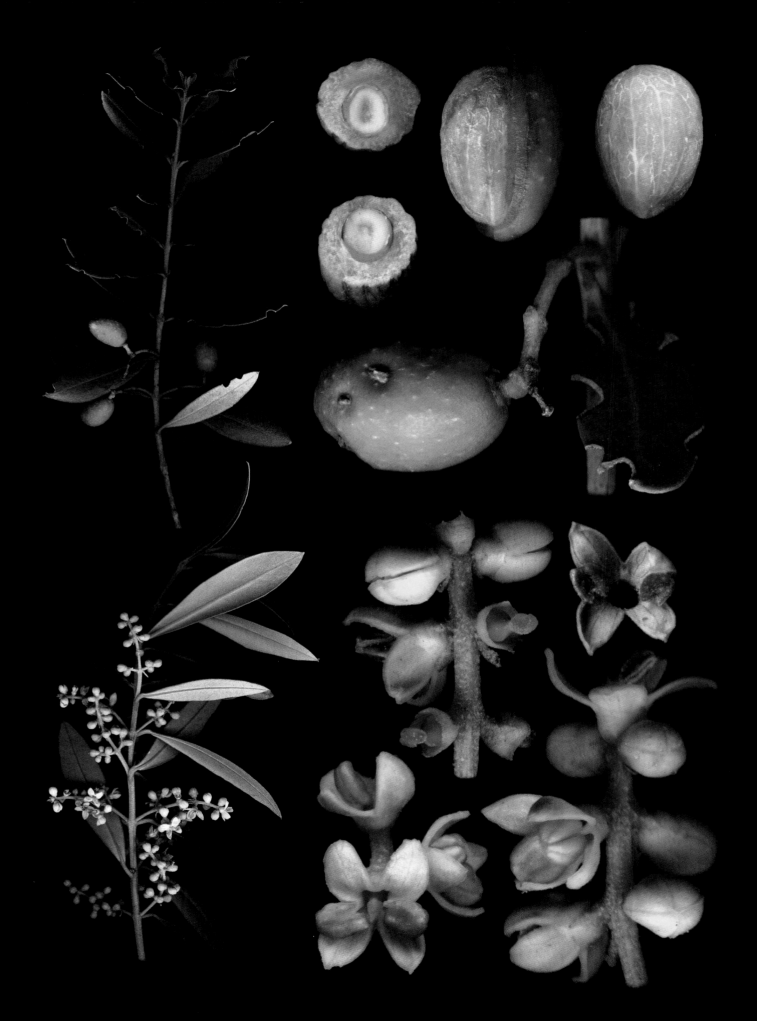

Olive

Olea europaea
FAMILY: OLEACEAE

Active elements:
Leaves: secoiridoids (including oleuropein, oleoside and ligstroside), triterpenes, flavonoids (including rutin). Fruits: fatty oil rich in oleic, linoleic and palmitic fatty acids, sterols, tocopherols, triterpenes, pigments, bitter principle (oleuropein) .

MAIN BENEFITS

★ Lowers blood pressure and sugar levels
★ Good for the circulatory system
★ Diuretic
★ Laxative, easy on the liver
★ Sooths sunburn

PARTS USED

★ Leaves, fruit, oil, extracted from fruit

• Olive oil works as an **antihelmintic (vermifuge)**. It is sometimes used to relieve irritation of the digestive tract in the case of certain types of poisoning.
• When applied externally, the oil **instantly soothes the pain of a burn** and aids healing. It is also effective in treating sunburn.
• Olive oil is recommended for the **prevention of receding gums**.
• The thin, penetrating quality of the oil makes it ideal as an **excipient (inert carrier) for a wide range of liniments**, ointments and pharmaceutical products.

In ancient times, the Olive leaf was used to treat injuries. It was used for many centuries as a tonic and to bring down a fever. It was used instead of the bark of *Cinchona* species to treat intermittent fevers. These qualities have now been eclipsed by the discovery of much more significant properties. In the 1930s it was demonstrated that the olive leaf had a hypotensive action, a property that has been widely confirmed since then.

A true oil of good health

• The Olive leaf **lowers blood pressure** (hypotensive) and improves circulation by softening and dilating the arteries.
• It works as a diuretic, **reduces oedema** and decreases urea levels in the blood. It is therefore recommended for people suffering from high blood pressure or heart or kidney failure.
• The Olive leaf also demonstrates **hypoglycaemic action**. This property is useful when people suffering from high blood pressure are also diabetic.
• Olive oil has a reputation as a true oil of good health. It is rich in monounsaturated fatty acids, and contributes to **protecting the cardiovascular system** and is said to help prevent certain cancers.
• It is an emollient and laxative, **stimulates bile production and activates intestinal functions**. It is also recommended for biliary colic and to aid the evacuation of gallstones.

METHOD OF USE

• **INTERNAL: Infusion.** Aside from the special extracts available from the pharmacy, two dozen leaves can be boiled in a large mug of water until reduced by half. Strain, add sugar and drink morning and evening. Good for high blood pressure and diabetes.
Olive oil. Administer 1 tablespoonful morning and evening (it can be mixed with citrus fruit juice). Use to enhance biliary and intestinal functions.
• **EXTERNAL: Enema.** A little squirt of Olive oil can be very effective in treating constipation.
  Massage oil. Mix Olive oil with an egg white, to treat burns and sunburn. Use on its own, to massage the gums.

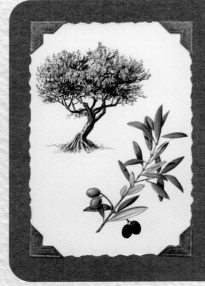

Description

A shrub or small tree originating in the Mediterranean basin, where it is cultivated on a widespread basis as it is in California and Chile. Its characteristic crooked trunk, bears opposite, evergreen leaves which are tough and lanceolate, green on top with a silvery underside. The small greenish flowers produce the universally recognized fruit, the olive, which changes from green to black as it ripens. The Olive tree is a symbol of Peace and Wisdom and was the subject of numerous legends. It was considered sacred by the ancient Greeks. Its leaves and oil are renowned for their medicinal properties.

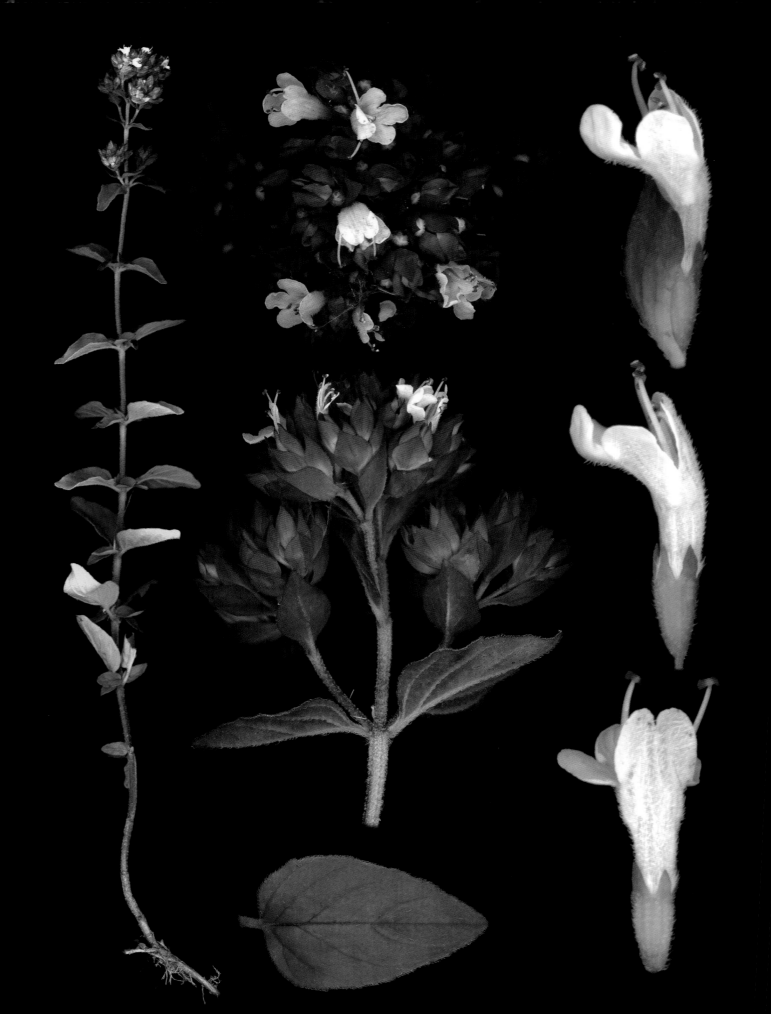

Oregano

Origanum vulgare

FAMILY: LAMIACEAE

Active elements:
Aromatic oil rich in thymol and carvacrol, tannins, phenolic acids and flavonoids.

Two thousand years ago, Dioscorides had already recorded that Oregano was one of the best remedies for appetite loss. A little more recently, just a century ago, Henri Leclerc, the French physician and renowned medical herbalist, recommended it especially for patients with atonic, dilated stomachs.

Anti-inflammatory

• Oregano has **remarkable aperitive** properties, while also **facilitating digestion** and stimulating a sluggish stomach, relieving constipation. It alleviates bloating, flatulence and belching, and remedies a sluggish liver or gall-bladder.
• Oregano flowering tops are renowned as a **treatment for acute or chronic inflammation of the bronchial tubes**. They have expectorant and **sedative properties which tackle coughs** and colds and are an excellent treatment for respiratory tract ailments, as well as being one of the most pleasant.
• The plant acts as a **stimulant** and even an excitant for people suffering an abnormal lack of energy (asthenia) and can **promote the onset of menstruation** (emmenagogic) in girls.
• It can relieve **acute or chronic rheumatism**, not only in the form of an infusion but also in warm applications directly on to the painful limb.

DID YOU KNOW? Oregano's pink and purple flower clusters merit its name, which means "mountain beauty", from the Greek *oros*, "mountain" and *ganos*, "beauty". Also known as Wild Marjoram, it is often confused with Marjoram (*Origanum majorana*), which is sometimes known as Sweet Marjoram. Marjoram is native to North Africa and western Asia and is grown as a herb in gardens.

OTHER USES: The flowering tops make a nice seasoning in cooking. Add right at the end of preparation as they lose their flavour quickly when heated. As a result, they are best used raw, for example in a pesto to go with pasta or potatoes. For the same reason, Oregano works better as a solar tea than as an infusion.

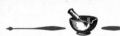

METHOD OF USE

• **INTERNAL: Solar tea.** 8 to 15g (½oz) of flowering tops per litre (quart) of water: place in a sealed container and leave to steep in the sun. Drink 2 or 3 cups per day for respiratory ailments.
Wine. 50g (1¾oz) of flowering tops per litre of sweet wine, such as Muscat or Banyuls. Leave to steep for 10 days. Drink 3 small coffee cups per day before meals for an aperitive effect, during or after a meal as a digestive and between meals for a stimulating, bechic effect (cough relief).
• **EXTERNAL: Poultice.** For rheumatic pain and stiff neck. Crush the fresh plant and wrap in a cloth; place on the lid of a saucepan containing boiling water. When the poultice is warm, apply it to the painful region. The plant can also be heated dry in a frying pan, but it is more difficult to apply.

Description

Attractive perennial growing to a height of 30 to 80cm (1 to 2½ft), forming appealing tufts in dry, exposed places. Oregano is found all over Europe and Asia and is sometimes grown as a herb. Its upright, reddish stems bear oval, opposite leaves and terminate in tight clusters of small pinkish, two-lipped flowers, among numerous purplish-red bracts. When crushed, the leaves, and in particular the flowering tops, give off a very pleasant, aromatic smell.

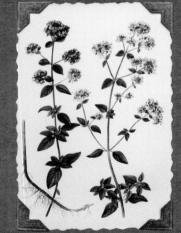

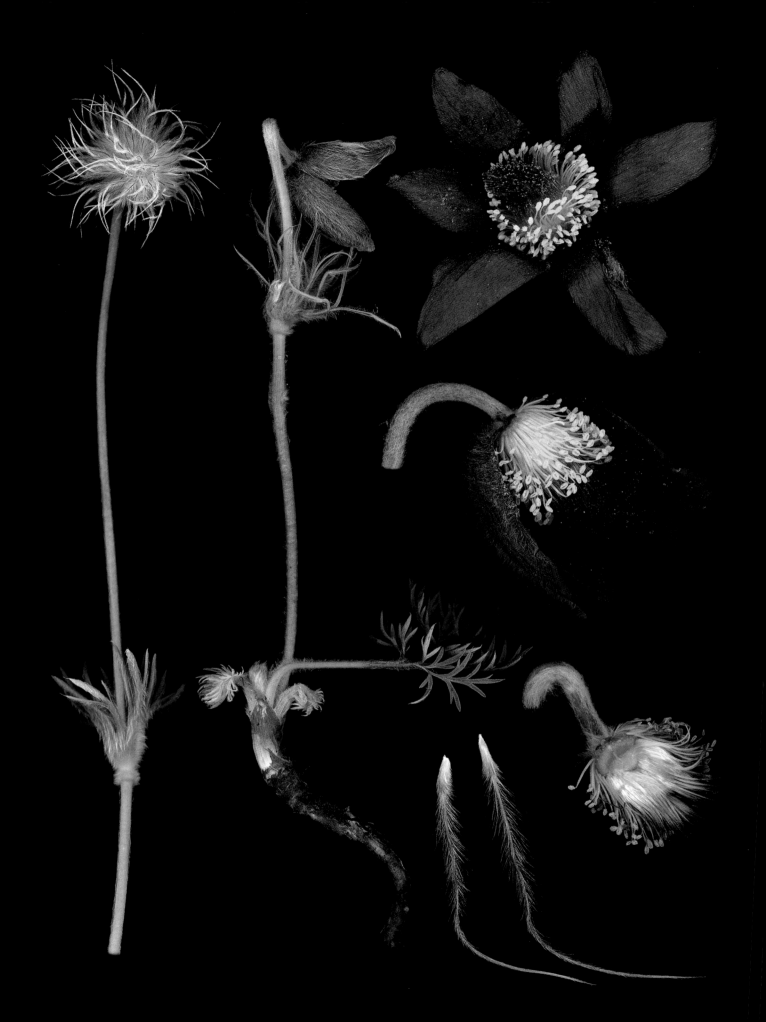

Pasqueflower

Pulsatilla vulgaris
FAMILY: RANUNCULACEAE

Active elements:
Tannins, triterpenic saponosides, protoanemonin (a lactone with rubefacient properties which transforms when dried into an inactive anemonin).

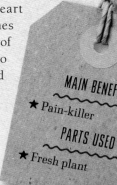

T he plant is highly caustic when fresh, so only the dried plant was used internally. This unfortunately meant that it lost a good proportion of its active ingredients, along with its pungency. It was nonetheless recommended for the treatment of nervous hyper-excitability, heart problems, headaches, migraines and painful spasms (especially of the genital organs). It was also used for spasmodic coughs and whooping cough, as well certain symptoms of syphilis (nerve root pain). The crushed plant was used externally, to produce a counter-irritant and thus a derivative effect on headaches, rheumatism and stitches.

TOXICITY

Pasqueflowers are irritants when fresh. Wrongful ingestion could lead to respiratory and heart problems. Use of the plant is not advised during pregnancy: the protoanemonin has been shown to cause abortions or malformations of the embryo in cattle.

A homoeopathic favourite

• Nowadays, Pasqueflower preparations made with the fresh plant are mainly used in homoeopathic medicine. They are used to **relieve pain** (the pain of varicose veins, or cramps, in particular of the uterus), **hyper-excitability and cardiac irregularity**.

• The protoanemonin of the fresh plant is said to have antibacterial and antispasmodic properties.

NOTE: The beautiful deep purple, almost black, colour of the petals of the Mountain Pasqueflower (*montana* subspecies), illustrated to the far left, differentiates it from the generic Pasqueflower (description on left). The two forms have the same properties.

Description

A perennial growing to a height of 10 to 30cm (4 to 12in), found on lawns and in dry meadows in Europe and northern Asia. It flowers from March to June, depending on altitude. The large, single purple flowers, with six hairy sepals, bloom from inside a crown of narrow, elongated bracts at the top of a thick stem covered in long silky hairs. The fern-like leaves, which grow from the base of the plant, are deeply dissected. When ripe, the fluffy heads are composed of numerous dried fruits (achenes) grouped together at the top of the stem, each with a long feathery ridge.

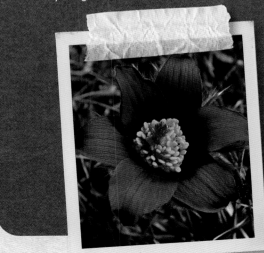

METHOD OF USE

• **INTERNAL:** In the past, the Pasqueflower was most commonly used for preparations based on the fresh plant, in particular **in the form of an alcoholature**. However, in the 19th century, François-Joseph Cazin, the French doctor and botanist, recommended the use of the dried plant in an infusion of 2 to 5g per 300g of boiling water, to be drunk over 24 hours, for the treatment of coughs.

• **EXTERNAL:** **Poultice** using the crushed plant. It has a counter-irritant effect against pain. Ensure that there are no abrasions in the area to be treated, exercise caution and never apply the poultice for too long.

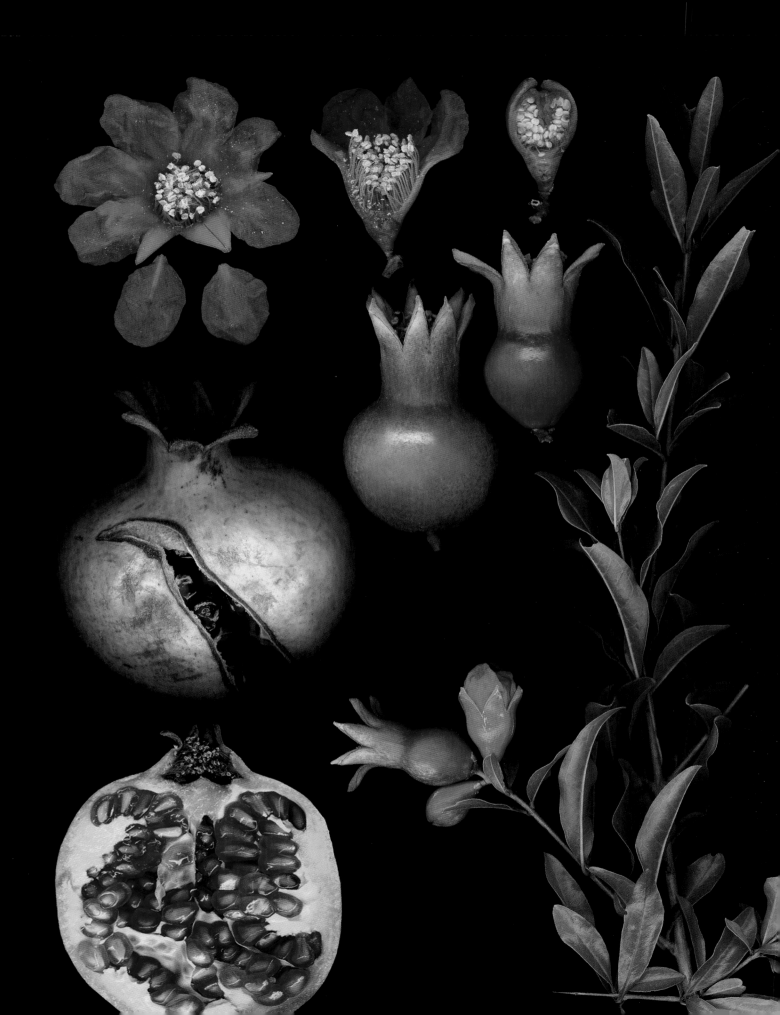

Pomegranate

Punica granatum

FAMILY: PUNICACEAE

Active elements:

Bark: piperidine alkaloids (including pelletierine and isopelletierine), ellagitannins, triterpenes.

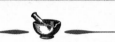

We know from ancient Greek, Arabic and Hebrew texts that the healing powers of Pomegranate were widely renowned. The Egyptians seem to have been the first to use it as a vermifuge (anthelmintic). The root bark was used for the same purpose in north India and by the Greeks in the time of Dioscorides (1st century AD). It fell out of use in Europe until 1807, when it was repopularized by Francis Buchanan, who observed its use in India in treating tapeworm.

METHOD OF USE

• **INTERNAL: Infusion of flowers.** 15 to 30g (½ to 1oz) per litre (quart) of water Allow to infuse for 10 minutes and then drink throughout the day for diarrhoea.

The root bark was once widely used to treat intestinal parasites in the form of "Tanret's pelletierine", but was abandoned due to its toxicity.

Root decoction. This foul-tasting preparation is not recommended because of the toxic alkaloids in root bark.

Fruit husk decoction. Dose equal to 30g (1oz) per litre of water as an anthelmintic, and only after medical advice.

• **EXTERNAL: Concentrated infusion of flowers.** In douches to treat white discharge (leucorrhoea).

Root bark decoction. Use in enema form to treat roundworm.

Astringent and anthelmintic

• The flowers are astringent. They are effective against **chronic diarrhoea, abdominal pains, leucorrhoea and haemorrhages**.
• The root bark is an **effective anthelmintic** but has a high toxicity risk. Its use is strictly prohibited in children, as well as pregnant and breast-feeding women. Overall, best avoided.
• The fruit husk is likewise an anthelmintic, but only in the case of roundworm.
• The Pomegranate juice is used **as a tonic** in cases of fatigue.
• Applied topically, the fruit can **treat skin problems** such as acne and skin inflammation.

OTHER USES: The juice from pressed Pomegranate pulp was traditionally used to make the famous grenadine syrup, which is nowadays based on the concentrated juice of a variety of red berries (not including Pomegranate) and flavouring. A black pigment was extracted from the bark that was used to make ink or to dye the wool used in carpet making.

Description

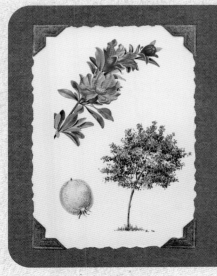

An elegant shrub originating in western Asia, cultivated in all countries with a warm, dry climate. Its trunk, often twisted and stunted, bears small, pointed, glossy leaves and bright orangey-red bell-shaped flowers. Pomegranate fruit are the size of an orange and contain seeds inside a bright, garnet-coloured pulp, which are slightly acidic and very refreshing.

TOXICITY

Pomegranate alkaloids are unequivocally toxic. They are more concentrated in the root bark, which should be avoided for internal use.

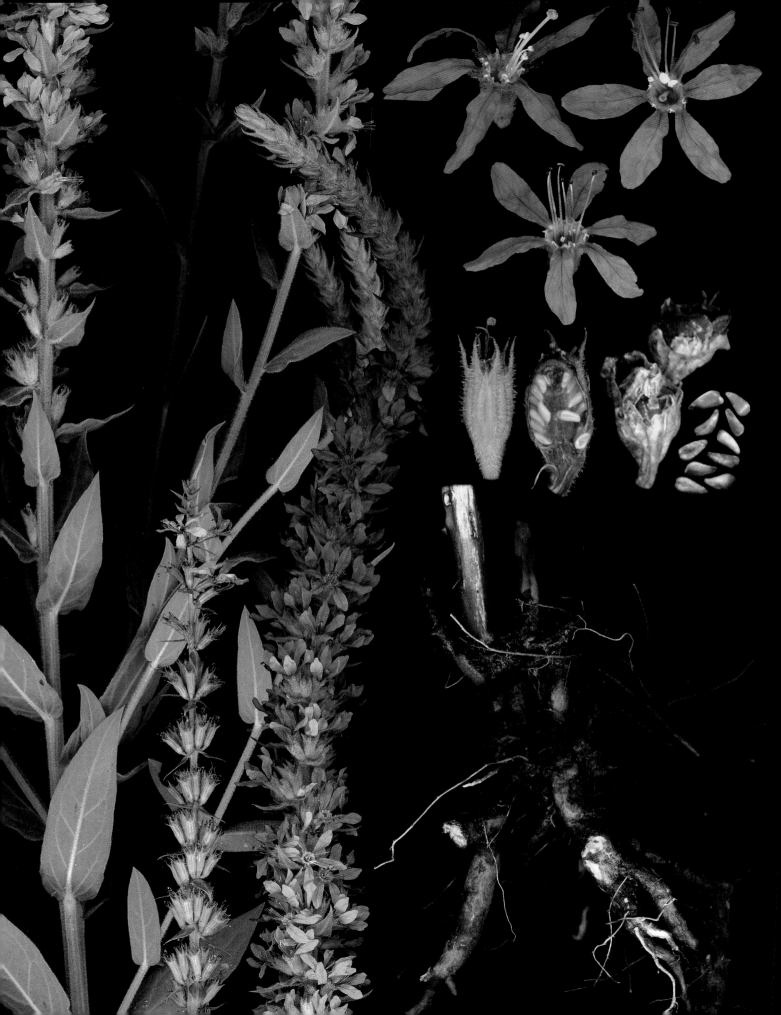

Purple Loosestrife

Lythrum salicaria
FAMILY: LYTHRACEAE

Active elements:
Tannins, flavonoid glycosides (including vitexin), anthocyanosides, phytosterols, mucilage, aromatic oil.

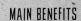
• Traditionally it is used (internally or topically) to **counter venous insufficiency**, by relieving heavy legs, varicose veins or haemorrhoids.

• It can also be used topically **as a pain-killer** for ailments affecting the mouth and/or throat. It likewise works as an analgesic on skin disorders such as varicose ulcers or eczema.

DID YOU KNOW? The botanical name for Purple Loosestrife, *Lythrum*, comes from the Greek word *lythron*, "thick, clotted blood", which evokes the colour of the corolla.

In ancient times, Purple Loosestrife was known for its astringent properties, but was often confused with other Loosestrifes of the *Lysimachia* sp., which are similarly astringent. It then fell out of common use until the mid-18th century, when it was hailed as a remedy for gastrointestinal inflammations and diarrhoea. It was also advocated for the treatment of varicose ulcers, acute vaginitis, itching of the vulva and certain other skin conditions (eczema, chafing rash).

Effective anti-diarrhoeal

• Purple Loosestrife, which is **highly astringent**, acts quickly on **diarrhoea**: diarrhoea in infants, intestinal flu. When administered to young children, it must be twinned with other suitable food (carrot, carob, grated apple, with which it can form an intestinal poultice).

• Purple Loosestrife is also used to **treat inflammation of the stomach and intestine**, leucorrhoea, blood in the urine and heavy periods.

• Fresh Purple Loosestrife **staunches nosebleeds and bleeding gums** and **promotes the healing** of wounds.

METHOD OF USE

• **INTERNAL: Infusion.** 20 to 30g (¾ to 1oz) per litre (quart) of water. Drink half a litre per day to treat diarrhoea and stomach inflammation.
Dried plant powder. 3 to 5g per day (take 1g at a time) for the same purposes as the infusion.
Syrup. Infuse 150g (5¼oz) of powder in one litre of boiling water. Leave to steep for 24 hours. Strain and mix with a litre of sugar syrup. Take from 50 to 100g (1¾ to 3½oz) of syrup per day. Use to treat blood in the urine and heavy periods.

• **EXTERNAL: Concentrated infusion.** 50g (1¾oz) of plant per litre of water. Infuse for 20 minutes. Use in douches, enemas or compresses.
Juice from fresh leaves. When applied to wounds, it tightens the tissue and promotes healing.
Maceration. 50g (1¾oz) of plant steeped in a litre of wine for 8 days. Used as a wash for varicose ulcers.

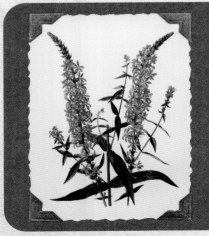

Description

A perennial growing to a height of between 50cm and 1m (1½ to 3¼ft), common around ponds and lakes and in wet places. Found throughout most of the northern hemisphere. Its four-cornered, upright stem bears opposite spear-shaped leaves reminiscent of the willow (*Salix* in Latin). From spring to late summer, the densely clustered flowers with their six purple petals form long, spectacular spikes.

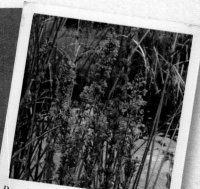

Purple Loosestrife is found around lakes and ponds and on river banks.

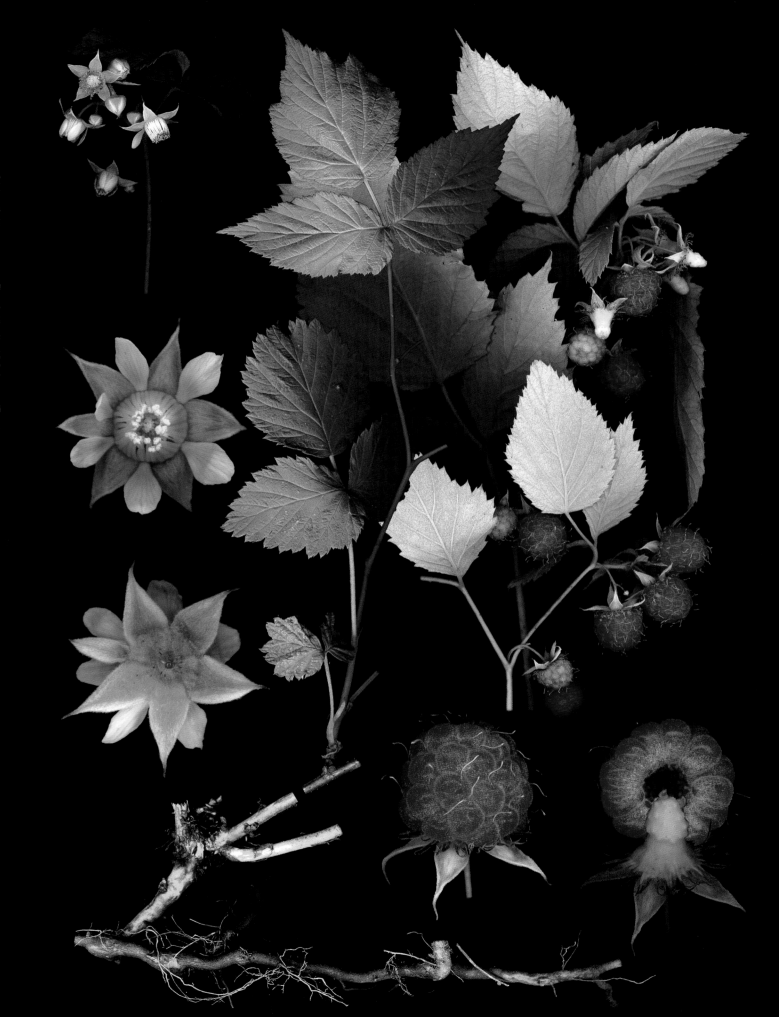

Raspberry

Rubus idaeus

FAMILY: ROSACEAE

Active elements:

Leaves: tannins, flavonoids, polypeptides.
Fruit: rich in sugar (levulose, fructose), organic
acids, pectin and vitamins (A, C, B9 and E).

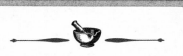

I n days gone by, Raspberry enjoyed an exalted reputation as a medicinal plant. It has been cultivated since the late Middle Ages. In Molière's time, one of its many properties was believed to be that a poultice of its crushed leaves on the abdomen could cure stomach ache.

Beneficial for pregnant women

• The leaves make a pleasant, **diuretic** infusion.
• Their astringency can be used **to treat gastrointestinal complaints**, in particular diarrhoea.
• They can act as the basis of gargles **for sore throats, mouthwashes to treat ulcers,** and a lotion for skin ulcers and irritated eyes.
• The leaves also have a fortifying effect on the **uterine muscle wall** and are prescribed as an infusion in preparation for labour. It is said to have a **tonic effect on the myometrium**, strengthening the contractions which serve to push out a baby.
• The tasty, refreshing fruit has **laxative and diuretic qualities**. It is low in saccharose so is **great for diabetics**.
• Its **significant folic acid** (vitamin B9) content, means the Raspberry is good for preparing the body for both pregnancy and birth. It may also help prevent Alzheimer's disease.

OTHER USES: The fresh fruit can be eaten raw in fruit salad, coulis, jam, jelly and syrups. The berries can be frozen. Young shoots are used in gemmotherapy (remedies made from buds and shoots of trees and shrubs). Raspberry seed oil is sometimes an ingredient in skin cream, bath oil, toothpaste and shampoo.

METHOD OF USE

• **INTERNAL: Infusion.** 40 to 50g (1½ to 1¾oz) of leaves per litre (quart) of boiling water. Steep for 10 minutes. Drink 3 or 4 cups per day for diarrhoea or before birth (drink from the 7th month of pregnancy).
Syrup. Simmer equal weights of sugar and fresh fruit until it reaches the desired consistency. A diuretic and very refreshing for febrile ailments.
Raspberry vinegar. Cover the fruits, arranged in an airtight container, with white vinegar (around a litre of vinegar for 1½kg (3¼lb) of fruit). Leave to steep for 10 days and strain. This vinegar can be sweetened with sugar or honey. Replace the vinegar with some colourless spirit for a home-made raspberry liqueur.
• **EXTERNAL:** All the above preparations: infusion of leaves, syrup, vinegar or syrup of raspberry vinegar can be gargled to treat sore throats.

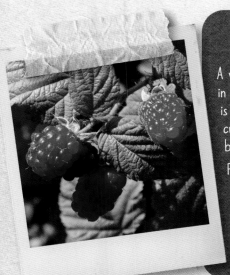

Description

A well-known perennial that grows wild on roadsides, in clearings and on mountain scree slopes. Raspberry is native to the whole northern hemisphere. It is widely cultivated in gardens for its red, delicately perfumed berries. Its stalks are profusely covered with fine prickles and bear large, composite leaves of serrated leaflets with whitish undersides. The white flowers produce fruit composed of many small, rounded segments known as drupelets, bursting with the tangy, characteristically reddish-pink juice.

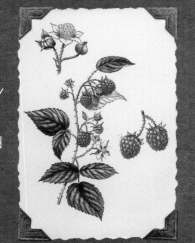

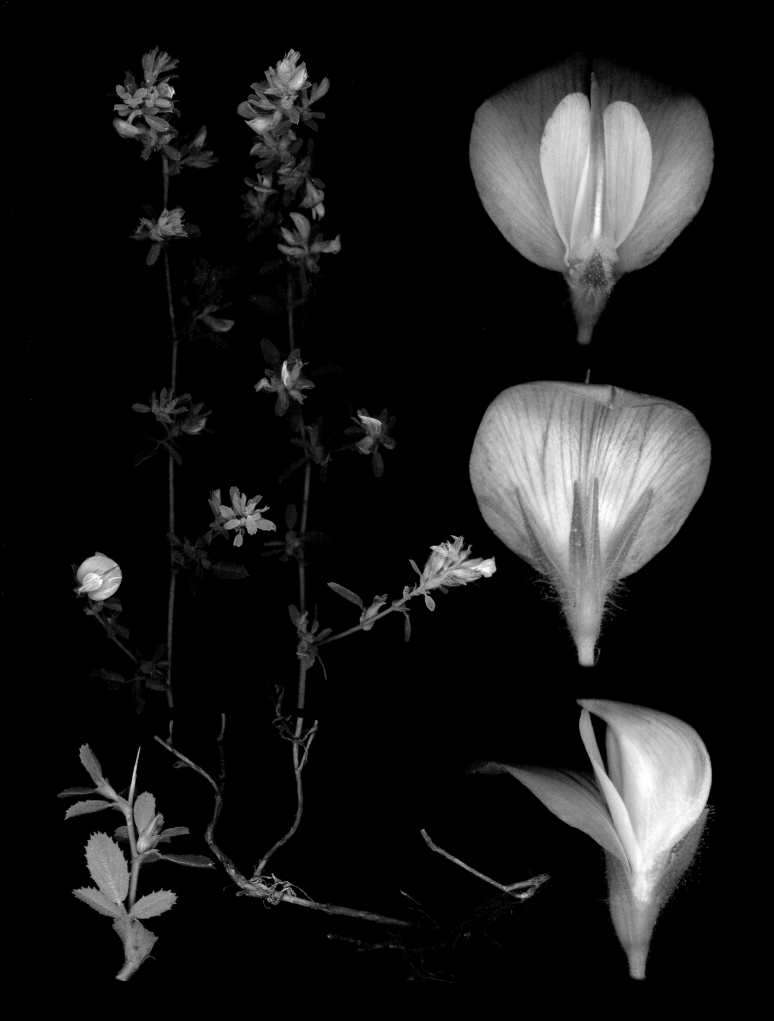

Rest-harrow

Ononis spinosa

FAMILY: FABACEAE

Active elements:

Roots: isoflavonoids, saponinosides, triterpene, onocerine, aromatic oil.

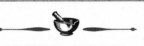

Rest-harrow has always been used to increase urine volume while soothing urinary system pain. In the 1st century, Dioscorides advocated Rest-harrow for reducing and expelling bladder stones. Henri Leclerc, the French physician and medical herbalist, used it in the early 20th century for chronic bladder inflammation, bladder stones and cystitis.

The urinary tract's friend

• The **diuretic and anti-inflammatory properties** of Rest-harrow root are renowned. It is advocated as a **depurative**, for inflammation of the bladder (**cystitis**) and the prostate (**prostatitis**), and to treat bladder stones. It can even prevent kidney stones from forming and unblock the bile ducts.

• The essential oil, as an infusion, boasts a powerful diuretic effect. It is sometimes recommended for the **treatment of generalized oedema** and is said to **relieve chronic rheumatism** (it decongests joints).

• A decoction of astringent Rest-harrow can be used as a gargle to **soothe sore throats** and mouth ulcers.

OTHER SPECIES: Yellow Rest-harrow (*Ononis natrix*), also known as the Shrubby Rest-harrow, has yellow flowers streaked with red. Although it is far less commonly used than *O. spinosa* (other than in homoeopathy), its root has similar diuretic properties. However, analysis of its seeds has revealed a much higher, and therefore more useful, content of essential fatty acids and antioxidants (proanthocyanidins and flavonoids such as quercetin).

DID YOU KNOW? Rest-harrow is said to have got its name from the fact that its tough stems would stop the harrow or plough. It is also sometimes known as Bugrane, which comes from the vulgar Latin *boveretina* (beef/cow) and *retinere* (to stop).

MAIN BENEFITS
★ Diuretic
★ Anti-inflammatory
★ Anti-oedemic
★ Anti-rheumatic
★ Sore throats and mouths

PARTS USED
★ Roots

METHOD OF USE

• **INTERNAL: Infusion.** 20g (¾oz) of Rest-harrow root per litre (quart) of water. Let it infuse for 20 to 30 minutes. Drink 2 to 4 cups per day for inflammation and stones.
Decoction. 20g (¾oz) of root per litre of water. Reduce to a third by boiling. Use as a gargle to soothe irritated throats and even in a compress to treat weeping eczema.

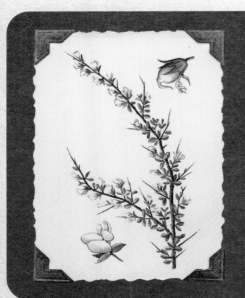

Description

A small perennial growing to between 20 and 50cm (8in to 1½ft) in height, commonly found along paths, in uncultivated fields and on dry land in Europe, western Asia and North Africa. Its stems, which slope upwards, are covered with fine, sharp spines, often in pairs, and small dark green leaves divided into three leaflets. In summer, its attractive flowers resemble pink butterflies, and grow in a leafy cluster.

ADVICE FOR USE

In order to preserve the diuretic effect, the root should be used in an infusion and not a decoction, as the aromatic oil, the main active principle, is volatile and evaporates when boiled.

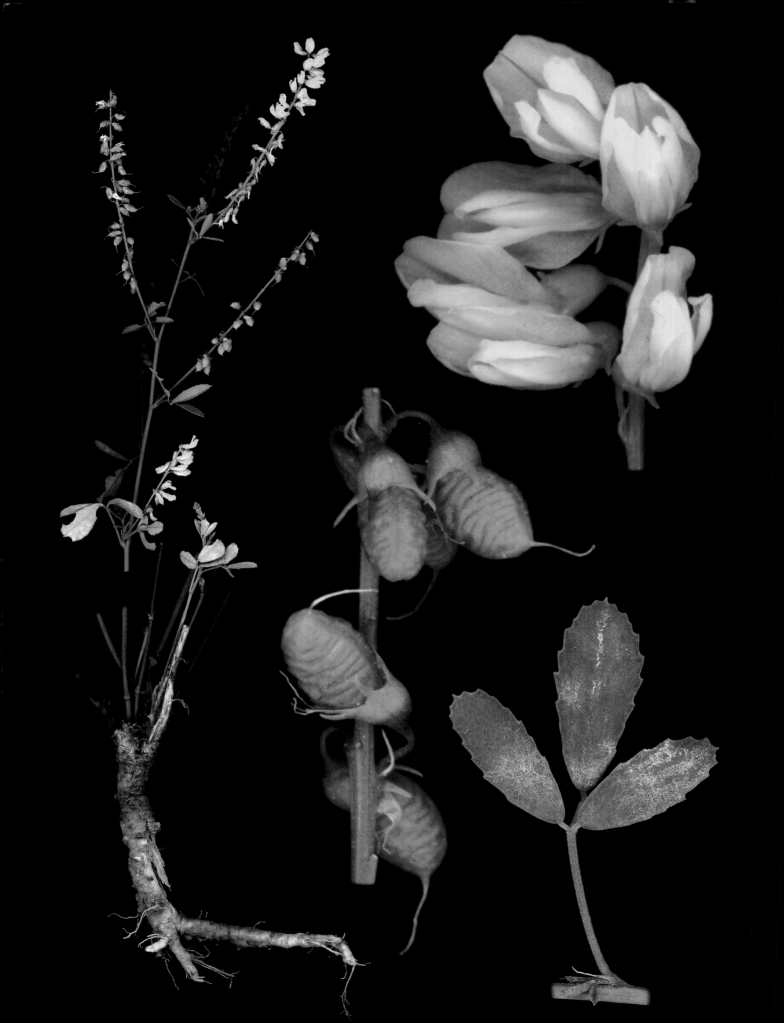

Ribbed Melilot

Melilotus officinalis

FAMILY: FABACEAE

Active elements:

Flavonoids, phenolic acids, triterpenic saponosides, melilotoside (which produces coumarin by hydrolysis).

G alen, the Roman philosopher and physician of the 2nd century AD, was the first to record the use of Ribbed Melilot for therapeutic purposes, as an antispasmodic and also as an anaesthetic in cases of dizziness and vomiting. Used externally, it has long been recommended in Central Europe for use in a bath, to treat rheumatism and gout. It was widely used in the Renaissance, to treat eye ailments (conjunctivitis, styes).

An acknowledged venous tonic

• Ribbed Melilot is mainly used as a venous tonic **to treat chronic venous insufficiency**. It is effective in the treatment of varicose veins and haemorrhoids. It reduces the risk of phlebitis and thrombosis. It is advocated for skin with fragile capillaries, for bruising and petechiae (small red or purple spots).

• Ribbed Melilot's coumarin content makes it a useful **antispasmodic, sedative and sleep aid**. It can be used for stress or anxiety and to **treat nervous excitement and mild insomnia**, as well as a sedative for headaches.

• It is good for soothing **coughing fits**, and quelling the fermentation that causes **bloating of the stomach and intestines**.

• The coumarin also gives it **diuretic** properties, and it is a good **antiseptic** of the urinary tract.

• Ribbed Melilot is used externally in Germany **to treat sprains, cuts and grazes**.

• It is also used to **treat knocks and bruises**.

• Distilled water of Ribbed Melilot, for swelling and **irritations of the eye**, forms the basis of some eye drops sold in pharmacies.

OTHER USES: Dried Ribbed Melilot, gathered in the wild, can be used to flavour creamy sauces, sorbets and drinks. In the past, the seeds were used as a spice, especially to flavour cheeses.

DID YOU KNOW? Its name comes from the Latin *mel*, "honey", because its flowers are full of nectar that is popular with bees.

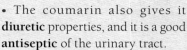

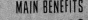

MAIN BENEFITS

★ Venous tonic
★ Antispasmodic
★ Sedative
★ Soporific
★ Diuretic
★ Relieves puffy eyes

PARTS USED

★ Flowering tops

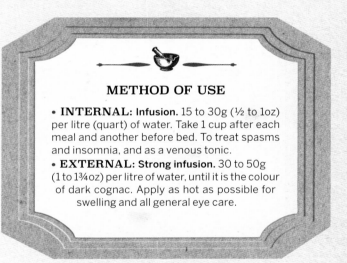

METHOD OF USE

• **INTERNAL: Infusion.** 15 to 30g (½ to 1oz) per litre (quart) of water. Take 1 cup after each meal and another before bed. To treat spasms and insomnia, and as a venous tonic.

• **EXTERNAL: Strong infusion.** 30 to 50g (1 to 1¾oz) per litre of water, until it is the colour of dark cognac. Apply as hot as possible for swelling and all general eye care.

TOXICITY

When Ribbed Melilot is attacked by mildew, the coumarin turns into dicoumarol. This is one of the ingredients of rat poison, which kills the rodents by causing internal haemorrhaging.

Description

A biannual growing to 40 to 80cm (16 to 31½in) in height, commonly found on uncultivated land and along pathways. Found throughout Europe and western Asia. Its leggy, truncated stem bears trefoil leaves like those of clover or lucerne. Its small, yellow flowers cluster along the tips of thin stalks like candles. Ribbed Melilot's modest appearance belies the fact that it gives off a sweet vanilla scent when dried.

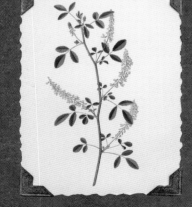

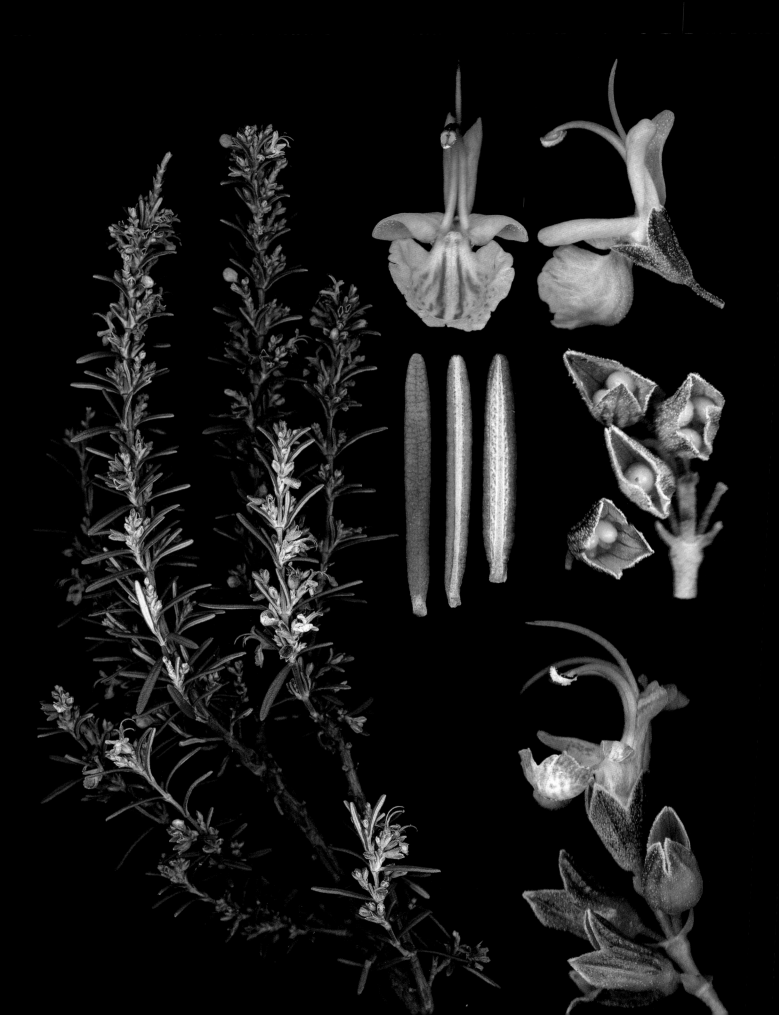

Rosemary

Salvia rosmarinus
(=Rosmarinus officinalis)

FAMILY: LAMIACEAE

Active elements:
Flowering tops: aromatic oil rich in camphor, cineole, alpha-pinene, borneol and camphene, flavonoids, tannins, tricyclic diterpenes, triterpenes, phenolic acids (including rosmarinic acid).

T his plant, beloved of medieval gardens, enjoyed great renown in days gone by. The famous "Queen of Hungary's Water", a simple alcoholate of Rosemary, gained unrivalled celebrity. The formula was given to Isabelle, the Queen of Hungary, by a hermit, and was said to have the power to restore youthful beauty. While it cured the rheumatism, gout and other conditions that she suffered, she also used it to wash her face "making it even more beautiful", according to the famous French medical writer Marie Fouquet in her book of herbal remedies published in 1678. She lived to the age of 80, after having experienced a second childhood.

Tonic, fortifying, digestive and analgesic

• Rosemary's attested **stimulant and tonic action** recommends it to improve circulation, particularly blood supply to the brain.

• Its stimulating action on gall-bladder function and **tonifying effect on the liver**, make it useful for a wide variety of conditions: congestion of the liver and inflammation of the gall-bladder; **a sluggish stomach**; and **abnormal lack of physical and mental energy** (asthenia).

• Rosemary has **antioxidant properties** due to its flavonoids and diterpenes.

• It also has an **anti-inflammatory** effect, in particular due to rosmarinic acid.

• Externally, it can be used as a **fortifying bath** for children and convalescents and can **relieve rheumatic pain**.

• Its external application is said to have healing properties, **relieve circulation problems** and **alleviate muscle pain**.

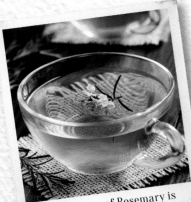

An infusion of Rosemary is a digestive and mental tonic.

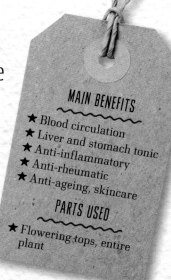

METHOD OF USE

• **INTERNAL: Infusion of flowering tops.** 20 to 30g (¾ to 1oz) per litre (quart) of boiling water.
Wine. Steep 30 to 60g (1 to 2oz) of flowers and leaves in 1 litre of wine. Add 100g (3½oz) of sugar and filter once fully dissolved. Very tonic.

• **EXTERNAL:** The wine can be used in compresses to treat a wide variety of skin problems, swelling of the joints, sprains.
Concentrated infusion. 50 to 60g (1¾ to 2oz) plant per litre of water in lotions or sprays, for fresh-looking, firm skin and to reduce the appearance of wrinkles. Added to the bath water, for an anti-rheumatic, fortifying and stimulating soak.
Tincture. Steep 80g (2¾oz) of the plant in 1 litre of alcohol (90% by volume) for 1 month. Excellent in a rub to alleviate rheumatism. To treat toothache, swill the infusion round the mouth, keeping it in contact with the painful tooth for as long as possible.

Description

A bushy shrub, rarely exceeding 1m (3¼ft) in height, common in arid areas of the Mediterranean basin. Commonly cultivated for use as a condiment or to create a hedge. Its woody stems are densely covered with tough, opposite, linear leaves. The large pale blue flowers have two distinct lips and cluster in the leaf axils towards the top of the branches. The whole plant exudes an aromatic scent reminiscent of both camphor and incense.

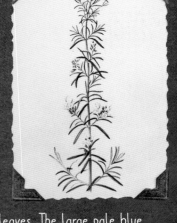

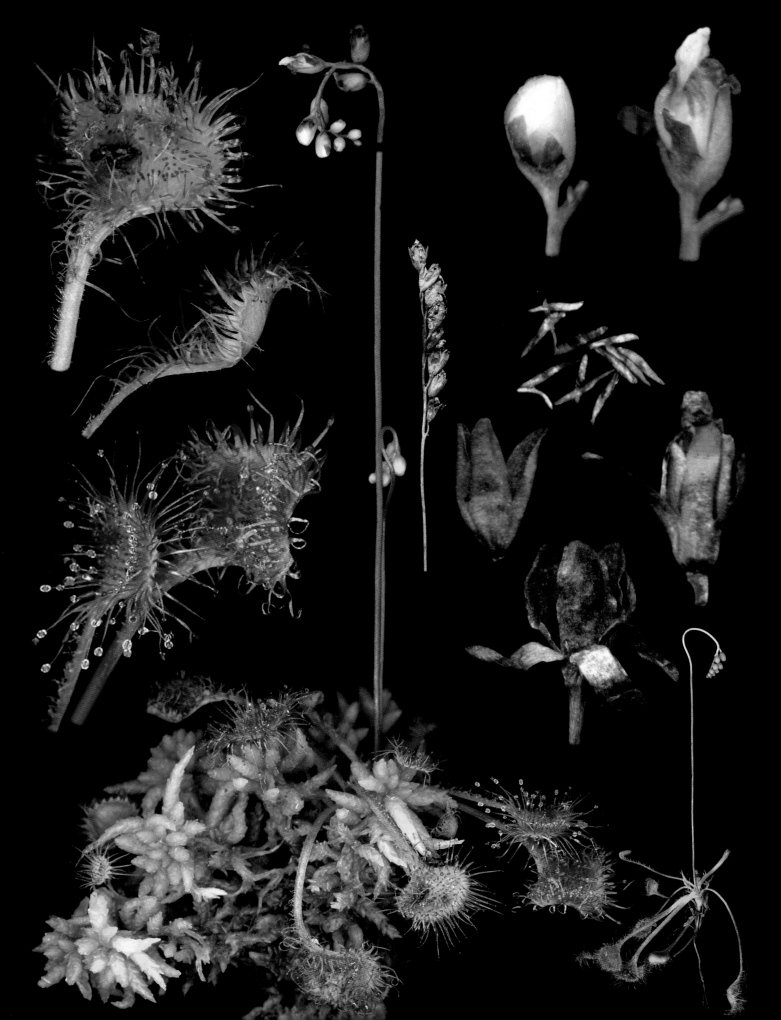

Round-leaved Sundew

Drosera rotundifolia

FAMILY: DROSERACEAE

Active elements:

A naphthoquinone (plumbagin), flavonoids, mucilage.

MAIN BENEFITS

★ Antispasmodic
★ Soothing
★ Antiseptic
★ Relieves coughing

PARTS USED

★ Whole plant

Described in the Renaissance by Clusius and Dodoens, the 16th-century physicians and botanists, this curious plant was also the subject of Darwin's attention. The fresh plant contains a principle with rubefacient properties, but present-day medicine no longer makes use of them.

Dew of the Sun

• Round-leaved Sundew is **antispasmodic and soothing**. It can be used to treat coughs, asthma and whooping cough.
• The plumbagin **destroys bacteria** as well as some pathogenic fungi and parasitic protozoa.

DID YOU KNOW? When an insect touches the open leaf, its tentacles close in, imprisoning the prey. The insect is then digested by the pepsin-rich acidic liquid, secreted by its glands, which earned this carnivorous plant the old poetic name *Ros Solis*, from the Latin *ros* and *sol*, meaning "dew of the sun" in reference to the drops of sticky liquid that form on the leaves. After digesting its victim, the trap reopens, ready for its next meal. *Drosera* comes from the Greek word *droseros*, meaning "dewy".

NOTE: Some species are dwarf, rare and officially protected. This does not stop unthinking people from collecting them anyway. Others import various species of flytrap from developing countries, especially Madagascar. While this may seem the best option, peatland plants cannot be cultivated and are harvested much faster than they can be renewed. The consequences are not hard to imagine.

METHOD OF USE

• **INTERNAL:** Antispasmodic **tincture** to treat whooping cough, prepared using the whole plant (5 to 20 drops, three to five times every 24 hours) to calm coughing fits, and decrease the frequency and duration of paroxysms. The remedy also has a sedative effect on whooping cough vomiting. Homoeopathy uses *Drosera* to treat pulmonary tuberculosis.

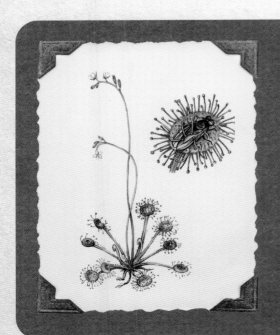

Description

A small insectivorous plant inhabiting peat bogs in temperate Europe, northern Asia and North America. The round leaves are arranged in rosettes of six to ten leaves that rest on the ground, their upper surface covered with long, glandular hairs. One or two reddish flowering stems grow from the centre of the rosette from which emerge white flowers, arranged in one-sided clusters.

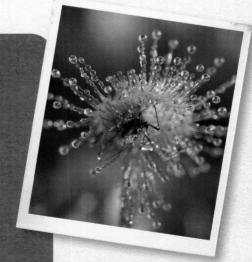

The sticky droplets that cover the leaves' hairs form a formidable insect trap, which earned the plant its name "Sundew".

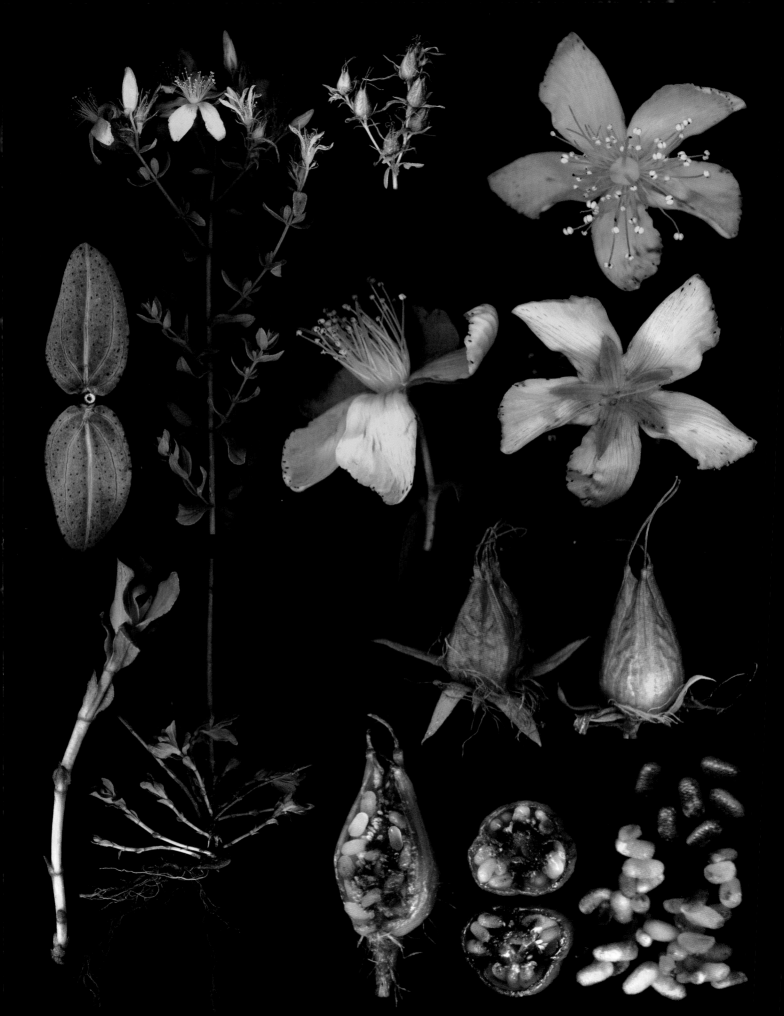

St. John's-wort

Hypericum perforatum

FAMILY: HYPERICACEAE

Active elements:

Aromatic oil rich in terpenic carbides, sterols, chlorogenic acid, condensed tannins, flavonoids (including hyperoside and rutin), biflavonoid, amentoflavone and a phloroglucinol, hyperforin. Red oil: naphtodianthrones (hypericin, pseudohypericin).

• The **antiseptic and healing (vulnerary) properties** of St. John's-wort come to the fore in the famous "red oil" which heals and sanitizes wounds, and soothes burns, irritation and sunburn (it should never be used as a sunscreen, however, as it renders the skin more sensitive to the sun).

• As a massage oil, it **relieves cramps and neuralgia**.

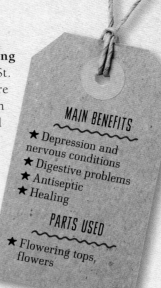

MAIN BENEFITS

★ Depression and nervous conditions
★ Digestive problems
★ Antiseptic
★ Healing

PARTS USED

★ Flowering tops, flowers

In the times of the Druids, St. John's-wort was considered sacred; its smell alone was enough to drive away evil spirits. François-Joseph Cazin, the 19th-century French doctor and botanist, used it to treat chest ailments such as asthma and bronchial catarrh. St. John's-wort is considered to have excellent healing properties, which 13th-century surgeons of Montpellier regarded as unparalleled. It was used in the form of a cordial for internal use and as a dressing externally.

An antidepressant, with healing properties

• St. John's-wort has a proven **antidepressant effect**. It is advocated for the treatment of mild to moderate depression. It can be used to treat a variety of nervous disorders causing tension and insomnia. The extract or a diluted tincture is used to achieve a sufficient dose of the main active ingredient.

• St. John's-wort is a **liver and gall bladder tonic**. It is recommended as an infusion to treat digestive disorders. It is said to have a positive effect on premenstrual syndrome and menopause-related problems.

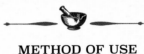

METHOD OF USE

• **INTERNAL:** Infusion. 15 to 30g (½ to 1oz) of flowering tops per litre (quart) of water (3 cups per day between meals) as a tonic for the liver.

• **EXTERNAL: Concentrated decoction.** It can be used in vaginal douches or for cleaning wounds. As a warm lotion, it can soothe irritation of thin and hypersensitive skin. To invigorate the skin, add 4 to 5 litres of this decoction to the bath. **Red oil.** Leave ½kg (1lb) of fresh flowers to steep for 3 weeks in a litre of olive oil. Strain, then pour the beautiful red oil obtained into small bottles. Apply to sunburn, or use to massage painful areas.

TOXICITY

St. John's-wort can decrease the effect of certain oral cardiotonic, antiretroviral, anti-asthmatic and contraceptive medicines when taken simultaneously. The hypericin in St. John's-wort can cause photosensitization, inflammation of the skin when exposed to sun. However, this has not been observed at usual doses of the infusion, as hypericin is not very soluble in water.

Description

A common perennial found in dry places, along paths. Its upright, branching stem has two ridges running its length. Its opposite, oblong leaves have black dots around the margins. The bright yellow flowers, with five large petals, grow at the end of the stems and bloom throughout the summer. When crushed, the flowers produce a few drops of purple liquid.

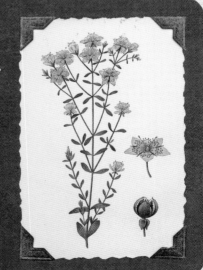

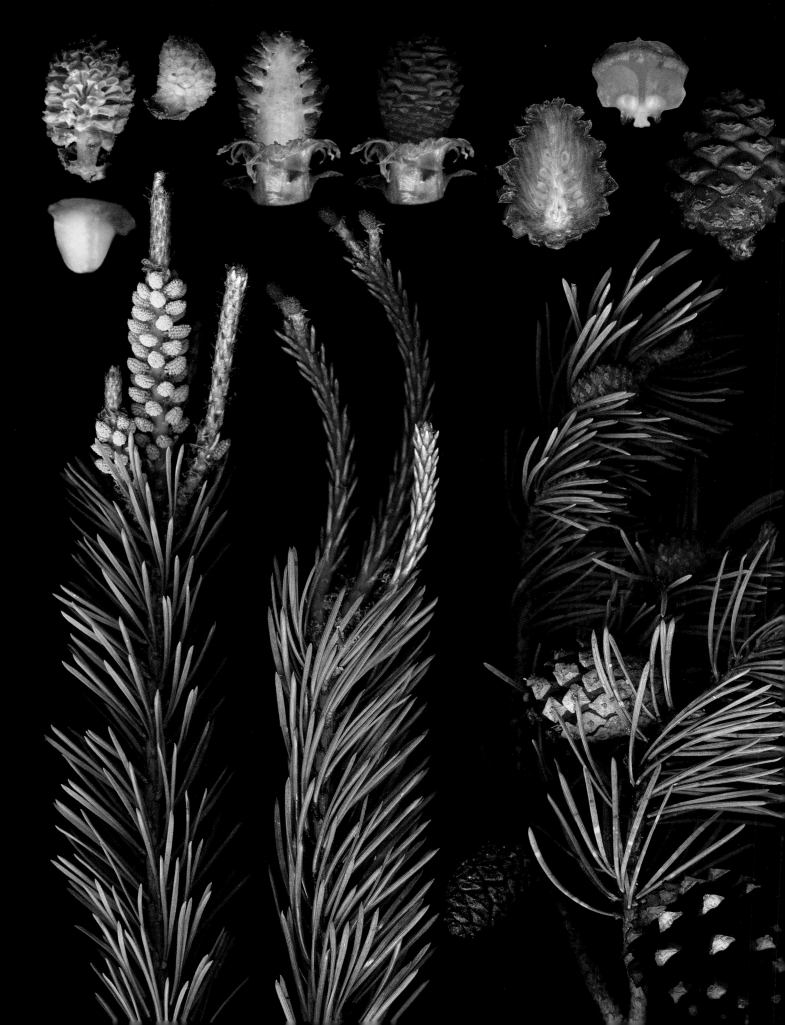

Scots Pine

Pinus sylvestris

FAMILY: PINACEAE

Active elements:

Leaves and buds: aromatic oil rich in alpha-and beta-pinene, limonene, carene and bornyl acetate. Sap: resin, bitter principle.

In Germany, the needles are used to make "forest wool" (*Waldwolle*), once much sought-after to make mattresses for rheumatism sufferers. The needles could also be boiled in alkaline water, from which "essential wood oil" was then skimmed off. This was used in baths to treat gout and rheumatism. Another common preparation was a balsamic, Pine needle syrup.

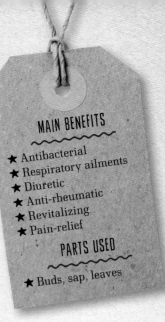

MAIN BENEFITS

★ Antibacterial
★ Respiratory ailments
★ Diuretic
★ Anti-rheumatic
★ Revitalizing
★ Pain-relief

PARTS USED

★ Buds, sap, leaves

METHOD OF USE

• **INTERNAL: Infusion.** Infuse 25 to 40g (¾ to 1¾oz) of buds per litre (quart) of water for an hour. Add plenty of sugar as the infusion is bitter. Use for respiratory ailments.

Syrup. Steep 60g (2oz) of buds in 50g (1¾oz) of colourless spirits for 1 hour. Then add a litre of boiling water. Leave to steep for another 6 hours. Then strain and add the same weight in sugar, and cook in a *bain-marie* until it has the consistency of syrup. Take 4 or 5 tablespoonsful per day for respiratory ailments.

• **EXTERNAL: Decoction.** 60g (2oz) of buds per litre of water. Used as a douche, an inhalation or a lotion for red, congested or irritated skin (a decoction of needles can also be used).

Remedy for colds and bronchial ailments

• Pine buds have proven **antiseptic and expectorant properties**. They are used in the treatment of respiratory tract ailments: bronchitis, flu, severe colds and chronic lung diseases.

• They are also recognized as having **excitant and diuretic** properties, and their usage extends to the treatment of inflammations of the bladder, leucorrhoea and skin ailments.

• Pine buds are also indicated for the treatment of rheumatism, to **relieve joint pain** and in cases of gout.

• They are also said to have **tonic and reinvigorating** properties, particularly in relation to sex drive.

• The distilled essential oil of leaves or resin (also known as turpentine essential oil) is an **antibacterial** and stimulates bronchial secretions.

• It is a **decongestant** for respiratory disorders.

• Used externally, Pine is effective **against a wide range of headaches**, rheumatic pain and muscle ache. The essential oil activates the circulation and is beneficial in cases of **venous insufficiency** (heavy legs, varicose veins, haemorrhoids).

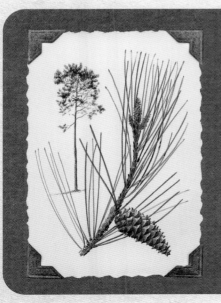

Description

Conifers vary in size (up to 30m (98½ft)) depending on the soil and the climate, and are common in the mountains. Found throughout Europe and northern Asia. The scaly bark of the trunk takes on a characteristic orange hue towards the top. The short, needle-like leaves are bluish-green, and have a small sheath at their base. The male cones are clustered in short yellow catkins. The female parts form small grey cones with woody scales. The leaf buds, wrongly referred to as "fir buds", are used in medicine.

TOXICITY

If Pine essential oil is taken internally it is toxic at too high a dose. It is counter-indicated in the case of whooping cough. It can also irritate the skin and mucous membranes.

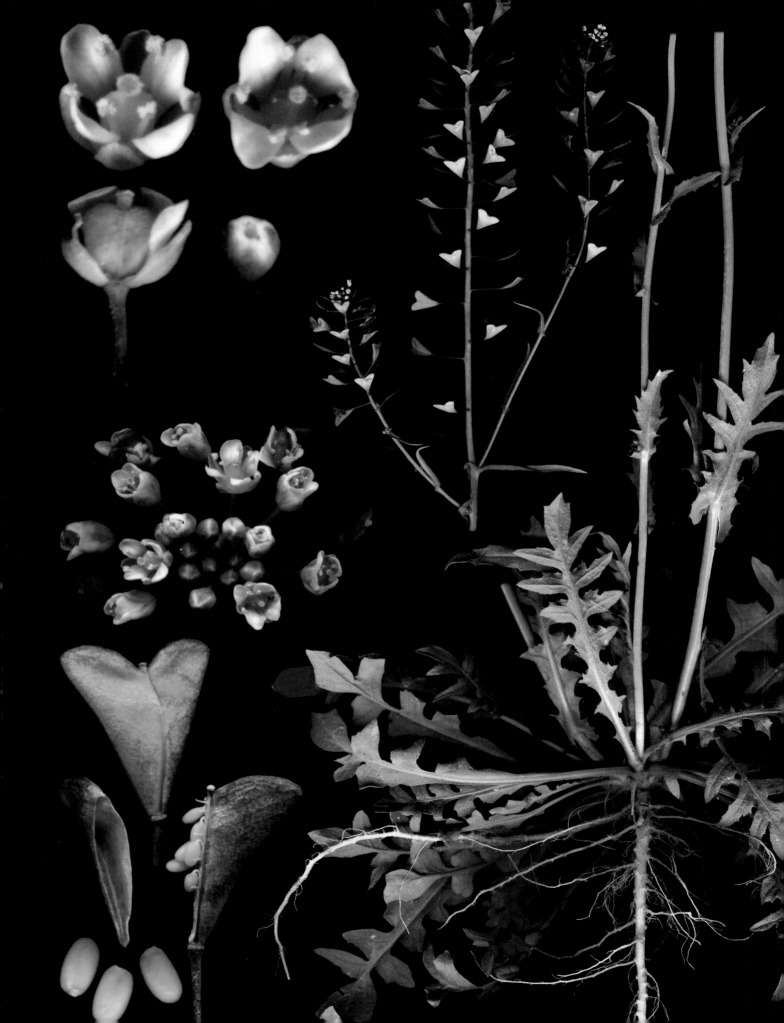

Shepherd's Purse

Capsella bursa-pastoris

FAMILY: BRASSICACEAE

Active elements:
Flavonoids, choline, acetylcholine, histamine, tyramine, sulphur heteroside.

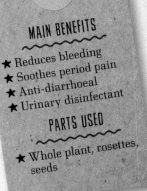

MAIN BENEFITS

★ Reduces bleeding
★ Soothes period pain
★ Anti-diarrhoeal
★ Urinary disinfectant

PARTS USED

★ Whole plant, rosettes, seeds

Popular medicine has long been aware of the blood-clotting properties of Shepherd's Purse. Dioscorides advocated its use to treat haemoptysis (coughing up blood). Throughout the Middle Ages, it was used as a remedy against haemorrhaging. In the early 1900s, Henri Leclerc, the French physician and renowned medical herbalist, prescribed its use for women suffering uterine bleeding, during puberty and the menopause.

A one-stop shop for bleeding

• Shepherd's Purse has widely acknowledged blood-clotting properties. It can be used to **treat most types of bleeding**: heavy or prolonged menstrual bleeding, bleeding between periods or nosebleeds.
• Used internally or externally, it **can relieve heavy legs and haemorrhoids**.
• Combined with Mugwort, Shepherd's Purse can relieve menstrual pain, especially during puberty and the menopause. The plant is also recommended for the **treatment of diarrhoea and as a urinary disinfectant** for cystitis sufferers.

OTHER USES: Shepherd's Purse flowers can be eaten raw in salad or cooked as a vegetable. In China and Japan, the plant is cultivated and sold in vegetable markets. The tiny, pungent yellow seeds can be used as a spice, crushed like mustard seed.

DID YOU KNOW? The botanical name *Capsella* comes from the Latin *capsa*, meaning "box". The fruit is reminiscent of a little box, such as may have been a farmer's leather bag or shepherd's purse of bygone times.

METHOD OF USE

• **INTERNAL: Decoction.** 30 to 50g (1 to 1¾oz) of dried plant per litre (quart) of water. Allow to boil for 10 minutes and drink 3 cups per day for the various ailments listed above.
Tonic wine. Same decoction as above, replacing the water with red wine and using 60g (2oz) of the plant. Take 2 or 3 small (100g (3½oz)) glasses per day, as a course of treatment.

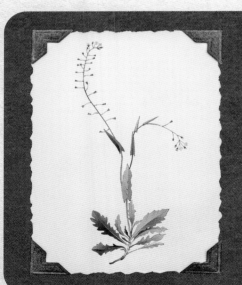

Description

Small annual plant found on cultivated ground and meadows, rarely exceeding a height of 30cm (12in). Its lobed leaves form a rosette at the base of which emerges a vertical stem bearing a few small leaves, with small groups of tiny white flowers at the end, producing long clusters of flat, triangular fruit, the shape of upside-down hearts.

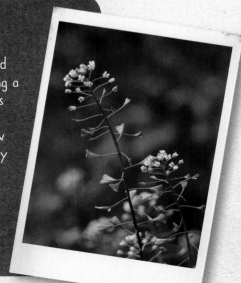

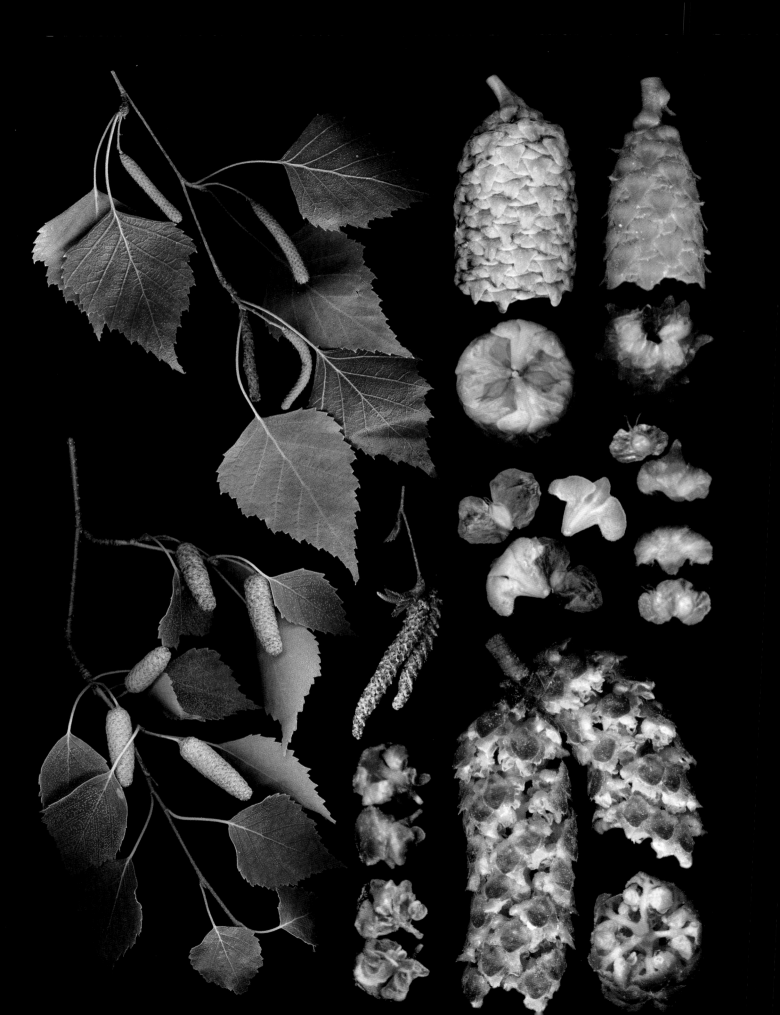

Silver Birch

Betula alba

FAMILY: BETULACEAE

Active elements:

Flavonoids (including rutoside), phenol acids, triterpenes, tannins, bitter principle, aromatic oil. The bark in particular contains betulinic acid.

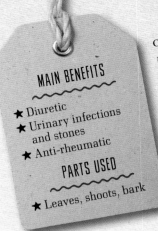

MAIN BENEFITS

★ Diuretic
★ Urinary infections and stones
★ Anti-rheumatic

PARTS USED

★ Leaves, shoots, bark

OTHER USES: Silver Birch bark was used by the American Indians to make containers, cover their huts and make lightweight canoes. It is an excellent fire lighter as its high resin content means it burns even when wet. The young leaves have a bitter, resinous flavour and can be added to salads. Birch pitch can be extracted from the bark using a dry distillation process and is used in Russia to tan leather in order to preserve it. This sticky substance has been used since Neolithic times to fill holes and repair cracks in jars and other vessels.

The 12th-century Saint Hildegard of Bingen was the first to record the healing power of birch flowers. In 1565, the Italian physician Mattioli described how, if a birch trunk was pierced with an auger, a large quantity of water was produced, which he held to have "great property and virtue in breaking down both kidney and bladder stones.... This water removes marks from the face.... When used to wash out the mouth, it heals ulcers".

A powerful diuretic

• Silver Birch has powerful **diuretic** properties. Its leaves are advocated for the treatment of inflammation and **infection of the urinary tract**, kidney stones and also as part of **treatment for rheumatism**.
• The buds have the same properties.
• The bark, likewise a diuretic, **stimulates digestion** and brings down fevers. It is **excellent for skin problems**, especially areas of dry skin.
• Silver Birch sap is a clear, slightly sparkling liquid that is said to have **diuretic and purifying properties**. It is drunk as a cure for arthritis and bladder stones.

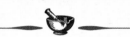

METHOD OF USE

• **INTERNAL:** Infusion. 30 to 40g (1 to 1½oz) of leaves per litre (quart) of boiling water. Wait until cooled to 40°C and then add 1g bicarbonate of soda, to ensure the resinous principle is fully dissolved. Drink 2 or 3 cups per day to treat urinary problems, calculi and rheumatism. **Decoction of buds.** 150g (5¼oz) per litre of water. Boil for 5 minutes. Use for the same conditions.
Decoction of bark. One teaspoonful of bark per cup of water. Boil for 5 minutes. Drink 3 cups per day before a meal to stimulate digestion.
Sap. Take 100 to 200g (3½ to 7oz) per day as a purifying treatment in springtime.
• **EXTERNAL: Decoction of bark.** Handful per litre of water. Simmer to three quarters liquid. Use as wash or compress, to treat areas of dry skin.

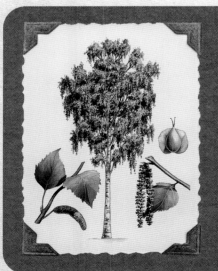

Description

A beautiful tree that grows in both forests and mountains, reaching a height of 15 to 18m (49 to 59ft). Common throughout Europe and Asia. Its smooth, slender trunk is covered in white bark. Its long, pendulous branches bear simple, diamond-shaped leaves. Its flowers (photo opposite) take the form of catkins.

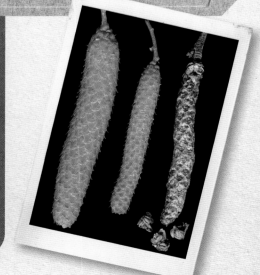

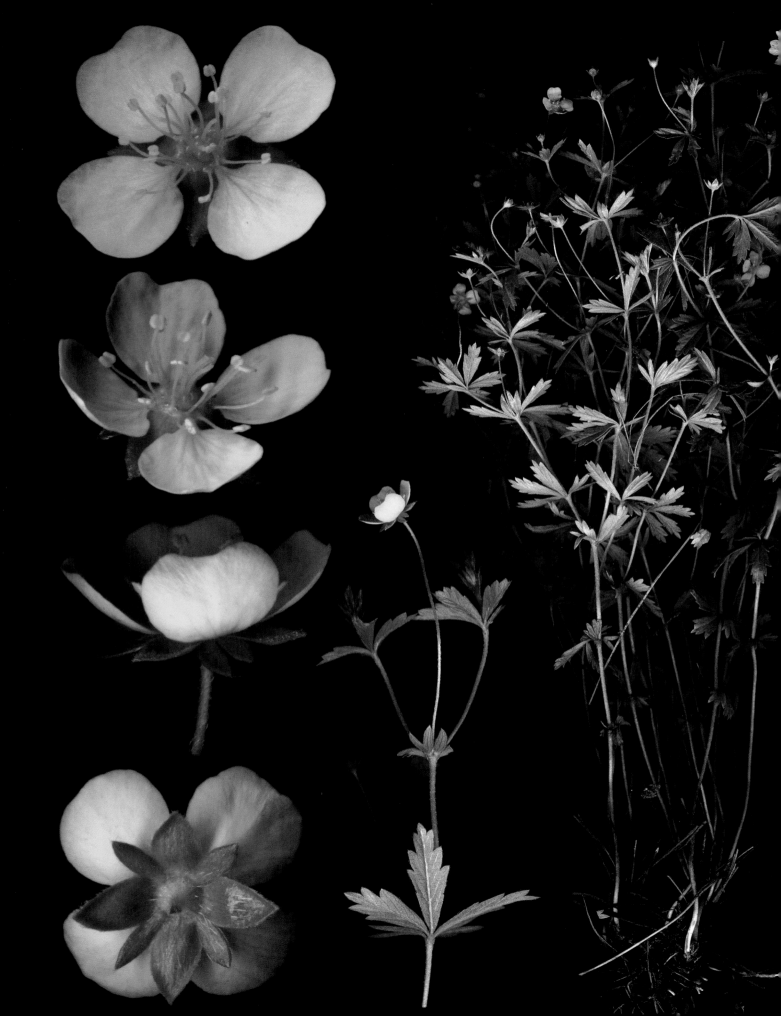

Silverweed

Potentilla anserina

FAMILY: ROSACEAE

Active elements:
Many hydrolysable and condensed tannins.

In the 16th century, Olivier de Serres, the French agronomist, recommended Silverweed for "torments of the teeth".

Powerfully astringent

• The roots are used for their **astringent** and stomachic properties. Generally administered internally to **treat benign diarrhoea and leucorrhoea**.

• Used in mouthwashes to treat inflammations of the mouth (**ulcers, gingivitis**), as a gargle for throat problems and in lotion form for skin ulcers.

• The leaves are used for the same purposes as the roots.

• Silverweed is sometimes used to relieve period pain.

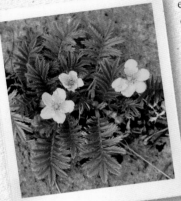

OTHER USES: Silverweed roots feature fleshy bulges that are rich in starch. They are nutritious but astringent so are only sometimes consumed. Once cooked, their flavour, akin to that of a parsnip, is not unpleasant. Canadian Indians ate Silverweed as a vegetable. They may also have used it as a currency to exchange for less common commodities. The plant was also eaten by the people of Siberia (the Yakuts and Tungus).

OTHER SPECIES: The roots of other *Potentilla*, all very high in tannins, are used for the same medicinal purposes: Creeping Cinquefoil (*P. reptans*), which looks much like Silverweed, Spring Cinquefoil (*P. verna*) and Tormentil (*P. tormentilla*). Tormentil root extract has been shown in clinical trials to be effective in treating rotavirus infections in babies and young children.

DID YOU KNOW? *Potentilla* comes from the Latin *potens*, meaning "powerful", an allusion to the (real, but perhaps slightly exaggerated) medicinal properties of these plants.

MAIN BENEFITS

★ Astringent
★ Stomachic
★ Anti-diarrhoeal
★ Inflammations of the mouth

PARTS USED

★ Roots, leaves

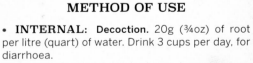

METHOD OF USE

• **INTERNAL: Decoction.** 20g (¾oz) of root per litre (quart) of water. Drink 3 cups per day, for diarrhoea.

Wine. 70g (2½oz) of crushed root, leave to steep for 8 days in a litre of fortified wine such as Banyuls or Muscat. Drink 1 or 2 cups per day, for diarrhoea. Do not use utensils made of iron as it will react with the tannins.

• **EXTERNAL: Decoction.** 30 to 60g (1 to 2oz) per litre for lotions, gargles, douches, enemas, compresses on ulcers.

Dried root powder. One of the best remedies for firming gums and preventing them from receding. Use on a toothbrush, in the same way as toothpaste, or steep in strong wine and rub directly on to inflamed gums.

Description

A tall perennial, with flower stalks growing to 20 to 40cm (8 to 16in). Common in ditches, wet meadows and along paths, it is found almost everywhere in the northern hemisphere. Silverweed covers the ground with a finely dissected silvery carpet. Its leaves are divided into numerous long leaflets, with sharp-toothed edges covered in long, silky hairs. The five-petalled flowers dot the foliage with gold. The creeping stem anchors its adventitious roots at leaf junctions and stretches into long runners.

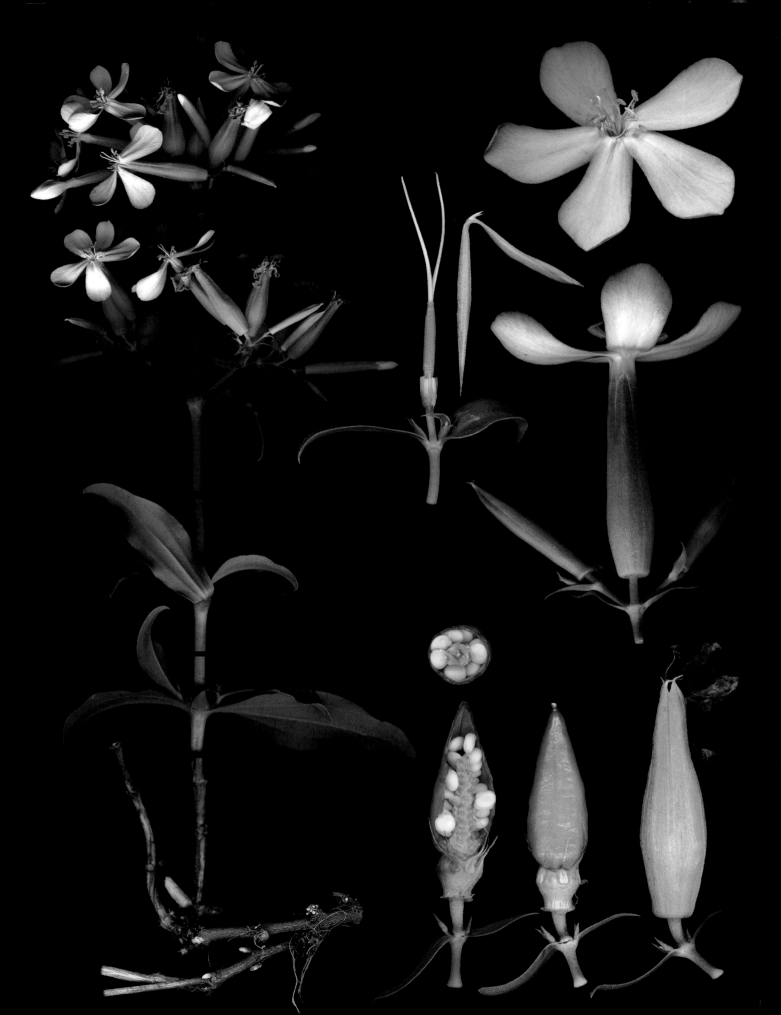

Soapwort

Saponaria officinalis
FAMILY: CARYOPHYLLACEAE

Active elements:
Roots, but also whole plant: saponosides (including gypsogenin), resin, aromatic oil.

• It is also recommended for the alleviation of jaundice, **chronic rheumatism, gout and lymphatic congestion**.

• In Germany, Soapwort roots are used as an **expectorant** to treat congestion of the respiratory tract as they act as a strong irritant of the mucosae.

OTHER USES: The plant contains saponosides (or saponins), which foam on contact with water: this property means it has long been used to wash both clothes and hair. It is sometimes still used for very delicate fabric which would be damaged by the soda in classic soaps.

While Soapwort has been widely used as a soap substitute for washing laundry or hair, its medicinal properties have been acknowledged since ancient times. The Romans added it to their baths to alleviate itching. In the early 18th century, Herman Boerhaave, the famous Dutch physician, advocated it for the treatment of jaundice.

Detoxifying plant

• A best-in-class **depurative** (detoxifying) plant, it combines **diuretic, sudorific, tonic** and aperitive properties. It combats liver failure and engorgement of the spleen. Both the leaves and roots can be used to **treat skin ailments** (acne, psoriasis and eczema flare-ups).

Description

A perennial growing to a height of 30 to 50cm (1 to 1½ft), commonly found in ditches and on river banks. Found in Europe, Asia and North America. Its upright stem, which rises from a creeping rhizome, bears opposite, lanceolate leaves with three to five clearly marked veins. The large pink, sweet-smelling flowers, with five petals, are arranged in terminal clusters at the top of the stem. The whole plant, in contact with water, foams like soap, from whence its name; other common names include Lather Root and Bouncing Bet.

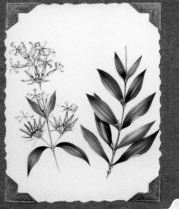

METHOD OF USE

• **INTERNAL: Decoction of leaves.** 30g (1oz) per litre (quart) of water. Boil for 5 to 10 minutes. Drink 3 small (100g (3½oz)) glasses per day before meals as a detoxifier.
Root decoction. 100g (3½oz) per litre of water. Boil for 5 to 10 minutes. Drink 2 glasses per day. For the same conditions as above. Do not boil for longer than the specified time and do not leave the plant to steep in the water. Strain the decoction as soon as it is made and do not prepare it in advance.

• **EXTERNAL: Decoction of leaves.** 100g (3½oz) per litre of water as a gargle for benign sore throats and painful inflammation of the gums and cheeks.
Poultice of crushed leaves. For lymphatic congestion, dry patches of skin, eczema-related conditions, herpes, and swollen ankles and knees.
Whole plant decoction. Produces a soapy water that is excellent for cleaning woollen fabric and fragile hair.
Scalp lotion. The root macerated in alcohol means you can leave longer between hair washes and keeps the hair wonderfully clean.

TOXICITY

Internal administration of Soapwort requires some precautions. The plant should not be left to steep in water before or after decoction, in order to avoid side-effects such as shaking or a dry mouth.

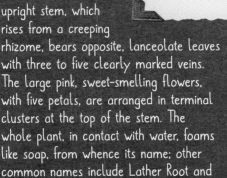

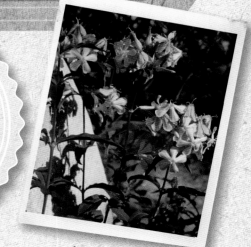

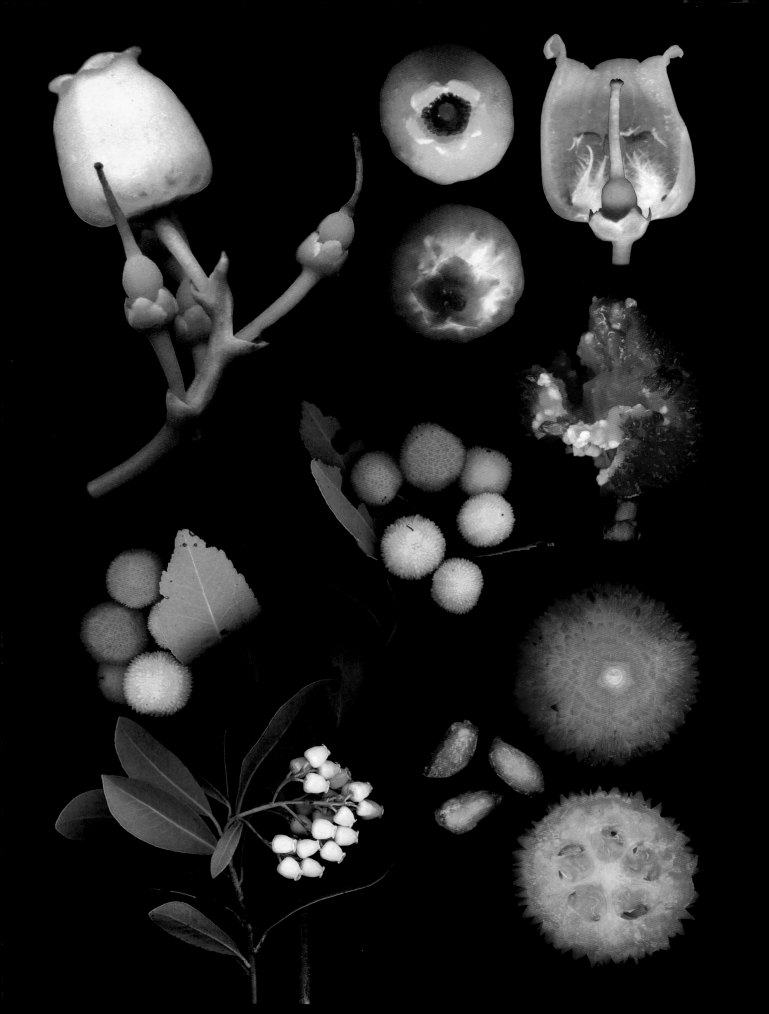

Strawberry Tree

Arbutus unedo
FAMILY: ERICACEAE

Active elements:
Tannins, phenolic heterosides (including arbutoside), bitter principle. Fruits: high in carbohydrates and organic acids.

According to Pliny the Elder the species name *unedo* comes from the Latin expression *unum tantum edo*, meaning "I eat only one", implying perhaps that having tasted one, you would not want to eat another. It would seem that the Strawberry Tree was not held in particularly high regard in ancient times.

people find them difficult to digest. This problem can be resolved by cooking. They are a good basis for jams and compotes.

Arbutus-berry jam is widely available in markets in the south of France. In Spain and North Africa, the fruits are used to flavour sorbets, and are also distilled into a perfumed alcoholic liqueur. They are rich in carbohydrates, which contributes to their high nutritional value.

DID YOU KNOW? The Roman goddess Cardea was said to ward off witches and heal sick or bewitched children with her Strawberry Tree wand. In Italy, during the struggle for independence (1848–1870), the patriots took the Strawberry Tree as their symbol: it bears green leaves, white flowers and red fruit simultaneously, the colours of the Italian national flag.

Diuretic and astringent

• The fresh leaves and young shoots are **diuretic and astringent**. The arbutoside they contain acts as **an antiseptic for the urinary tract**, useful for treating cystitis and urethritis.
• The leaves are also used to **treat diarrhoea** and dysentery.
• They can be gargled to **soothe sore throats**.
• The astringent root was sometimes used to treat arthrosclerosis, poor blood circulation and high blood pressure.
• The fruit, the arbutus berry, is considered a **diuretic** and is also used as an **astringent** to treat diarrhoea.

OTHER USES: The fruit are aromatic, creamy and sweet, but their orange pulp contains small hard lumps, like some varieties of pear. They have a pleasant taste when eaten raw and are best slightly before they fully ripen, when they are orange in colour. Some

METHOD OF USE

• **INTERNAL:** Infusion. 10g (¼oz) of fresh leaves per litre (quart) of boiling water, to be drunk throughout the day as a diuretic, anti-diarrhoeal or to treat urinary tract disorders.
Arbutus-berry jam. Make from an equal weight of sugar and fruit. Use for mild diarrhoea.

Strawberry Trees are much more famous in Spain than elsewhere.

Description

The Strawberry Tree is common throughout the Mediterranean basin, particularly to the west. It is an elegant shrub with rough brown bark revealing a smooth, reddish-orange wood. The dark green, leathery, evergreen leaves look a little like bay leaves, but have serrated edges. The greenish-white bell-shaped flowers bloom from October to January. The shrub often continues to flower while it is bearing fruit. The fruits are large green spheres covered with small bumps, which turn yellow, orange and finally red as they mature.

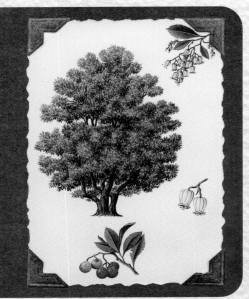

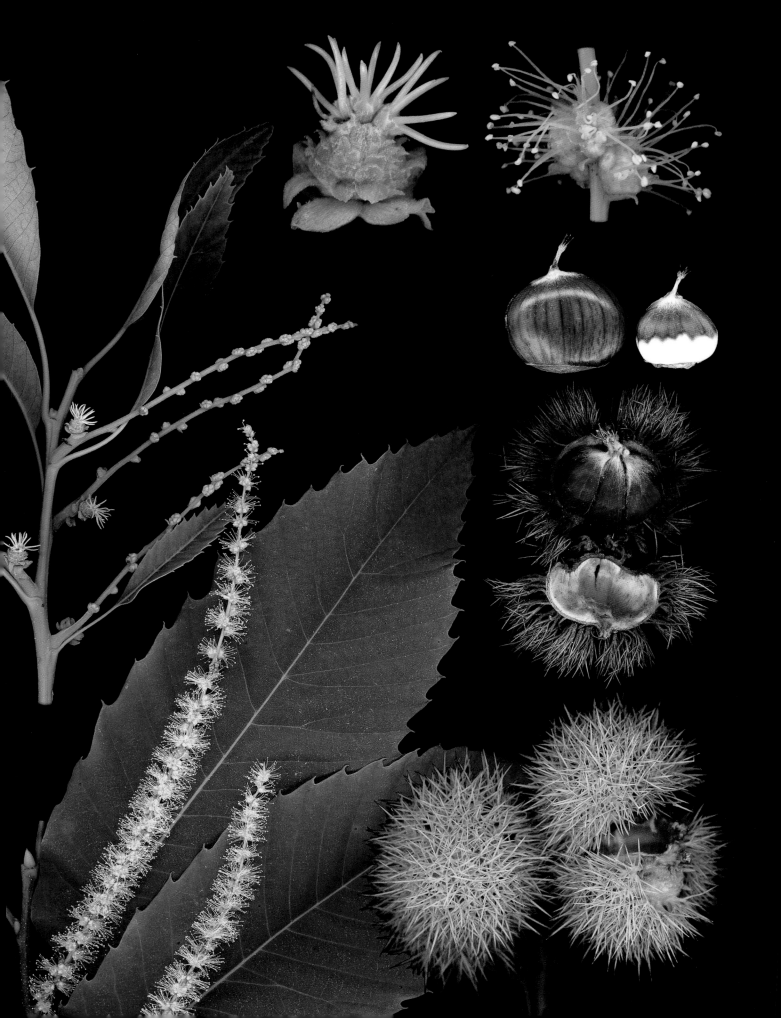

Sweet Chestnut

Castanea sativa
FAMILY: FAGACEAE

Active elements:
Tannins.

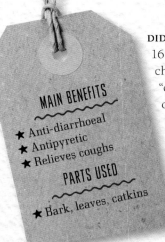
DID YOU KNOW? According to a 16th-century Italian poet, the chestnut tree was named after "chaste Nea" (Casta-Nea), one of Diana's nymphs. Separated from her companions, she was assiduously pursued by Jupiter, but chose virtue over passion and killed herself rather than submit to his advances. The God transformed her body into a Sweet Chestnut.

I t was the Romans who first cultivated the Sweet Chestnut tree, which for centuries provided the staple food of many peoples in European regions where the soils were too acidic for successful cereal cropping.

Rich in tannins

• Sweet Chestnut (bark, leaves and catkins) is a great astringent that was used in the past to **treat dysentery**.
• The bark was also popularly used to reduce fever (**antipyretic**) in days gone by.
• In North America, treatment using Sweet Chestnut leaves is advocated as a **cough sedative**, for bronchitis and especially whooping cough.

OTHER USES: Tannins form stable compounds with proteins which gives them the ability to tan hides, thus making them rot-proof. Sweet Chestnut has one to three large shiny seeds (known as chestnuts) contained in a rounded, spiny cupule. It superficially resembles the Horse-chestnut fruit (called conkers) but the Sweet Chestnut fruit is prickly and partitioned into seeds. The two species are not related.

METHOD OF USE

• **INTERNAL: Decoction of catkins.** 15 to 20g (½ to ¾oz) per litre (quart) of water, to treat diarrhoea. Put the catkins in cold water and bring to the boil for 2 minutes. Then leave to infuse for 15 minutes and drink throughout the day.
Infusion. 30g (1oz) of leaves per litre of water. Use for whooping cough.
Tincture. For adult bronchitis, steep the leaves for 15 days in an equal volume of clear brandy. Take a teaspoonful when a cough comes on.
Pureed or braised the **chestnuts** are delicious, nutritious and very well tolerated by delicate stomachs. They can be used to treat mild diarrhoea.

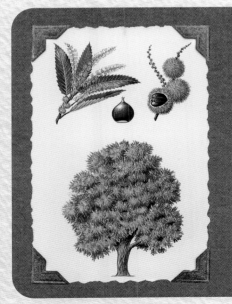

Description

Sweet Chestnut trees can grow to 30m (98½ft) in height. Native to the siliceous mountains of southern Europe, from Portugal to the Caucasus, the Sweet Chestnut is easily identified by the smooth, grey bark of its young trunk; its large, boldly toothed leaves; its long, hanging catkins; and its characteristic fruit formed by a spiny sheath containing large brown fruits.

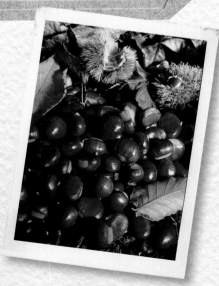

The chestnut can be candied (*marron glacé*), roasted or cooked as a vegetable. It is possibly the only fruit that is always harvested in its wild setting.

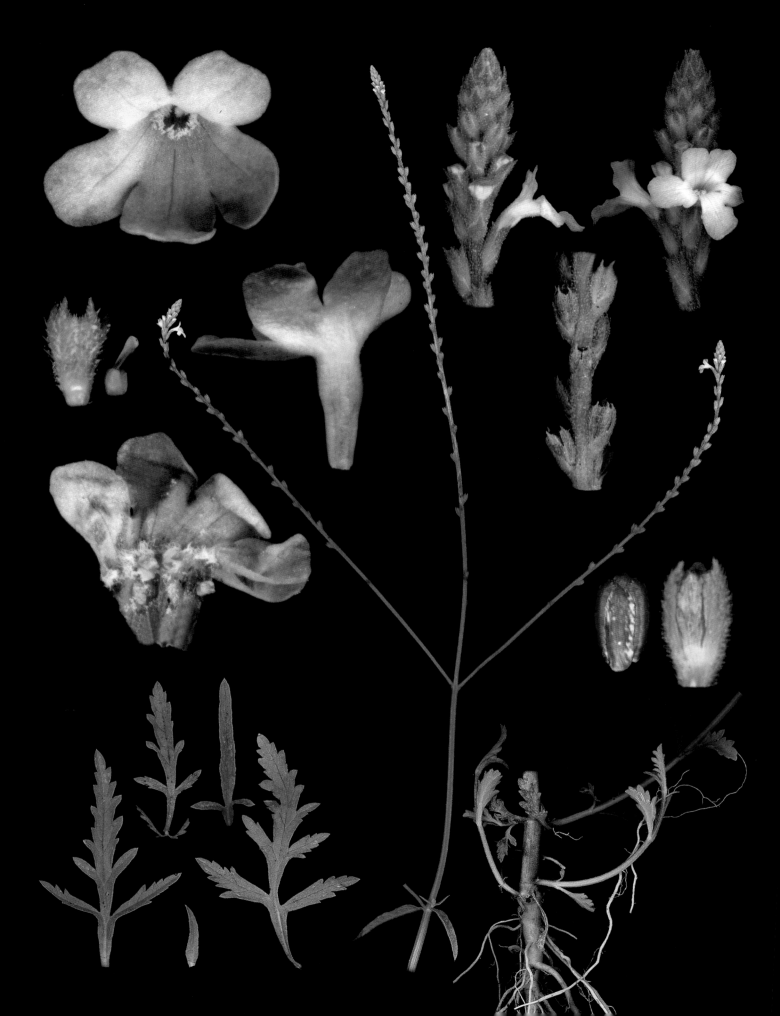

Verbena

Verbena officinalis

FAMILY: VERBENACEAE

Active elements:

Tannins, mucilage, iridoids (including verbenaloside and hastatoside), phenylpropionic heterosides (including verbascoside and eukovoside).

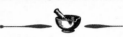

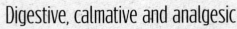

METHOD OF USE

- **INTERNAL: Infusion.** 15 to 30g (½ to 1oz) of plant per litre (quart) of boiling water. Drink 3 cups per day before meals as an aperitif. It is also possible to drink a cup after each meal to relieve anxiety-related stomach cramps.
- **EXTERNAL: Decoction.** 40 to 50g (1½ to 1¾oz) per litre of water. Used in compresses for injuries including knocks and bruises.
Poultices of fresh flowering tops boiled in vinegar. Apply this mixture as hot as possible to the areas of pain arising from pleurisy or stitches, or to soothe pain or reduce swollen veins after knocks, blows or a fall.

Verbena was sacred to the Gauls (its name is said to come from the Celtic *Ferfaen*). Druids washed their altars with an infusion of Verbena flowers before making sacrifices, while the ovates drank it before predicting the future or casting spells. It was ascribed countless properties, in particular, the power to cure epilepsy, fevers, sore throats, skin ailments and bruising.

This reputation as a "herb for all ills" lasted many centuries, if Mattioli, the eminent 16th- century physician and naturalist, is to be believed, "Magicians [...] say that those who are rubbed with it will obtain all that they desire, believing that this herb cures fevers and causes persons to fall in love and, in short, that it cures all illnesses and others besides".

MAIN BENEFITS

- ★ Aperitive
- ★ Digestive
- ★ Calmative and sedative
- ★ Anti-rheumatic
- ★ Analgesic

PARTS USED

- ★ Leaves, flowers

Digestive, calmative and analgesic

- Verbena is used above all to **facilitate digestion**. It is both aperitive and digestive and is effective in treating dizziness, headaches and sleeplessness linked to poor digestion.
- Its **anti-rheumatic and analgesic properties** means it works on stitches and bumps, knocks and bruises of all kinds.
- Anxiety-sufferers find it a **calmative which aids sleep**.
- Verbena is sometimes used externally to treat **day-to-day skin problems**. It soothes superficial burns, sunburn, nappy rash and itchy insect bites.

DID YOU KNOW? Lemon Verbena (*Lippia citriodora*) is not related in any way to Common Verbena (*Verbena officinalis*). Little Lemon Verbena, with white flowers, whose leaves exude a pleasant lemon scent is used in cooking to add flavour to shellfish and ice-creams and sauces that accompany chicken and fish. Lemongrass (*Cymbopogon citratus*) is a tropical grass used in southeast Asian cuisine, and can be used to make infusions tasting similar to those of Lemon Verbena.

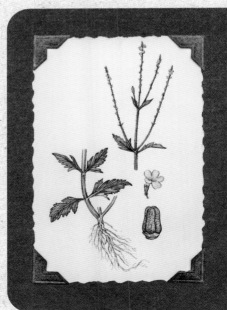

Description

A perennial growing to between 40 and 80cm (16in to 2½ft), commonly found along pathways and roadsides and on uncultivated land throughout Europe, Asia and North Africa. Its upright, branched stem bears opposite, deeply dissected leaves and small mauve flower clusters on long filiform spikes. It is not aromatic.

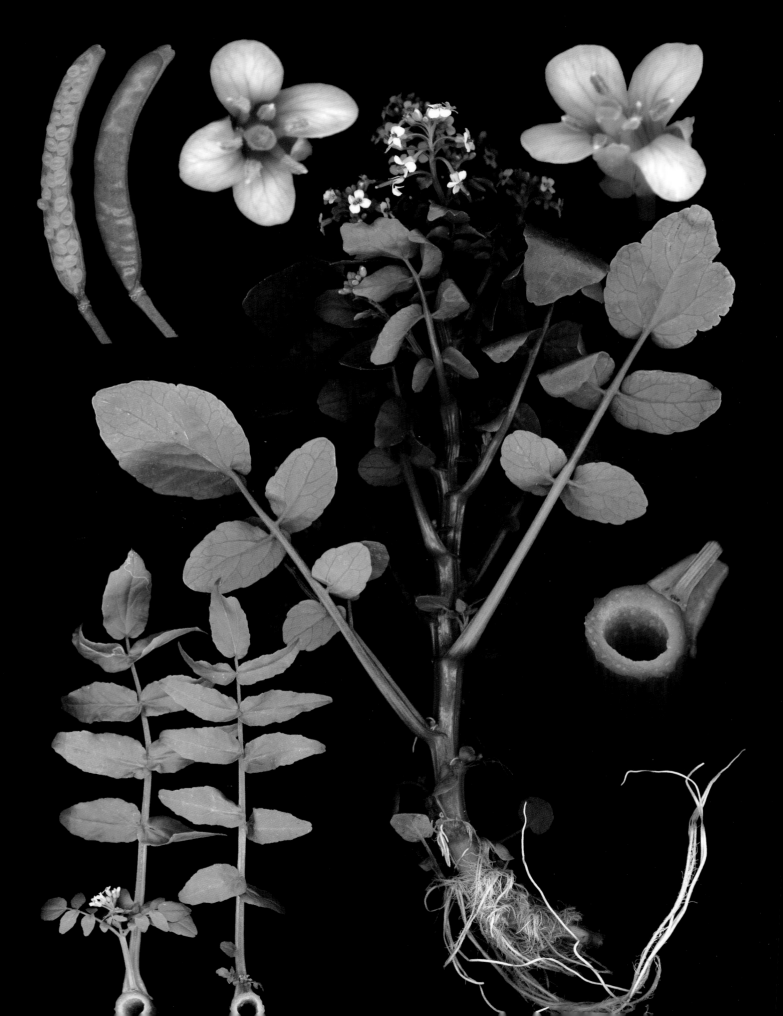

Watercress

Nasturtium officinale

FAMILY: BRASSICACEAE

Active elements:

Minerals, vitamins (including a high level of vitamin C), sulphuric heterosides, including phenethyl glucosinolate (which gives, among other derivatives, gluconasturtiin).

Viewed generally in antiquity as a stimulant, Watercress was used by Hippocrates as an expectorant and by Dioscorides as an aphrodisiac. In the Renaissance, it was rightly attributed with numerous properties, including the power to cure sciatica and headaches. Récamier, the illustrious 19th-century French physician, treated patients suffering from tuberculosis with two handfuls of Watercress to be taken each morning, topping off their unusual breakfast with a nice glass of milk. It was used to treat diabetes by Constantin Paul, and for pulmonary ailments and chronic bronchial catarrh by Henri Leclerc. François-Joseph Cazin, the 19th-century French doctor and botanist, advocated its revitalizing properties for people lacking in energy and for the treatment of all visceral diseases (liver, spleen, bladder, kidneys and urinary tract), also prescribing it for gout and rheumatism.

MAIN BENEFITS

★ Detoxifying
★ Diuretic
★ Expectorant

PARTS USED

★ Juice, whole plant

TOXICITY

Over-consumption of raw Watercress can lead to painful cystitis as it contains an irritant sulphurous essential oil.

Aperitive and purifiying

• Watercress **stimulates the appetite** and is recommended for people suffering from lymph-node problems or rickets, and convalescents in general.

• It is recommended as a **depurative for skin ailments**.

• As a **diuretic**, it is beneficial to the kidneys and bladder, and is useful in treating generalized oedema and kidney or bladder stones

• Its **expectorant properties** make it useful for people suffering bronchitis or whooping cough.

• Used externally, crushed Watercress is sometimes recommended for **curing ulcers** and painful gum and cheek inflammations. Crushed Watercress leaves are excellent for improving gum health.

• It is highly regarded in the form of a hair lotion for **slowing down hair loss**.

NOTE: As heat causes the evaporation of its highly volatile, active principle, Watercress must always be used raw if its benefits are to be enjoyed. However, it is essential to know the origin of the plant: never eat raw, wild watercress (and in general, any wild aquatic plant), because it could be contaminated by the larvae of a dangerous parasite, the liver fluke. The controlled conditions under which farmed watercress is grown ensure that this risk is eliminated. Note that while cooking kills the contaminating liver fluke larvae, it also means that the plant's desirable properties are lost.

Description

A perennial of 20 to 50cm (8in to 1½ft), found in running water and ditches. Sometimes cultivated by market gardeners in beds fed by spring water. The aquatic stems grow upwards, bearing compound leaves of rounded leaflets, the terminal leaf larger than the others. The small, white flowers have four petals in a cross formation that produce long seed pods. The whole plant has a strong, spicy flavour.

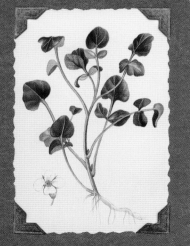

METHOD OF USE

• **INTERNAL: Watercress juice.** Crush the plant with a pestle and mortar or using a mixer. Strain and drink 60 to 150g (2 to 5¼oz) per day of the juice as an aperitive and depurative.
• **EXTERNAL:** Daily morning rubs with a suede cloth using **Watercress juice,** either neat, or mixed in equal parts with rum, to prevent hair loss and encourage regrowth.
Restorative **Watercress poultice.** Crush a bunch of Watercress, and mix with a stiffly beaten egg white to obtain an even paste which can then be applied.

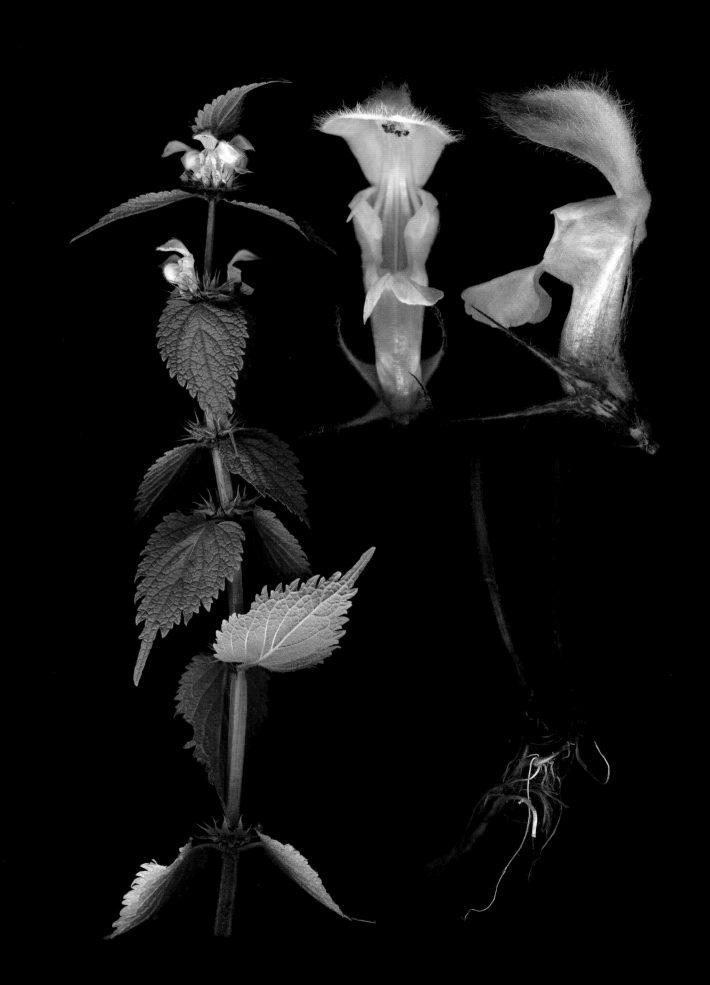

White Deadnettle

Lamium album
FAMILY: LAMIACEAE

Active elements:
Tannins, mucilage, chlorogenic acid,
flavonoids, iridoids, saponosides.

MAIN BENEFITS

★ Astringent
★ Soothing
★ Regulates periods
★ Anti-diarrhoeal
★ Expectorant

PARTS USED

★ Leaves, young shoots, flowering tops, whole plant

• Their expectorant properties make them useful in treating **respiratory problems**.
• Effective as a gargle, to treat **throat inflammations** and runny noses.
• It can be used on the scalp to tackle **flaking skin, irritation or dandruff**.

OTHER USES: Young shoots can be added raw to salads. The leaves can be cooked and eaten as tasty vegetables.

DID YOU KNOW? The name *Lamium* comes from the Greek *lamia*, meaning "Ogress", a reference to the flowers that look like wide open mouths. Its common name, White Deadnettle, references flower colour and that it does not sting.

The White Deadnettle has long been a popular remedy for leucorrhoea or white discharge. As early as the 16th century, Dodoens, the Flemish physician and botanist, advocated its use for this purpose. Others used it to treat haemorrhages. Henri Leclerc, the French physician and renowned medical herbalist, recommended it for both leucorrhoea and abnormal vaginal discharge.

The good ogress

• The flowering tops are both **astringent and soothing**. They were traditionally used in vaginal douches.
• Internally, their use was advocated **for heavy periods** in young women with anaemia, for diarrhoea and for coughing up blood.

OTHER SPECIES: There are many other common species of deadnettle. The Spotted Deadnettle (*Lamium maculatum*), found in the same habitats as the White Deadnettle, is identifiable by its pink flowers and the white and purple markings on its lower lip. The Yellow Archangel (*L. galeobdolon*) is more commonly found in woodland. Its attractive yellow flowers smell strongly of weasel (*galea* in Greek). Red Deadnettle (*L. purpureum*, below left) is found in fields, gardens and on ploughed soil. Its small purple flowers bloom from the end of winter.

METHOD OF USE

• **INTERNAL: Infusion.** 10 to 30g (¼ to 1oz) of flowering tops per litre (quart) of water. Drink a cup in the morning on an empty stomach and one before the two main meals of the day to regulate menstrual flow.
• **EXTERNAL: Decoction.** 50g (1¾oz) of the whole plant, chopped, per litre of boiling water. Boil for 10 minutes, then cool slightly to use as a warm vaginal douche or gargle.

Description

A perennial, growing to 20 to 60cm (8 to 24in), commonly found along walls, in hedgerows and on the edge of woodland. Common throughout Europe and temperate Asia. The shape and the leaves of the White Deadnettle are similar to the Common Nettle, but it does not sting. Its stems are square and upright, bearing broad opposite leaves with serrated margins. Its double-lipped flowers are grouped in whorls in the leaf axils.

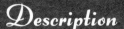

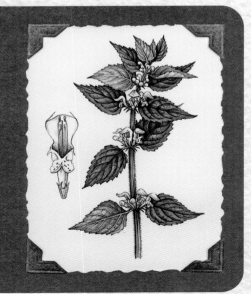

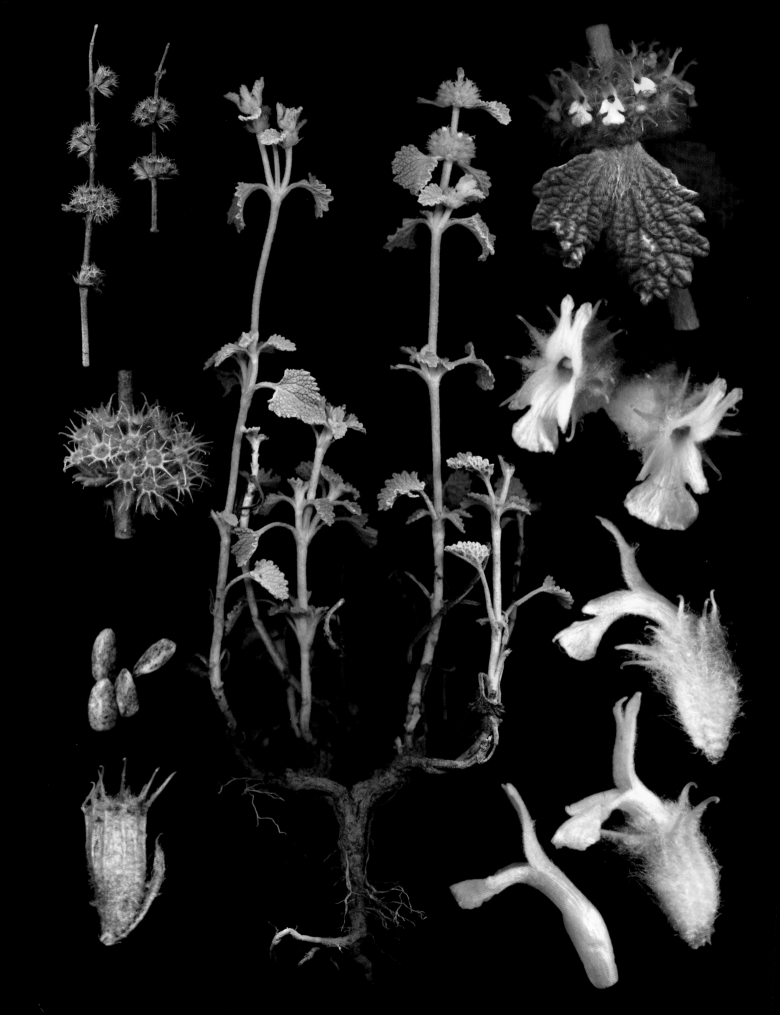

White Horehound

Marrubium vulgare

FAMILY: LAMIACEAE

Active elements:
Flavonoids, diterpenoid lactones (including marrubin), mucilage, aromatic oil.

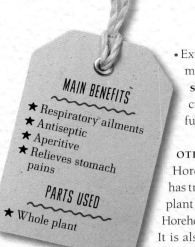

Both the ancient Egyptians and Greeks used White Horehound to treat respiratory tract ailments. In the 1st century, Dioscorides advocated its use for asthma, coughs and tuberculosis. White Horehound has remained an important part of the herbalist's medical chest ever since, particularly for lung conditions.

Valuable for the respiratory tract

• White Horehound **soothes coughs** and can alleviate respiratory difficulties, especially in cases of non-chronic inflammation of the bronchi and airways. It also makes the heart more robust.
• It is a first-rate **expectorant and antiseptic** for bronchial secretions, **thinning mucus and bringing down fevers**.
• Active element marrubin has demonstrated a **choleretic** affect (stimulating the secretion of bile by the liver).
• The plant's **bitterness stimulates the appetite**, which is valuable in cases of flu or bronchitis, when appetite is diminished.
• White Horehound is a good **stomach tonic**, relieving heaviness. It also has a beneficial effect on digestive problems: it relieves bloating by stimulating the evacuation of gas.

• Externally, its **antiseptic** properties make it useful **for cleansing the skin** in the case of ulceration, cuts or sores with swelling, and fungal diseases.

OTHER SPECIES: The wild Silver Horehound (*Marrubium incanum*) has traditionally been used as a herbal plant in the same way as the White Horehound in the Mediterranean basin. It is also used as an anti-arrhythmia agent, to regulate the heartbeat. Other Horehounds are used throughout the world for their medicinal properties. This is the case, for example, with Peregrine Horehound (*Marrubium peregrinum*), originating in Asia Minor, advocated for the treatment of vascular problems.

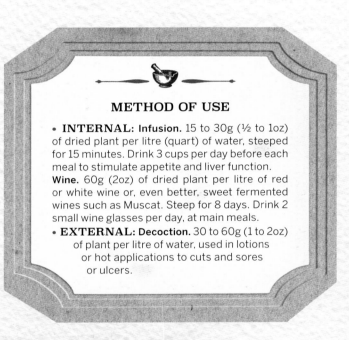

METHOD OF USE

• **INTERNAL:** Infusion. 15 to 30g (½ to 1oz) of dried plant per litre (quart) of water, steeped for 15 minutes. Drink 3 cups per day before each meal to stimulate appetite and liver function.
Wine. 60g (2oz) of dried plant per litre of red or white wine or, even better, sweet fermented wines such as Muscat. Steep for 8 days. Drink 2 small wine glasses per day, at main meals.
• **EXTERNAL:** Decoction. 30 to 60g (1 to 2oz) of plant per litre of water, used in lotions or hot applications to cuts and sores or ulcers.

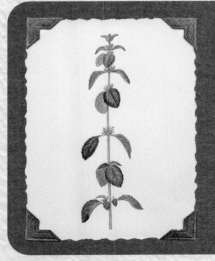

Description

A perennial growing to 30 to 80cm (1 to 2½ft) in height, commonly found on wasteland along pathways. Found in Europe, Asia and Africa and naturalized in America. Its upright, square stem bears round, downy, whitish leaves, and small white flowers grouped in whorls in the leaf axils, that bloom from May to September. The plant gives off a strong, rather unpleasant smell, when crushed.

TOXICITY

Do not exceed the stated doses, White Horehound can cause irregular heartbeat problems if taken to excess.

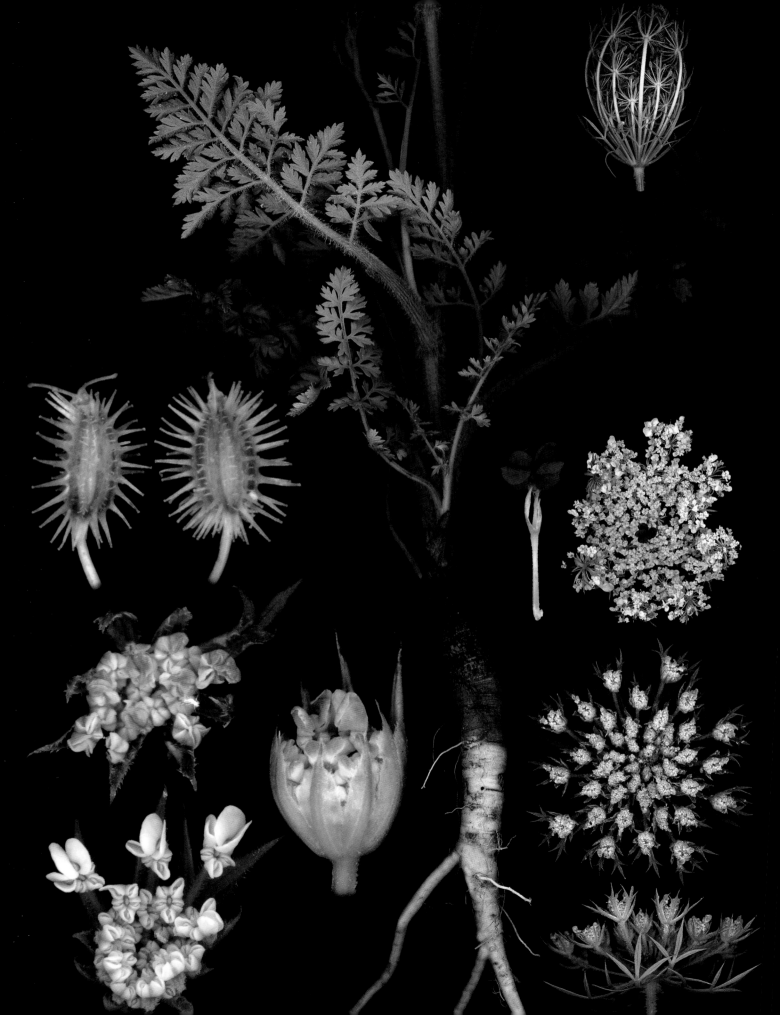

Wild Carrot

Daucus carota
FAMILY: APIACEAE

Active elements:
Root: carbohydrates, pectin, minerals, vitamins (including provitamin A), asparagine. Leaves: falcarinol. Fruits: flavonoids and an aromatic oil rich in asarone, carotol, pinene and limonene.

I n the time of the Gauls, the Wild Carrot was the national vegetable of the French, referred to by Pliny as *pastinaca gallica*, the "food of Gauls". However, it was not until the Middle Ages that the Wild Carrot became a staple in every household. Dioscorides advocated its use to ease menstruation and as a diuretic.

Good digestion and glowing skin
• Wild Carrot is said to **accelerate growth, increase resistance to infections and improve eyesight**. It boosts the action of the liver, so is recommended as a popular remedy for jaundice.

• It **regulates intestinal functions**, treating both constipation and diarrhoea (especially good for children).

• It is also a **diuretic** (increasing the volume of urine and the quantity of uric acid eliminated by 10%). Its juice can be used to alleviate rheumatism, gout and arthritis.

• It **stimulates skin regrowth** and healing and treats skin diseases such as children's impetigo and burns.

• It rejuvenates the skin and **reduces age spots**.

• The leaves have **diuretic properties**.

• Wild Carrot seeds are **aperitive, digestive, carminative and promote lactation**.

• They can also be used to **treat intestinal worms** and promote menstruation.

TOXICITY
The seeds should not be consumed during pregnancy. Wild Carrot juice must be organic, as herbicides and insecticides can be concentrated in the root.

METHOD OF USE
• **INTERNAL:** Carrots should be an essential part of your day-to-day menu, either raw or cooked.
Carrot juice in a blender. Drink the juice of 100g (3½oz) of Carrot in the morning on an empty stomach, as a diuretic, purifier and anti-anaemic.
Carrot soup for babies suffering diarrhoea. Cook 500g (17½oz) of finely chopped Carrot in a litre (quart) of water for at least an hour. Pass through a fine sieve to get rid of the lumps and top up with boiled water to obtain 1 litre of liquid. Bottle-feed with it alone until normal stools return.
Infusion of seeds. One teaspoon per cup to facilitate digestion and lactation.
• **EXTERNAL:** Fresh, finely grated **pulp poultice** on burns, to sooth the pain.
Lotion made with the juice is the best thing to use on dry patches of skin. In terms of beauty treatment, use either face masks made from grated pulp, or daily lotions of carrot juice.

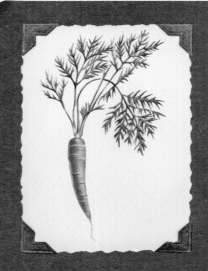

Description
The carrot we use as our day-to-day root vegetable was obtained by selectively planting varieties with orange roots. The only difference between the Wild Carrot and its cultivated relative is the former's thin, white root. Both have hairy, finely divided leaves and small white flowers clustered in umbels which are sometimes pinkish in the centre, and numerous long, divided bracts beneath. At the end of the season, the small, hooked fruit come together in a characteristic "bird's nest". When rubbed between fingers, they give off a strong smell of pear.

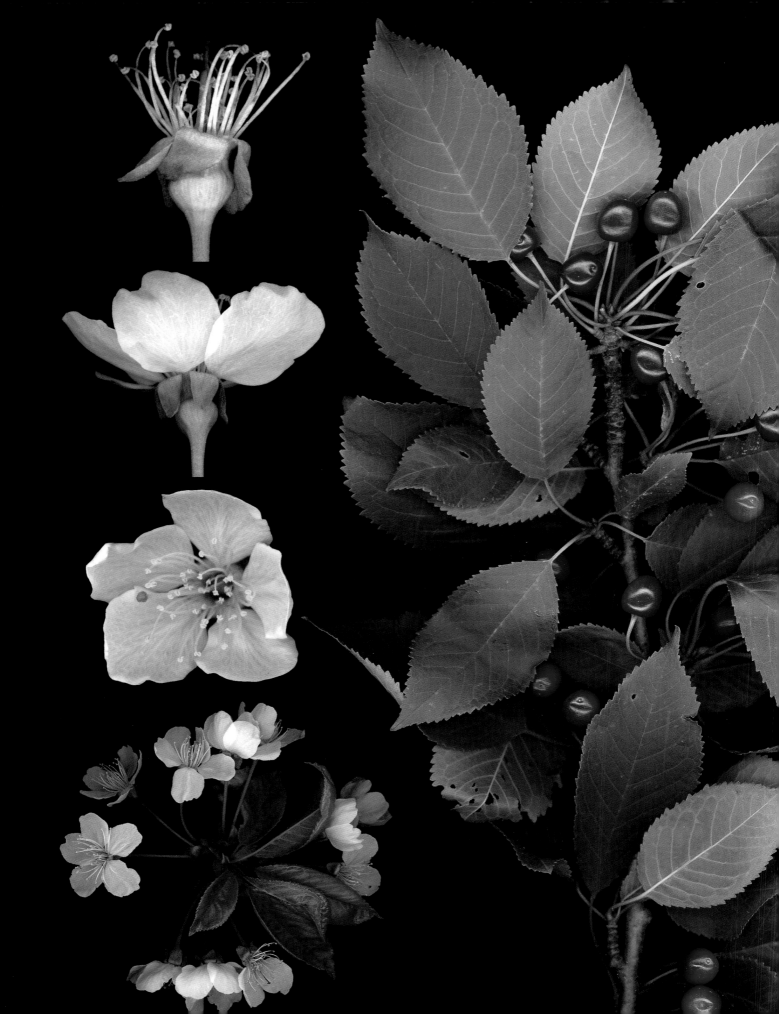

Wild Cherry

Prunus avium

FAMILY: ROSACEAE

Active elements:
Stalks (cherry stalk): tannins, isoflavone glucoside, phenols (salicylic acid in particular). Cherries: rich in organic acids and vitamins.

In the past, bark from the Wild Cherry tree was used to reduce fever or relieve gout. The gum exuded from the trunk and branches was held to be good for arthritis. When dissolved in water, it made a lotion used to treat patches of dry skin.

Delicious and good for you

• The cherry is a **refreshing** and **thirst-quenching** fruit popular in cordials.
• The fruit is recommended for people who are overweight or obese, as well as those suffering from high blood pressure, gout or rheumatism.
• It has a slightly **laxative** effect which makes it **useful in cases**

TOXICITY

Cherry pits, like apricot stones and almonds, contain a cyanogenic heteroside which, when hydrolysed during digestion, produce hydrogen cyanide. This makes them toxic.

of constipation. However, it is not recommended for enteritis sufferers. Some people suffering intestinal problems may have difficulty in digesting cherries. Diabetics can eat them in moderation.
• The **antioxidant** properties of cherries are more marked in acidic varieties than sweet ones.
• The stalks of the fruit have long been used **as a diuretic** in the case of cystitis, nephritis or arthritic problems.

OTHER USES: Cherry stone cushions are a traditional Swiss remedy. When the cushion is heated, the dry cherry pits retain the heat and can be used to relieve aches and pains, and soothe stomach aches, colic in babies or a cricked neck.

VARIETIES: There are many varieties of Cherry. The flesh of the early-fruiting Morello cherries, used to make Kirsch, is less firm than that of the Bigarreau cherry. This appellation (which comes from the streaky appearance of their flesh, described as *bigarré* in French) covers some diverse varieties: Burlat, Napoleon and *Coeur de Pigeon* (Pigeon Heart). The Wild Cherry, or Bird Cherry, is just the wild form of the Sweet Cherry.

OTHER SPECIES: The Sour Cherry (*Prunus cerasus*) produces Morello and other sour cherries; an infusion of its stalks is a diuretic. Maraschino is a liqueur made from the Marasca variety.

METHOD OF USE

• **INTERNAL: Cherry cure. U**sed to lose excessive weight and relieve arthritis. Consists of replacing meals by a pound of cherries for a few days in a row, or for one day a week during the season.
Cherry syrup. Mix 1¼ to 1½kg (2¾ to 3¼lb) of sugar with 1kg (2lb) of cherry juice and heat until boiling. The syrup can then be filtered and kept in a bottle: use as a cordial; simply add water for the perfect drink on a hot day. A great thirst-quencher for anyone with a fever.
Cherry stalk decoction. Soak 220g (8oz) of cherry stalks in cold water for 12 hours to soften, then boil for 10 minutes in a litre (quart) of water. Drink over 1 or 2 days. To add flavour, boil the infusion and pour over 250g (9oz) of fresh cherries, or the same amount of sliced apples. Infuse for 20 more minutes and strain.

Description

This well-known tree, cultivated in all temperate countries, can grow to a height of 8m (26¼ft). It originated in western Asia. Its dark green leaves are oblong and serrated. Its white, five-petalled flowers grow in clusters of three to ten blossoms. The juicy, sweet, aromatic fruit can be used in a variety of preparations.

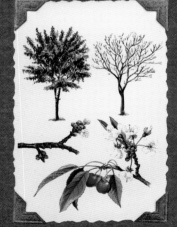

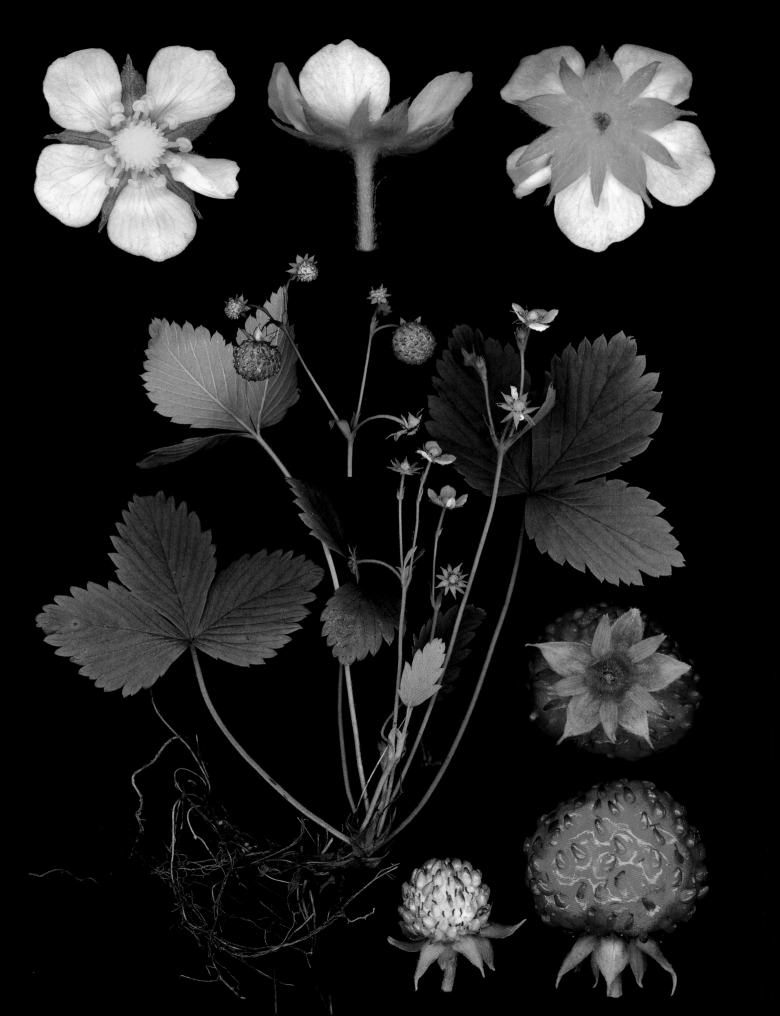

Wild Strawberry

Fragaria vesca

FAMILY: ROSACEAE

Active elements:
Tannins, flavonoids and lots of vitamin C (in the leaves), various sugars and vitamins (in the fruit).

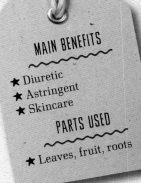
• When used externally, the Wild Strawberry's **skin-beautifying properties** are well renowned.

DID YOU KNOW? The strawberry plant does not bear a fruit in the botanical sense of the word, namely a ripe, fertilized ovary. Instead it produces a "false fruit" formed by the growth of the fleshy base of the flower, covered in "seeds" which are in fact the real fruits.

From Roman times onwards, we know that the Wild Strawberry was a popular fruit, gathered in woodlands throughout Europe. It was cultivated for the first time in the 14th century when Charles V of France had 1,200 Wild Strawberry plants grown in the gardens of the Louvre for the decorative value of their flowers. It was a later royal gardener, Jean de La Quintinye, in the reign of Louis XIV, who "domesticated" the succulent fruit.

Protector of the kidneys and bladder

• The **diuretic** properties of the roots and leaves mean they have long been used to **treat kidney and bladder ailments**. They are also effective in treating rheumatism and gout.

• Their **astringency** renders them an excellent treatment for diarrhoea and enteritis and they can be gargled to **soothe sore throats**.

• As strawberries have a simultaneous **diuretic and laxative** effect, they are recommended for arthritis, rheumatism, stones and other liver-related conditions. Care should be taken as people with a predisposition to hives can suffer itchy welts. Desensitization may be possible by taking a small mouthful of mashed strawberry every day for a week.

METHOD OF USE

• **INTERNAL: Decoction of crushed roots and leaves**. 25g (¾oz) per litre (quart) of water. Boil for 10 minutes and drink freely throughout the day for urinary problems and diarrhoea.
Infusion of leaves alone (same proportions), gathered in spring and dried. Excellent alternative to tea, with diuretic properties.

• **EXTERNAL: Concentrated decoction.** 30 to 50g (1 to 1¾oz) per litre of roots and leaves. Gargle to relieve sore throats or use for diarrhoea.
Strawberry face mask. Simply apply crushed strawberries to the make-up free skin of the face and hold in place with gauze. After 10 minutes, rinse off with rose water. For greasy skin, add a beaten egg white to the strawberry purée. For dry skin, add a teaspoon of sweet almond oil.
Strawberry scrub. An astringent scrub made with strawberry juice, an equal quantity of fresh milk and a few drops of *Eau de Cologne*.

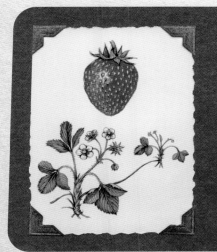

Description

A small perennial which grows in its wild state in woodland and on sunny banks across much of Europe. Found almost everywhere in the northern hemisphere. A hybrid of the North American strawberry and a Chilean strawberry is currently grown for its large berries, which do not match the Wild Strawberry for flavour.

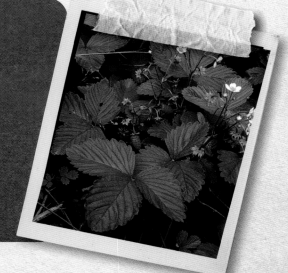

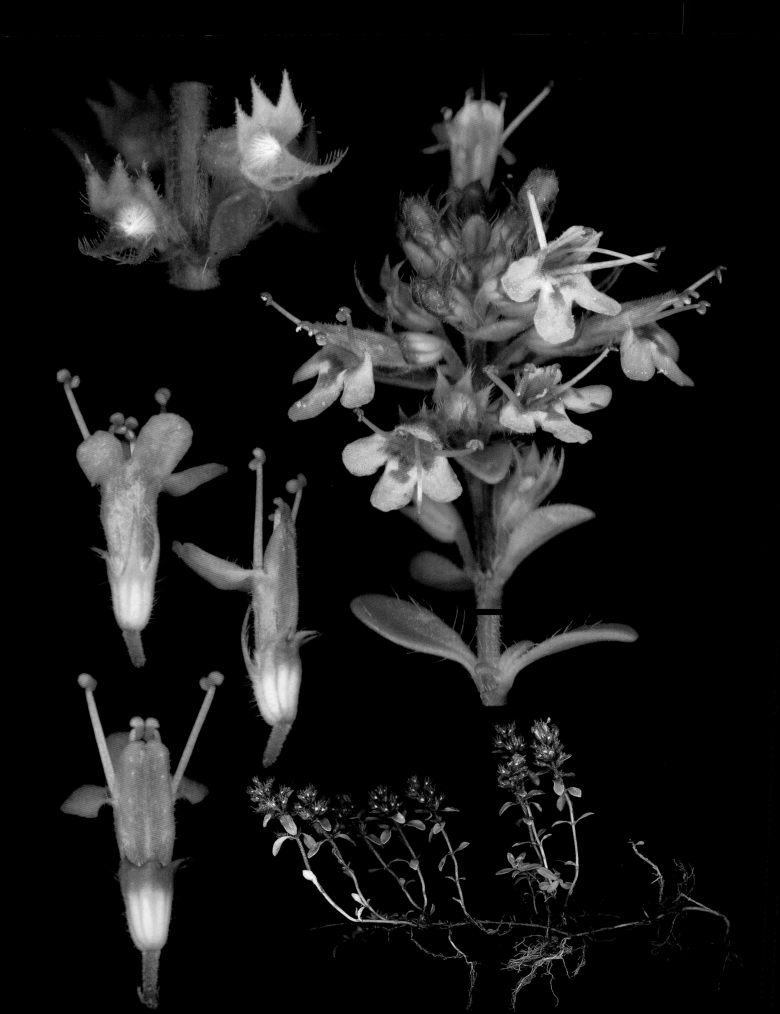

Wild Thyme

Thymus serpyllum

FAMILY: LAMIACEAE

Active elements:

Tannins, flavonoids, caffeic acid and aromatic oil with a composition that varies depending on the chemotype (dominated by thymol, carvacrol, linalool).

W ild Thyme, a close cousin of Garden Thyme, has been used in popular medicine since time immemorial. Culpeper, the 17th-century English botanist, recommended it for coughs, vomiting and internal haemorrhages. In the following century, Linnaeus, the Swedish botanist and physician, used it to relieve headaches.

Kickstart the body

• Wild Thyme is a **stimulant which boosts energy** and physical strength, lifts the spirits and awakens digestive functions. Consequently, it is recommended for nervous asthenia, depression-related fatigue and to treat anaemia in girls as they reach puberty.

• It is both aperitive and **sedative for digestive cramps** and causes expulsion of intestinal gas.

• It provides relief from period pain.

• In addition, it acts as an **antiseptic on the airways and soothes coughs**. It can be used freely to treat convulsive, hacking coughs and asthma. As an expectorant it thins bronchial secretions, so is useful for bronchitis sufferers.

• Essential oil of Wild Thyme is **antibacterial and antiviral**. It can be diffused to purify the air.

• Used externally, Wild Thyme oil (or its essential oil diluted in a massage oil) relieves inflammatory pains, such as those related to **sciatica or headaches**.

• The **antiseptic** infusion is used to treat ulcers, irritations and white discharge (leucorrheoa).

OTHER USES: Wild Thyme is a useful condiment, but pick only those that smell good, and use them raw at the end of cooking.

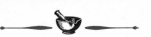

METHOD OF USE

• **INTERNAL: Infusion.** 10 to 20g (¼ to ¾oz) per litre (quart) of boiling water. Drink 3 or 4 cups per day. To stimulate the body and promote digestion. This pleasant infusion is sometimes known as "shepherds' tea" in France.

• **EXTERNAL: Concentrated infusion.** 30 to 50g (1 to 1¾oz) of plant per litre of boiling water. Used in lotions, compresses and douches to treat irritation, ulcers and white discharge.

Wild Thyme oil is prepared by steeping a handful of flowering tops in a litre of olive oil for 3 days in the sun. Strain then add sufficient fresh plant to ensure that the oil is perfumed. Use to treat aches and pains.

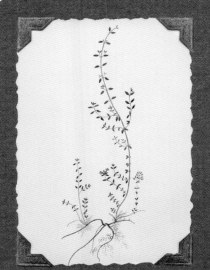

Description

This small, creeping plant, growing to a height of 5 to 20cm (2 to 8in), is similar to Garden Thyme (described earlier) and is commonly found on dry and stony soil, especially limestone. Its thin woody stems creep along the ground, then send up erect shoots, bearing small, opposite leaves that are round and green, and pale or deep-pink flowers, grouped in terminal spikes. The plant gives off a fairly varied smell (ranging from the fresh scent of lemon or *Eau de Cologne* to the smell of rancid butter or earthy mushrooms). It also occasionally has no smell at all.

TOXICITY

The essential oil of Wild Thyme is an irritant in contact with skin and mucosae. It should always be diluted with a vegetable oil (sweet almond, avocado, wheatgerm).

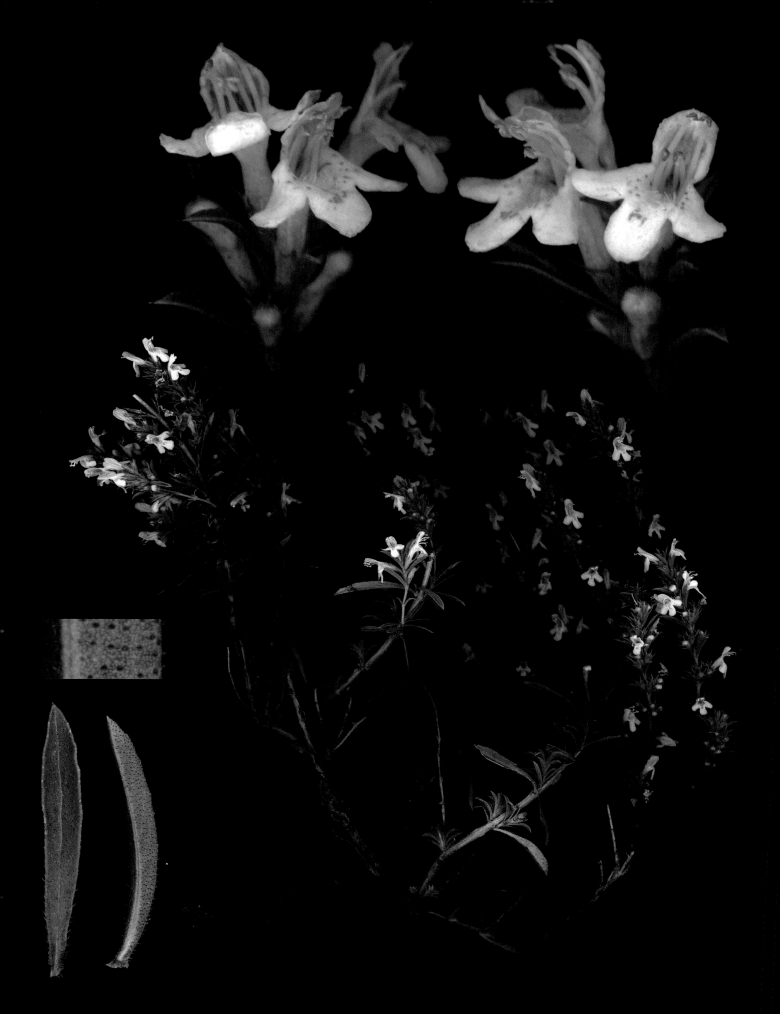

Winter Savory

Satureja montana

FAMILY: LAMIACEAE

Active elements:
Aromatic oil rich in carvacrol and sometimes thymol.

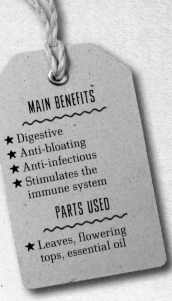

The leaves of Winter Savory have been used as a condiment since ancient times, to add flavour to grilled meat, sauces and vegetables, especially peas and pulses such as haricot beans, as it prevents bloating and gas. Its name in German is *Bohnenkraut*, "bean herb".

Light digestion

• In terms of more specifically medical use, it has digestive properties that help **alleviate painful digestion, stomach cramps** (it is antispasmodic) and nervous contractions, and stimulates a sluggish stomach.
• It is carminative, eliminating flatulence, **promoting the evacuation of gas** and preventing gut fermentation.
• In Germany, Winter Savory is a popular **remedy for diarrhoea**. It is sometimes also used to treat respiratory tract infections.
• Winter Savory can be used to **treat small sores and wounds**, and it makes a good mouthwash for oral hygiene.
• It can also be beneficial **in cases of erectile dysfunction**.
• The essential oil has **anti-infectious properties** and **stimulates the immune system**. It is prescribed for bacterial or parasitic intestinal, pulmonary or cutaneous infections. It is also an antioxidant.

• Winter Savory, along with a number of other aromatic plants, is one of the ingredients of the "vulnerary alcoholate" known as "Arquebusade Water".

OTHER USES: Winter Savory is used in Provence, France, under the name *pebre d'aï* (donkey pepper), to flavour rabbit, beans and peas, crayfish and fresh goat's cheese.

OTHER SPECIES: Summer Savory (*Satureja hortensis*) is mostly grown in gardens and is an annual plant, originating in the eastern Mediterranean region. It can be distinguished from Winter Savory by its herbaceous stems, softer more downy leaves, pink flowers and less pronounced flavour. It is likewise used in cooking and infusions.

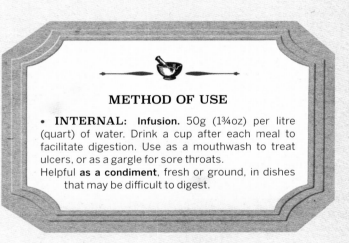

METHOD OF USE

• **INTERNAL:** Infusion. 50g (1¾oz) per litre (quart) of water. Drink a cup after each meal to facilitate digestion. Use as a mouthwash to treat ulcers, or as a gargle for sore throats.
Helpful **as a condiment**, fresh or ground, in dishes that may be difficult to digest.

TOXICITY

Essential oil of Winter Savory should not be used pure because it is caustic. Contact with skin and mucosae are to be avoided. It is also toxic for the liver: always mix it with another essential oil that protects the liver (such as lemon oil).

Description

A sub-shrub growing to a height of between 10 and 40cm (4 to 16in). Found in southern Europe and North Africa. It is sometimes grown as a condiment. Its woody stems bear small, lance-shaped leaves which are tough and glossy. The corolla of its flowers is white, or occasionally pink, gathered on long terminal spikes, interspersed with leaves. Simply brushing against the plant is enough to release a strong, aromatic scent. The leaves sting the tongue if chewed.

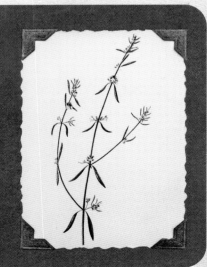

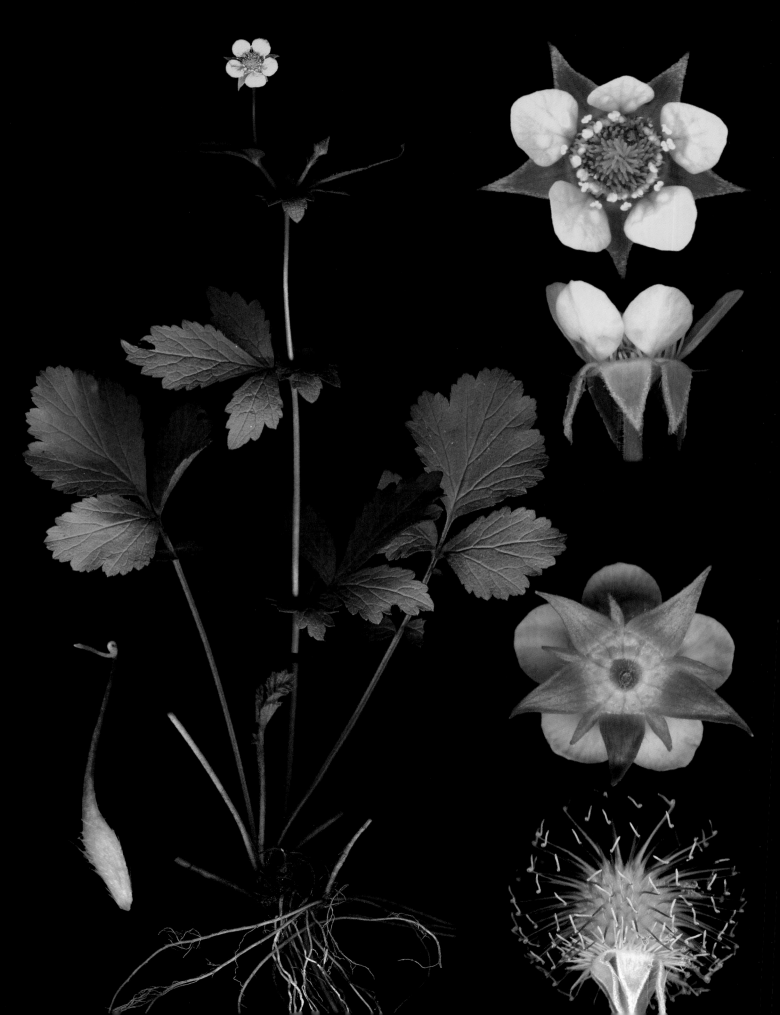

Wood Avens

Geum urbanum

FAMILY: ROSACEAE

Active elements:
Tannins, phenolic heterosides (such as gein) and an aromatic oil rich in eugenol (the principal component of the distilled essential oil of cloves).

W ood Avens was used in the 17th century to treat chest pains and to flush out the stomach. It was subsequently used as an astringent, tonic and antipyretic (against fever). Henri Leclerc, the French physician and renowned medical herbalist, particularly advocated its use for stomach pains accompanied by flatulence and for the treatment of diarrhoea. It was also used to treat haemorrhages, the coughing of blood and involuntary ejaculation.

Extraordinary powers

- The **astringent** powers of Wood Avens are due to its tannins and make it useful in treating diarrhoea and dysentery.
- The rhizomes and roots can be used to **soothe gastric ulcers**.
- They can also be used as a **mouthwash** to treat ulcers and to strengthen gums, as a **gargle** for sore throats, and in the form of a **douche** to treat vaginal discharge.

- The roots contain an oil that is rich in eugenol (a substance used in the production of dental wound dressings) which endows them with **antiseptic and anaesthetic properties** that are effective in soothing toothache, like cloves.

OTHER USES: Wood Avens root is an extraordinary condiment, which can be used as the basis of sauces for cereals, fish or game. It spices up vegetables and adds flavour to syrups, sorbets and drinks. In northern Europe, its roots were used to flavour beer, or steeped in wine with orange zest. Only the smaller roots are used, not the thick rhizome, which is astringent.

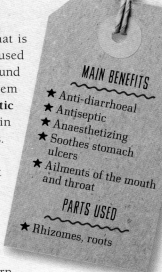

MAIN BENEFITS
- ★ Anti-diarrhoeal
- ★ Antiseptic
- ★ Anaesthetizing
- ★ Soothes stomach ulcers
- ★ Ailments of the mouth and throat

PARTS USED
- ★ Rhizomes, roots

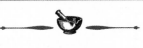

METHOD OF USE

- **INTERNAL: Infusion.** 30 to 40g (1 to 1½oz) of root per litre (quart) of water. Drink ½ litre per day between meals for diarrhoea. **Wine.** Infuse 500g (1lb) per litre of wine. Drink 3 small glasses (100g (3½oz)) per day for the same conditions.
- **EXTERNAL: Decoction.** 50g (1¾oz) of root per litre of water boiled for 10 minutes. In mouthwashes, gargles or enemas.

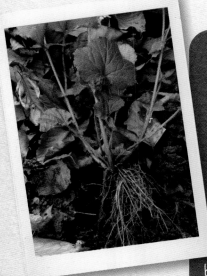

The main active ingredients of Wood Avens are concentrated in the roots.

Description

This perennial plant growing to 40cm (16in) is commonly found in cool woodlands, roadsides and hedgerows. Its dissected leaves bear small leaflets interspersed with larger ones, and end in a large lobe with a serrated margin. Its yellow flowers, colour aside, are similar to those of the strawberry plant. The fruit has burrs which aid its dispersal by catching onto the fur of passing animals and sticking to clothes. The short, thick rhizome (horizontal stem) is covered in light-brown root hairs, which when crushed between the fingers, exudes a strong smell of cloves mixed with smoke, with some delightful floral notes.

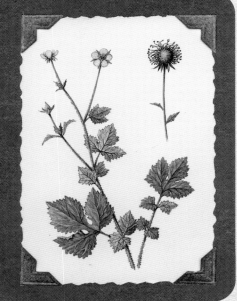

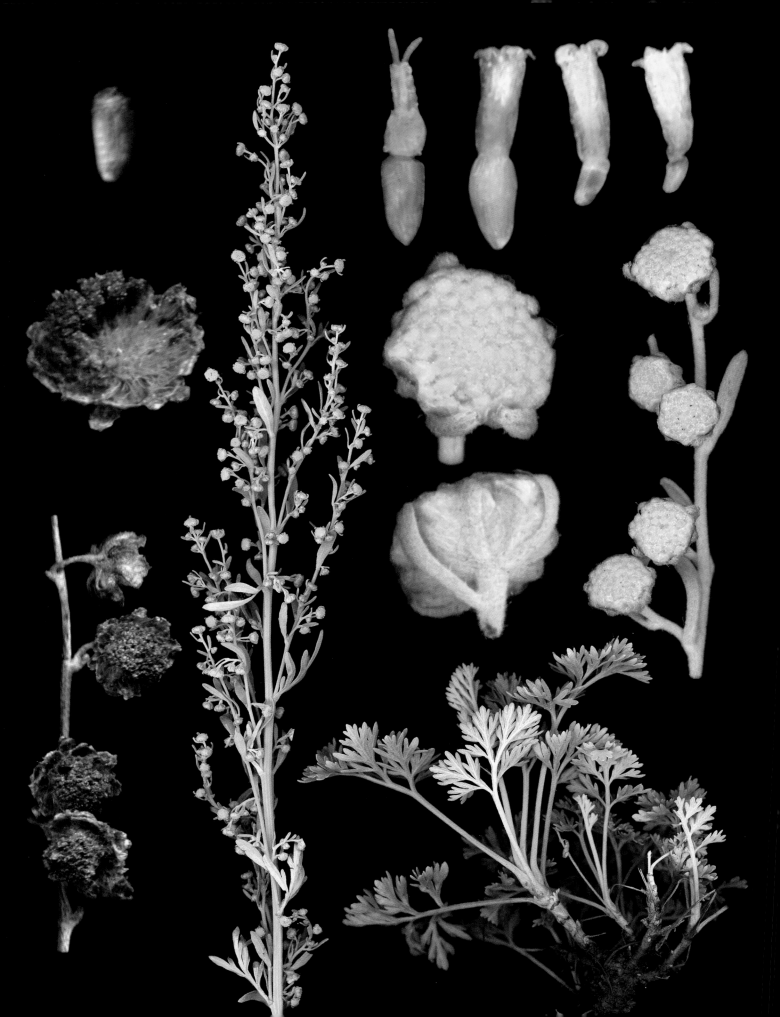

Wormwood

Artemisia absinthium

FAMILY: ASTERACEAE

Active elements:

Aromatic essence which is generally rich in thujone, a compound that exists in numerous chemotypes: *o*-cymene, beta-thujone, sabinyl acetate and chrysanthemyl acetate. Wormwood also contains flavonoids and sesquiterpene lactones, including absinthin.

While historically considered a symbol of bitterness —*absinthium* means "without sweetness"—the plant was once considered a panacea. Cuneiform tablets recounting the Epic of Gilgamesh found in Assyria and Babylonia testify that Wormwood was used to tackle a sluggish stomach. The Ancient Egyptians used it as an anthelmintic and to treat gastric diseases. The Druids were also aware of Wormwood's anthelmintic properties, and made it an offering to the Gods. In the time of the Gauls, the men used it to treat rheumatism, while the women took it to promote menstruation.

METHOD OF USE

- **INTERNAL: Infusion.** 5 to 6g of flowering tops per litre (quart) of boiling water. As a tonic, drink 2 or 3 cups per day. As an anthelmintic, take in the morning on an empty stomach, half-an-hour before breakfast, for 4 or 5 days.
Wine. Steep 20 to 30g (¾ to 1oz) per litre for 8 days. Drink a liqueur glassful before each meal, as an aperitif and digestif.
Beer. Steep 10g (¼oz) of Wormwood in a large glass of beer for 12 hours. Take in the morning on an empty stomach, 5 days in a row, as an anthelmintic.
Powder. Grind the dried plant in a mortar. Take 2 to 3g of this powder as an antipyretic or anthelmintic in a hot drink, mixed with honey, or a prune compote. This dose can also be mixed with 2g of liquorice powder and 0.5g of green aniseed powder.
  - **EXTERNAL:** Use the infused plant in a warm **poultice**. Place on the stomach as an antihelmintic for children.

Tonic, stimulant and digestive

- Wormwood leaves and flowers make an excellent, stimulating tonic which **piques the appetite while enhancing digestion**; it is therefore recommended for people with anaemia and for convalescents.
- In the past, Wormwood was widely used to treat sea sickness, and is a valuable **anti-vomiting agent**.
- Like many bitter plants, Wormwood helps to reduce fevers (antipyretic), and was used in the past to treat bouts of malarial fever, either on its own or in combination with Common Centaury, Gentian and Willow bark.
- Wormwood **promotes menstruation and reduces period pain** when caused by uterine inertia. This property, together with its tonic action, means it has traditionally been recommended to pale and weak women, and adolescents tired out by their studies.
- Wormwood is an effective **treatment for worms**, especially roundworm and pinworm; however, its bitter taste must be masked before it can be tolerated by children.

TOXICITY

Wormwood is the basis for the famous absinthe drink so dear to the painter Verlaine. The disastrous effect on drinkers of the "green fairy" was said to be the plant's thujone content. However, that the liqueur's toxicity was due to thujone is now contested. The anti-absinthe campaign was in fact orchestrated by French winemakers to bring down this competitor. The aniseed-based aperitifs that took its place contained anethole, a substance whose neurotoxic effects are now widely known. Thujone does give Wormwood essential oil a convulsive and abortive effect.

Description

A perennial plant growing to a height of 40cm (16in) to 1m (3¼ft), commonly found in uncultivated areas. It is native to Europe, northern and central Asia and North Africa. The stems grow in dense tufts. The divided leaves have a silvery tinge. The numerous small, greenish-yellow flower heads, arranged in clusters, appear from June to September. The whole plant gives off a strong aromatic scent. Its taste is extremely bitter.

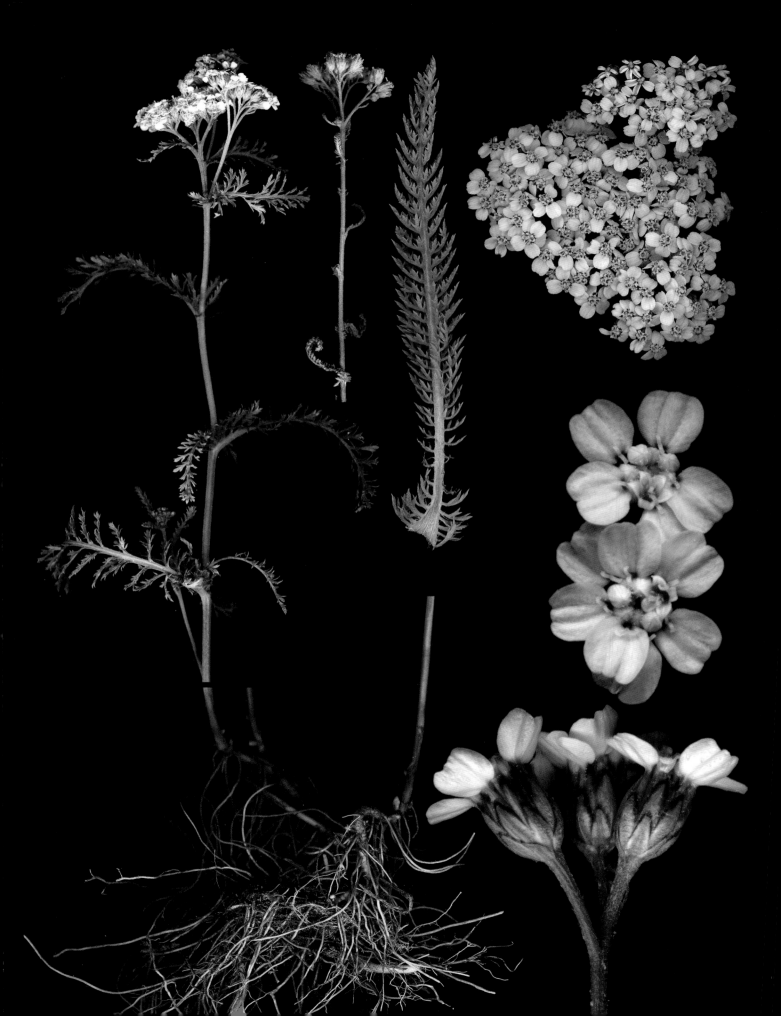

Yarrow

Achillea millefolium

FAMILY: ASTERACEAE

Active elements:

Tannins, flavonoids, sesquiterpene lactones, alkaloids (including achillin), triterpene, polyine, coumarin, salicylic acid, aromatic essence (including camphor, linalool, sabinene and proazulene).

Yarrow's medicinal reputation dates back to prehistory. A strong concentration of Yarrow pollen was discovered in the Shanidar cave, in Iraq, along with the remains of several Neanderthal people. This plant must, therefore, have formed part of the rudimentary pharmacopoeia of the Neanderthal people more than 50,000 years ago. Much later, the Greek herbalist Dioscorides wrote that Yarrow demonstrated, "incomparable effectiveness in staunching wounds, and old or recent ulcers". In turn, Hippocrates recommended it for treating bleeding haemorrhoids. Yarrow's main medical use over the years has been for the treatment of both internal and external bleeding. In the 19th century, Jean-François Cazin and Teissier, also advocated it for conditions affecting the venous system (varicose veins) and uterine cramps.

Healing and soothing

• The leaves are astringent making them suitable for **healing injuries of all kinds**, especially grazes and chapped skin. Their anti-inflammatory properties soothe itching.
• They can also be used to **reduce heavy menstrual flow**, treat haemorrhoids and coughing up of blood.

• The flowering tops can be used as a bitter tonic, **aperitive and digestive**. They are recommended by the German Commission E to treat lack of appetite, digestive disorders such as bloating, trapped wind, flatulence and abdominal pain.
• Like the leaves, they help regulate the menstrual cycle and **relieve painful periods**. Yarrow is recommended in sitz baths for women's pelvic pain.

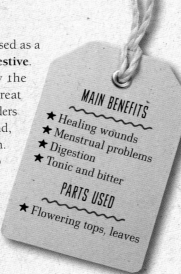

METHOD OF USE

• **INTERNAL: Infusion.** 30 to 50g (1 to 1¾oz) of flowering tops per litre (quart) of boiling water. Drink 2 or 3 cups per day for digestive problems or painful periods.
• **EXTERNAL: Juice** from a well-washed plant applied to a recent cut. Staunches blood flow and activates the healing process.
Decoction. 60g (2oz) of flowering tops per litre of boiling water. Excellent for cleaning wounds or soaking poultices for haemorrhoids.
Wine. Boil 40 to 50g (1½ to 1¾oz) of plant per litre of wine. It acts as a powerful disinfectant and can be used to heal chapped skin, chilblains and cracks, and to dress skin ulcers.

OTHER USES: Tender young Yarrow shoots add texture to mixed salads. The leaves can be chopped as a condiment in the same way as parsley or blanched in water and then quickly sautéed in butter, as was customary in England. They add flavour to *cervoise*, the traditional French barley beer. The flower heads can be used to perfume desserts.

DID YOU KNOW? The Latin name for Yarrow, *Achillea*, is borrowed from Achilles, the hero of the Trojan War in Greek mythology. He is said to have used Yarrow leaves to heal the wounds of Telephus, the King of Mysia.

Description

A perennial plant growing to a height of 20 to 70cm (8in to 2¼ft) very commonly found in meadows, wasteland and along paths. Found in Europe, Asia and North America, where it is naturalized. Its straight, stiff, almost woody stem bears many finely segmented leaves, reminiscent of a scruffy-looking marigold. The white flower heads (sometimes pink in mountainous areas) are in fact mini-florets growing in a flat-topped cluster. When crushed, the foliage gives off a pleasant but powerful smell of camphor.

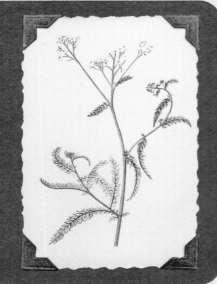

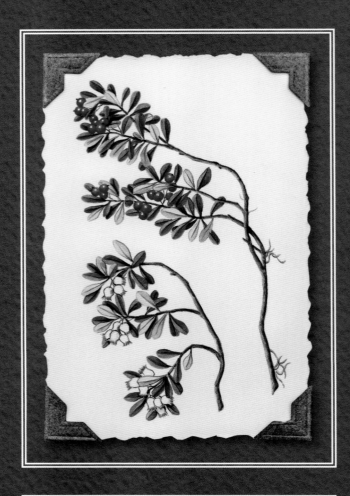

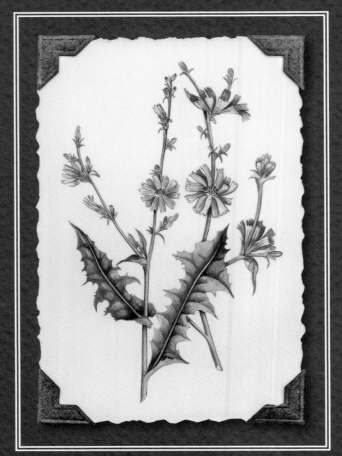

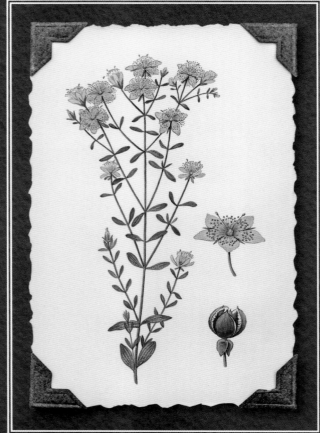

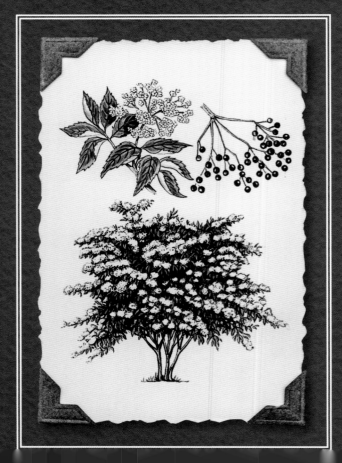

A SMALL PRACTICAL GUIDE

FOR BUDDING HERBALISTS

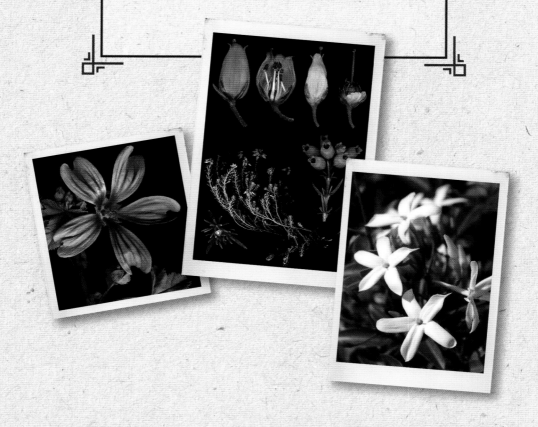

Gathering medicinal plants

Cultivate or collect?

Medicinal plants can be cultivated or gathered in the wild. The former category might include Lavender or Garden Thyme, while St. John's-wort and Chaste Tree generally belong to the second category. Nettle could belong to both categories. Having your own garden of medicinal plants means you have fresh herbs at your disposal, of trusted provenance. However, there is little point in growing your own medicinal plants if they are going to bring traces of fertilizers and pesticides into your body. Therefore it is important to follow the rules of organic growing. In turn, collecting medicinal plants in the wild is a unique and thrilling experience for anyone with an interest in plants. You may sometimes have to walk for hours, far from the noises of civilization to find the plant you are looking for.

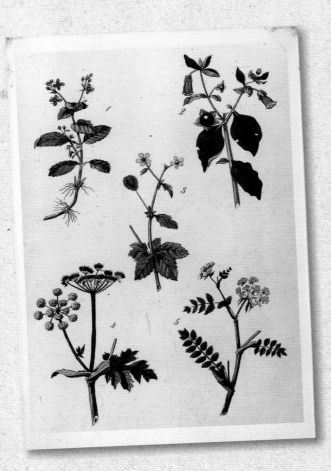

Ethical guidance for responsible plant hunters

• Nature is not a supermarket! Many medicinal plants are becoming rare, or are even on their way to extinction due to thoughtless picking. Consequently, any collecting of medicinal plants must be done in a framework that respects others and the environment.

• If it is a **public** place (a park or nature reserve), make sure that you are legally permitted to gather plants. National parks often have very specific regulations governing the picking of plants.

• If the place where the plants are growing is **private**, make sure you seek permission. If you are polite, most people will be more open to the idea than you might imagine. Some may even take an interest.

• Make sure you are well aware of **protected species** in your region. Regional parks often display a list on their websites. You must likewise learn to recognize **dangerous plants**. Any medicinal plants that you pick should be growing at a safe distance from harmful ones.

• Pick **well away from footpaths** where possible. First and foremost this is because plants are often soiled by dogs and other animals (both wild and domestic) in places where there is higher footfall. Some edible plants can become poisonous when infested with parasites such as liver fluke (often found in wild Watercress) or echinococcosis, a parasitic disease that can be transmitted via dog or fox faeces. On this basis, Bilberry and other berries should not be picked below a height of 80cm (2½ft). For wild flowers that you are planning to eat raw, only pick those that grow above ditches, for example, where foxes and dogs would find it difficult to access.

• The place where you pick should not be visible to other people: bear in mind that most walkers do not leave the path. They should be allowed to enjoy the untouched biological and aesthetic diversity of the flora in your region.

• If the same medicinal indications are given for several plants, **make sure you choose the most common among them locally**. This means not turning your nose up at plants found in abundance, such as Dandelion, Nettle and Yarrow.

• **Be methodical and moderate** in your collecting. It is not worth picking huge amounts of plants if they are just going to end up in the compost. Take a few and come back for more if you need them. Only pick the useful parts: such as leaves, flower or bark, without damaging the rest of the plant. For example, if you only need the flowers, do not cut entire stalks.

• **Do not pull up plants** unless you specifically want to use the part that grows underground. Only do so for species that are widespread and abundant locally.

• Always leave at least **a third of the plants that you find** *in situ*. Just pick a few leaves from each plant, depending on how big it is. By contrast, you can collect as much Dandelion and Nettle as you like, as they are robust species that grow in abundance.

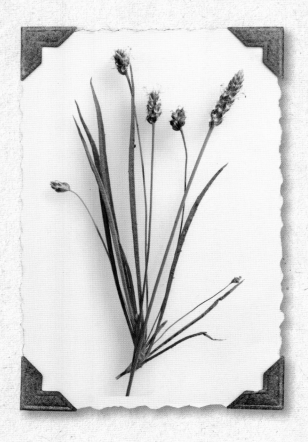

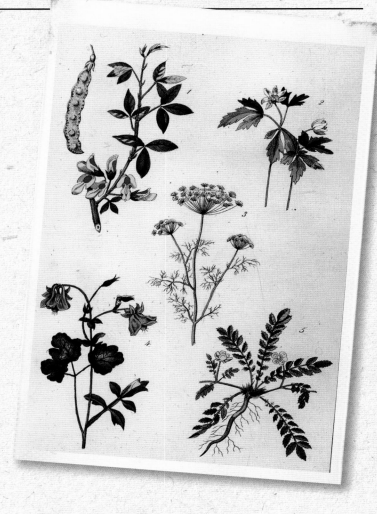

The harvesting calendar

Some plants, such as Rosemary, can be gathered practically all year round, but most should be harvested at a specific point in their life cycle in order to be used immediately or preserved. This optimum moment varies, naturally, depending on the plant species, but it also depends on the part of the plant that is to be gathered.

Some medicinal plants, where it is the flower that is used, have a very brief flowering period (Wild Cherry blossom, for example). By contrast, others might flower for two months or more (such as Great Mullein).

Some factors might amend the harvesting calendar: periodically, for example, a year might be exceptionally warm and vegetation in general may be more "advanced" than what would normally be expected. This is becoming more and more common as a result of global warming. Some regions also enjoy their own mild microclimate, where everything blooms earlier and for longer than in colder areas, where winter starts early and ends late.

Harvesting different parts of the plant

The following are general guidelines only.
Wood can be gathered throughout the winter.

Roots, tubers, rhizomes and bulbs can be gathered in autumn for annual plants and in springtime for others, in other words after the plant has accumulated its reserves and before they have been mobilized.

Stems should be gathered in autumn, when they are still tender, but the leaves are no longer in an active phase.

Leaves should be gathered at the height of their development, but before flower buds form as this will reduce their content of active principles (for example, Mint, Nettle, Dandelion).

Flowers are best harvested just before they fully bloom and certainly before they are fertilized (for example, Arnica, Cornflower, Garden Nasturtium, Colt's-foot).

Flowering tops should be harvested just as flowers start to bloom and always before the seeds have formed (for example, Wormwood, Mugwort, Hyssop).

Buds should be gathered at the end of the winter or in early spring, as soon as the sap starts rising in the tree's branches.

Fleshy fruit should be harvested just as it ripens (for example, Bilberry, Raspberry).

Seeds should be gathered when they are fully ripe, when the plant begins to dry out. This is not always easy to judge as in general they fall quite quickly (for example, Caraway, Fennel).

Collecting
MONTH BY MONTH

The following calendar is
a general guide for European regions.

JANUARY

roots: rest-harrow (can be gathered all year round)

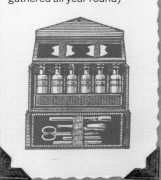

FEBRUARY

buds: silver birch, oak
bark: silver birch
flowers: colt's-foot

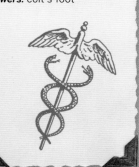

MARCH

buds: poplar, pine
bark: oak
leaves: dandelion
branches, young shoots: strawberry tree

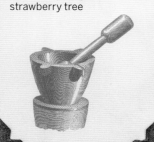

APRIL

buds: pine
leaves: cowslip, bearberry, ivy, hogweed
flowers: cowslip
whole plant: fumitory, white deadnettle

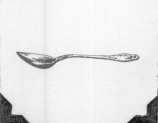

MAY

roots: wood avens, gentian (regulated)
leaves and flowers: herb robert
flower heads: wormwood, white horehound, watercress
leaves: lemon balm
flowers: pasqueflower, borage

JUNE

leaves or flowers: mugwort, arnica, borage, chicory, poppy, dog rose, fennel, germander, lavender, mallow, ribbed melilot, common hazel, plantain, rosemary, elder, thyme, verbena
fruits: cherries, strawberries, raspberries

JULY

leaves and flower heads:
flowers: common agrimony, common centaury, greater celandine, hyssop, immortelle, lavender (from mid-June to late August, depending on variety and region), marjoram, lemon balm, mint, yarrow, St. John's-wort, oregano, meadowsweet, rosemary, winter savory, garden or wild thyme, lime
flowers: great mullein, cornflower, borage, poppy, mallow
seeds: oat, hogweed, glandular plantain

AUGUST

Many of the plants listed for July can also be gathered in August, with the addition of the following:
leaves: common agrimony, mint, bogbean
flowers: borage
fruits and seeds: caraway, fennel, nuts
cones: hops

SEPTEMBER

roots: chicory, fennel, butcher's broom, gentian (harvesting regulated), soapwort, silverweed
flowers: heather
fruits: bilberry, dog rose (rose hips), figs, pomegranate, sweet chestnuts, hazelnuts, grapes, elder

OCTOBER

roots: comfrey, wild strawberry, soapwort
fruits and seeds: almond, strawberry tree, garden nasturtium, sweet chestnuts, flax, juniper, blackseed

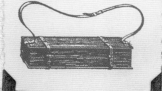

NOVEMBER

bark: oak
roots: butcher's broom, silverweed

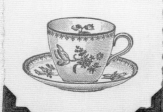

DECEMBER

roots: rest-harrow (can be gathered all year round)

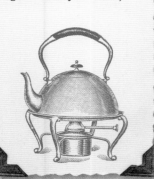

Harvesting and preserving

There are rules to follow that ensure the plant's optimal content of active principles is preserved to the greatest extent possible, so that they retain all their medicinal properties.

When to harvest plants

Plants are best collected when the weather is dry and warm: those that are wet from rain or dew can spoil, moulder and ferment, losing their medicinal value in the process. Morning is the best time, but evening, before it gets cooler, is also fine.

How to harvest plants

As far as possible, it is best to harvest wild plants from the least frequented places. Plants that are to be dried **should under no circumstances be washed**; so those that gather dust on busy roadsides, or which could have been inadvertently sprayed with fertilizer on field edges, should be avoided. Gather wild plants **well away from any sources of pollution**: avoid roadsides, industrial or urban wasteland, stagnant or polluted water, as well as non-organic fields (rapeseed fields, orchards) because of pesticides and fertilizers. Remember that medicinal plants grown under conventional rather than organic farming, such as commonly sold vegetables, have been chemically fertilized and may have undergone a range of phytosanitary treatments, sometimes even after they have been harvested.

While harvesting, **remove extraneous material** (moss, leaves, twigs) as you go, so you only keep the plant matter that you want: it is far more difficult to separate it at a later stage. Check that you have not got any other plants that you have picked by mistake (the accidental inclusion of a dangerous plant can have serious consequences).

Where possible, try and avoid mixing plants of different species as you are collecting. The best solution is to ensure you have a number of different bags, preferably made of paper or cloth. **Make sure you do not crush plants** by cramming them into bags or containers: this may cause them to wilt or trigger fermentation. Once the bags are full, it is better to put them in a large wicker basket than risk crushing them in a backpack. **The roots** are the only parts of the plant that can, and must, be washed carefully under running water, to remove all traces of soil.

How to dry plants

Other than plants that are used fresh, those that you wish to preserve need to be dried carefully. This drying process must be done quickly to ensure that the plants do not spoil, by starting to ferment and losing their active principles. Plants can be laid out to dry on trays or racks (of a fine nylon mesh, for example) so the air can circulate freely. You can also hang them up in garlands by threading them onto yarn or string, however this is time consuming. Ideally, they should be dried in shade during warm weather, somewhere large and well-ventilated like an attic, barn or shed. In rainy areas, the drying process can be started in a very low oven, with the door slightly open, then leaving the plants to desiccate fully on racks or trays in a dry, well-ventilated attic or shed. The fleshy organs of a plant would ideally be dried by this process, but to ensure they do not spoil, or indeed cook, the temperature of the oven must not exceed 20 to 40°C.

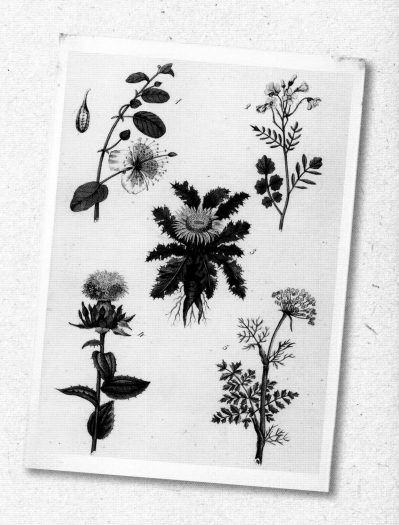

The **drying process** will vary according to the different parts of the plant. Water is not distributed in the same way, or in the same proportions, across the plant's different organs.

• *Roots and rhizomes*: remove any damaged parts, wash carefully, then wipe dry; cut into slices, chunks or chips. Leave to dry in the sun, or in a low oven.

• *Stems, bark and wood*: leave to dry in the sun, in fresh, dry air, or in a low oven.

• *Leaves and whole plants*: spread out on trays, in the shade, in a warm, well-ventilated location. Remove stalks from leaves; this job can be done before or after drying.

• *Flowers and flowering tops*: the drying process can be tricky (as is the case with some aromatic leaves: Verbena or Mint, for example). It is best to dry them on trays in the shade, at temperatures of 20 to 25°C, taking care to cover them with greaseproof paper, to preserve their colour.

• *Fleshy fruit* (such as Juniper berries): leave to dry for a long time in the sun or a low oven.

• *Seeds*: spread out on a sheet of paper to air dry, turning frequently.

How to store dried plants

When all trace of humidity has gone, lay the dried plants separately in containers marked with the name of the plant and the date. Ensure that the containers are clean, do not retain any smell from previous contents and are air-tight. Plants bought in bulk, which are in simple paper bags, should be stored in the same way, in air-tight containers.

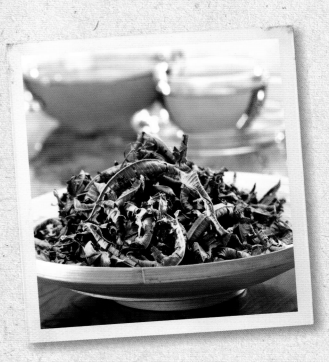

How to use medicinal plants

Traditional preparations

The three basic preparations are **infusion**, **decoction** and **maceration**.

The infusion and the decoction generally use water as the means of extraction and therefore mainly contain water-soluble substances.

INFUSION. Involves pouring boiling water over plants (or placing plants in the recipient containing the boiling water) at the precise moment when the water starts boiling. The container should then be covered and the contents left to infuse: the result is an infusion. Infusion time varies, depending on the type of plant: from 10 minutes to 1 hour.

DECOCTION. The plant is chopped into small pieces and heated in the water until it boils. The length of time it will then be left to boil will depend on the species, but in general between 10 and 30 minutes. It is then strained, pressing hard to extract the maximum active principles. Decoction works best with the bark, roots, stems and fruit.

MACERATION. Very simply, this preparation is obtained by immersing plants in some kind of liquid, without heating. This liquid may be an alcohol (for example, Rosemary alcoholate), oil (for example, oily maceration of St. John's-wort), or even wine (Gentian wine). Contact time is generally longer, up to a month.

IMPORTANT. These different means of preparing plants have different effects. It is important to learn to distinguish between them as the composition and concentration of the various active principles will vary. For example, an infusion of Lime flowers, which makes the most of their aromatic oil has a calmative, sedative effect, while the decoction releases flavonoids which in turn thin the blood. The difference in effect is significant, but the only difference in preparation is the extra boiling time.

Uses

The above three basic preparations, which are the ones most commonly given in recipes, can be used in different ways.

ORAL ADMINISTRATION. The usual way of taking infusions and tinctures.

GARGLE AND MOUTHWASH. Holding a few sips of the lukewarm liquid in the mouth, then swilling it around or gargling it to ensure contact with the necessary parts: throat, tonsils, lining of mouth. Always spat out, never swallowed.

LOTION. Rubbed lightly on the area requiring care, using a soft cloth or a piece of cotton wool soaked in the prepared liquid.

COMPRESS. Applied to the area requiring care in the form of a compress soaked in the liquid and held in place for a few minutes. A compress differs from lotion in that the latter is just wiped over the area in question, while a compress is held in place.

BATH. Immersion of the whole body, or relevant part of the body, in a liquid prepared for this purpose. For example, a soothing Lime bath is a full-body bath, while a sitz bath or foot bath are for specific areas of the body. A cold bath is one where the temperature is approximately 10 to 20°C; a tepid bath is 25 to 30°C; while a warm bath (which should only be administered with great care), is 30 to 40°C. To prepare a plant-based bath, first make a concentrated decoction comprising at least 3 to 4 litres (quarts) of the plant in question or a specific mixture of plants. Leave to infuse for around an hour, then strain the decoction, pressing down hard, and pour it into the bath water, having first checked the temperature.

DOUCHE. The liquid is administered directly into the natural cavities using a syringe (ear) or a douche (vagina). The liquid used is an infusion or decoction made with astringent, emollient or aromatic plants; it should be administered at close to body temperature, namely approximately 37°C.

Other means of preparation and traditional uses

In addition to the three classic methods of preparing medicinal plants, by infusion, decoction and maceration, plants can also be used in the form of powder, poultices, fumigation, tinctures and extracts.

POWDER. Dried plants (whole plants or leaves, seeds, stalks, roots and bark) are crushed in a pestle and mortar, or in a mill, then sifted. The powder obtained can be added to food (jam or other conserves, for example), processed into tablets, or put into capsules to be swallowed. Plant powders still contain almost all the plant's active principles, with the exception of any volatile substances which disappear. They are easy to administer but are less stable and less resistant to oxidation than the whole plant. They also contain cellulose which can attenuate the activity of the active principles.

POULTICE. Consists of applying wet preparations, in the form of a soft paste (a Flax flour poultice, for example) or poultices of grated or crushed plants (Carrot pulp poultice, for example), directly to the skin. Poultices can also be made with the plants used in an infusion or decoction, placing them between two pieces of cloth to form a pad that is then applied directly to the area requiring treatment. Poultices can be emollient, maturative (accelerate suppuration), restorative, calmative and rubefacient (skin reddening). They are generally applied warm, at 35 to 40°C. However, soothing poultices can be applied tepid or cold when the area to be treated is painful or inflamed.

FUMIGATION AND INHALATION. The plants are boiled or burned so their therapeutic properties can be enjoyed in the form of the vapours or fumes produced. The vapours from aromatic plants that are boiled or placed in boiling water (Eucalyptus, Lavender, Thyme, for example) are strong antiseptics. These beneficial vapours can be inhaled directly by bending over the saucepan, once removed from the source of heat, placing a towel over the head to form a tent and inhaling.

TINCTURES are obtained by macerating the dried plant in alcohol, in proportions of approximately 1g of dried plant to obtain 5g of tincture. In some cases, the soluble components of a dried plant powder are extracted by steeping it in warm alcohol (or at room temperature), then straining.

MOTHER TINCTURES are the basis of homoeopathic drug preparation. On the whole they are macerations of a tenth fresh plant in 65% alcohol. The relevant amount of fresh plant is dried, and then made up in a proportion of 1g of dried plant to obtain 10g of tincture.

ALCOHOLATURES are the result of macerating a fresh plant in a more diluted alcohol than that used for the mother tincture. The enzymes they contain are still active so alcoholatures do not keep well and must be used quickly.

ELIXIRS are obtained by macerating plants, or plant extracts, in an alcohol solution with sugar or honey. This traditional form, which is not given any official legal classification, is barely used these days.

EXTRACTS are obtained by evaporating a decoction or tincture. These are classified, according to the resulting consistency, as liquid, semi-solid or dry (in which almost all the water has been evaporated, leaving only a powder).

Modern processes

Other processes have been developed to facilitate the taking of herbal medicines and to ensure their effectiveness. They are used by laboratories.

NEBULISATES or dry nebulized extracts, take the form of a fine powder. The active principles are extracted by maceration of the crushed plant in alcohol or water. The liquid is then sprayed with an atomizer in a puff of warm air, in an enclosed space. The liquid is transformed into a mist, each drop of which immediately dries out as it leaves the solvent. A dry extract is obtained which is easy to package; its composition is very close to that of the fluid extract from which it is taken, except for the more volatile molecules which have disappeared.

INTEGRATED FRESH PLANT SUSPENSIONS (SIPF) seek to preserve the integrity of the fresh plant, and thereby its effectiveness. They are obtained from an innovative process of stabilization by freezing, which prevents the reactions that would naturally destroy the enzymes as the plant dries out. As a result, the plant retains all its active principles in their original state. These suspensions are then kept in alcohol, at a strength of about 30%, which continues to preserve the properties of the plant that were retained by the freezing process.

STANDARDIZED HERBAL EXTRACTS are obtained by the phytostandard process which uses "gentle" techniques. The plants are crushed at a very low temperature. Their active molecules are then recovered by hydroalcoholic multi-extraction and preserved in a glycerine solution without either sugar or alcohol. Standardized Herbal Extracts are raw materials which can then be used in preparations formulated by a doctor or pharmacist.

GELS may contain either: a powder obtained by drying and classic pulverization or cryogenic grinding (grinding the frozen plant); or a nebulisate. To find out whether it is a dry powder or a nebulisate, simply open the gel and pour the contents into water: dry powder will float, while a nebulisate mixes in.

ESSENTIAL OILS are used in aromatherapy. They are obtained by distilling an aromatic plant in water or by using steam. They have a high concentration of the active principles and should be used with care. Failure to do so can be dangerous. Directly squeezing the juice from citrus fruit obtains "essences" rather than essential oils.

ALCOHOLATES are the result of distilling a plant macerated in alcohol.

HYDROLATES are distilled water or aromatic water which is the sub-product of distilling a plant in water after the essential oil has been recovered. They contain the hydrosoluble fraction of the distillation and the part of the essential oil that is in suspension in the water. Other than rose water and orange blossom water, they are not sold on a major scale, but in therapeutic terms, the benefits of hydrolates should not be ignored. However, they are difficult to preserve.

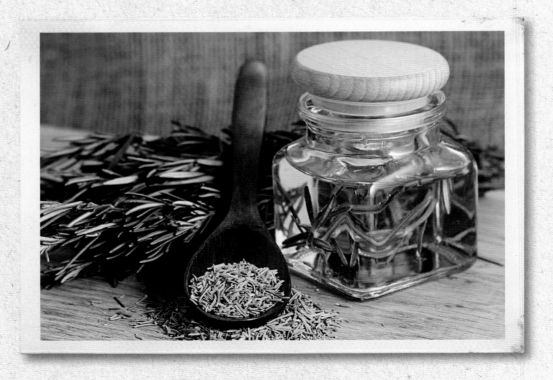

Healing properties of plants

❦ ─ ❦ ─ ❦

Medical herbalists have traditionally classified plants according to their particular properties and the action they have on the body. Each plant has one or more properties defined by specific terminology, characterizing their healing properties and the effect they have on the body. Some of the following classifications are somewhat outdated, others are very much in current usage.

ACIDULOUS
The tangy flavour of these plants quenches thirst; for example, Cherry.

ADAPTOGENIC
Adaptogens have an all-round tonic effect on the body and promote its resistance to stress while stimulating the immune system; for example, Siberian ginseng.

ANALEPTIC
Softening plant substances used as restorative food for the sick; for example, Almond and roasted acorns (Oak).

ANALGESIC
Plants that soothe, reduce or eliminate pain; for example, Pasqueflower.

ANAPHRODISIAC
Plants that reduce libido, the opposite of *aphrodisiac*; for example, Common Hop and Chaste Tree.

ANTHELMINTIC
SYNONYM of **Vermifugal**

ANTI-ALLERGENIC
By modulating immune system response, these plants decrease symptoms associated with allergies, such as pain, inflammation and swelling; for example, Black Elder (flowers).

ANTIBACTERIAL
These plants have properties that kill bacteria or prevent their establishment and propagation; for example, Common Centaury.

ANTIFUNGAL
The *antiseptic* action of these plants works on the infectious fungi responsible for fungal diseases; for example, Blackseed.

ANTI-INFLAMMATORY
Plants used to reduce inflammation and related symptoms (swelling, pain, and heat); for example, Common Agrimony, Glandular Plantain and Nettle.

ANTIPERSPIRANT
Plants used to reduce the excessive secretion of sweat; for example, English Walnut and English Oak.

ANTIPYRETIC
SYNONYM of **Febrifugal**

ANTISCORBUTIC
Initially intended to cure scurvy (disease caused by lack of vitamin C), antiscorbutic plants are high in vitamin C; for example, Blackcurrant, Watercress and Bogbean, along with numerous wild vegetables.

ANTISEPTIC
By helping to prevent the development of microbes (bacteria, virus and microscopic fungi), these plants enable the body to fight infection. Generally used externally, but can also be taken internally. Often *aromatic* plants; for example, Eucalyptus.

ANTISPASMODIC
These plants prevent spasms, involuntary contractions of the muscles and organs of nervous origin; for example, Lemon Balm and Lime (Linden).

ANXIOLYTIC
Plants used to reduce anxiety and panic; for example, St. John's-wort.

APERITIVE
These plants stimulate the appetite for food by acting on the digestive organs and glands. These are often *bitter* plants; for example, Chicory, Gentian and Common Hop.

APHRODISIAC
Excitant or generally stimulating, these plants are considered—rightly or wrongly—to boost libido and enhance sexual desire; for example, Hogweed.

AROMATIC

Plants with pleasant fragrance and strong taste due to essential oils and essences from glands in leaves and stems. *Tonic* and *stimulating* and invigorate digestive function. Also used in baths and lotions. Frequently Lamiaceae (Hyssop, Lavender, Lemon Balm, Mint, Oregano, Rosemary, Thyme), Apiaceae (Fennel), or Asteraceae (Wormwood, Mugwort).

ASCARICIDES

Plants with *anthelmintic/vermifugal* properties that attack roundworm and pinworm, but are not effective in treating tapeworm; for example, Wormwood and Mugwort.

ASTRINGENT

The high tannin content of these plants causes tissue, capillaries and orifices to contract, inhibiting mucous and glandular secretions. Used to treat diarrhoea, haemorrhages, white discharge (leucorrhoea) and sore throats; for example, Bilberry, English Oak, English Walnut and Purple Loosestrife. They are also *fortifying*.

BALSAMIC

The plants contain natural aromatic substances such as balms and resins. They act by stimulating the digestive and respiratory tracts; for example, Eucalyptus and Scots Pine.

BECHIC

Plants used to relieve coughs and irritations of the respiratory tract; for example, Hyssop and Colt's-foot. The term *pectoral* is also used.

BITTER

These plants pique the appetite, stimulate the digestive glands and facilitate digestion. They are also *febrifugal* and *tonic*. They should ideally be taken before a meal. For example, Fumitory.

CALMATIVE

Plants that act on the nervous system, to reduce excessive activity and irritability, and induce sleep. Those that calm coughs are *bechic*; those that relieve or suppress pain are *sedative* or *analgesic*; those that decrease spasms are *antispasmodic*; those that cure headaches of nervous origin are *cephalic*; those that induce sleep are *somniferous*, *narcotic* or *hypnotic*.

CARMINATIVE

Plants that assist in expelling gas from the intestine. These are *aromatic* and *stimulant* plants; for example, Fennel and Lemon Balm.

CATHARTIC

Plants that purge more energetically than *laxatives*, but do not cause inflammation.

CEPHALIC

Calmative plants that specifically treat headaches of nervous origin; for example, Lavender, Thyme and Lime.

CHOLAGOGIC

These plants assist in evacuating the bile ducts and consequently have a positive effect on the liver and digestive tract as a whole; for example, Chicory root, Dandelion and Rosemary. Cholagogic plants are very similar to *choleretic* plants.

CHOLERETIC

Plants that increase and stimulate bile secretion from the gall bladder; for example, Dandelion and Rosemary.

CICATRISANT

SEE **Vulnerary**

CORDIAL

These plants, which act on the heart and stomach, are comforting because of the "warming" effect they have on the body. They include *aromatic* and *stimulating* plants; for example, Fennel, Lemon Balm, Mint and Thyme.

COUNTER-IRRITANT

When applied to the skin, these plants cause redness with a feeling of heat. They create local irritation or mild inflammation in order to lessen discomfort in another location. They are used to decongest an internal organ; for example, garlic and chilli. Also referred to as *rubefacient* or *vesicant*.

DECONGESTANT

Decongestant plants can reduce congestion in the respiratory system. They help reduce the pressure that causes pain in the facial area when colds affect the sinuses; for example, Eucalyptus.

DEPURATIVE

Plants used to purify the blood and rid the body of the principle harmful toxins, by causing them to be sweated out (*sudorific*), or flushed from the kidneys (*diuretic*) or the gut (*purgative* and *laxative*); for example, Chicory, Fumitory, Dandelion and Soapwort.

DIGESTIVE

Plants that facilitate digestion by assisting the stomach in its work; for example, Gentian, Lemon Balm and Mint.

DIURETIC

These plants promote the emission of urine by acting on the urinary tract. Some diuretic plants simply increase the volume of urine (Cherry stalks and Leek); others eliminate chlorides from the body and reduce oedema (Silver Birch, Fennel and Butcher's Broom); others flush out urea and uric acid and are indicated when there is too much urea in the blood or for gout- or rheumatism-sufferers (Blackcurrant and Meadowsweet); others, in addition to their diuretic effect, are highly effective in treating urinary ailments and the resulting discomfort: cystitis, prostatitis, nephritis (Heather, Bearberry and Juniper berries).

EMETIC

Such plants cause vomiting, thus emptying the stomach of its contents in the case of indigestion or poisoning.

EMETOCATHARTIC

These plants cause both vomiting and bowel movements. They should be used with caution, carefully monitoring individual reactions; for example, Black Elder bark.

EMMENAGOGIC

Plants used to bring on, facilitate or increase menstrual flow; for example, Wormwood and Mugwort.

EMOLLIENT

SEE **Softening**

EXCITANT

SEE **Stimulating**

EXPECTORANT

Pectoral plants that facilitate expectoration, namely promote the evacuation of mucous blocking the trachea and bronchial tract; for example, Eucalyptus, Hyssop, White Horehound and Colt's-foot.

FEBRIFUGAL

Plants that reduce fevers and prevent them taking hold; for example, Wormwood, Common Centaury, Gentian and Bogbean. Also known as *antipyretic*.

FORTIFYING

These plants give strength, courage and energy. They are *bitter* (Common Centaury, Chicory, Gentian and Bogbean), *astringent* (Common Agrimony and Blackcurrant) or *analeptic*. They are also referred to as *tonic*.

GALACTOGENIC

Plants that contribute to increasing the production and flow of milk; for example, Fennel.

HAEMOSTATIC

Astringent plants. Their principal qualities are staunching bleeding; for example, Shepherd's Purse, Comfrey and White Deadnettle.

HEPATIC

Plants that facilitate liver function; for example, Common Centaury and Rosemary.

HYPNOTIC

These *calmative* plants induce restorative sleep; for example, Common Poppy and Common Hop. Also known as *somniferous*, *narcotic*, or *soporific*.

HYPOGLYCAEMIC

Plants that reduce blood sugar with an antidiabetic effect. For example, Herb Robert and Common Agrimony.

IMMUNOMODULATORY

Plants that moderate the activity of the immune system and regulate its functioning.

IMMUNOSTIMULANT

Plants that stimulate immune defences; for example, Hemp Agrimony, Gentian and Greater Celandine.

INSECTIFUGE

Plants used to repel insects, thus protecting from the consequences of insect bites and stings; for example, Lavender.

LAXATIVE

These plants act to gently promote evacuation of the bowels, without irritating or tiring the intestine; for example, Sweet Almond oil, Fig, Chard, Dog Rose.

LIPID-LOWERING (and CHOLESTEROL-LOWERING)

Plants used to reduce concentrations of fatty acids in the blood and lower cholesterol, thereby protecting against cardiovascular diseases; for example, Oat, Leek, Flax.

NARCOTIC

SYNONYM of **Hypnotic**

PECTORAL

Pectoral describes all plants that relieve chest ailments affecting the bronchial tubes, lungs and larynx. They help to evacuate, through the mouth, substances that could obstruct the bronchial tubes. *Bechic* plants, which soothe coughs, and *expectorants*, which facilitate expectoration, are also *pectoral* plants.

PURGATIVE

Purgatives are more energetic than *laxatives* and cause the vigorous evacuation of the bowels, by stimulating the secretions and peristalsis of the intestine; for example, Black Elder.

REFRESHING

Refreshing plants quench thirst and reduce body temperature and inflammation. They are *acidulous* plants (Cherry); or *softening* plants (Mallow).

RESOLUTIVE

Plants used to relieve blockages (accumulations of fluid obstructing particular parts of the body) and inflammation and allow the tissue to return to its normal state; for example, Chicory, Common Hop, Hyssop and Soapwort.

RUBEFACIENT

Rubefacient plants, as their name indicates, "redden" the skin; for example, Round-leaved Sundew. Also, *counter-irritant*.

SEDATIVE

These plants alleviate pathological manifestations (pain, anxiety, insomnia) or moderate the way an organ functions. This qualifier is often used in a narrower sense of "pain sedative". For example, Black Horehound. Also *analgesic* and *calmative*.

SOFTENING

These plants soften and relax the skin, and relieve inflammation (for example, Sweet Almond and Comfrey). Plants with this property are also known as *emollients*. They have the opposite action to *tonic* or *astringent* plants.

SOMNIFEROUS

SEE **Calmative** and **Hypnotic**

SOPORIFIC

SEE **Hypnotic**

STERNUTATORY

In powder form and administered via the nose, these plants cause sneezing and stimulate secretion from the mucosa; for example, Lavender and Thyme.

STIMULANT

Such plants increase activity and vitality by stimulating the nervous and vascular system, and the whole body in general (Wormwood, Mugwort and Rosemary). They are also known as *excitants*. Aromatics and spices (Scots Pine and Winter Savory) tend to contain substances that stimulate the digestive tract, their effect often spreading to other parts of the body. Herbal physicians of old distinguished "diffusible stimulants", which work fast but do not have a long-lasting effect (Wormwood), and "persistent stimulants", which are slower to act, but longer lasting.

STOMACHIC

Plants that stimulate and regulate stomach function; for example, Common Centaury, Fennel, Gentian, Hop and Rosemary.

SUDORIFIC

These plants cause perspiration and promote the secretion of sweat; for example, Black Elder, Borage and Blackthorn

TENIFUGAL

Describes vermifugal plants that expel tapeworm; for example, Pomegranate.

TONIC

These plants have a general invigorating effect on the body: they increase the activity of organs involved in the digestive process and repair damaged tissue. For example, Blackcurrant. Also known as *fortifying*.

VERMIFUGAL

Plants that expel worms from the intestine. *Vermifugal* plants include *ascaricides*, which destroy roundworm and pinworm, and *tæniafuges*, which rid the body of tapeworm. Also known as *anthelmintic*.

VESICANT

SEE **Counter-irritant**

VOMITIVE

SEE **Emetic**

VULNERARY

Applied topically, these plants aid the body in healing wounds, sores, cuts and bruises; for example, Arnica. In the past, "vulnerary plants" also included *antiseptic* and *aromatic* plants that were administered internally to revitalize people who had suffered a fall or injury, or revive them if they were feeling faint or weak; for example, Wormwood, Fennel, Hyssop, Rosemary, Garden Thyme and Wild Thyme.

Short glossary of botanical terms

—❦—

Plants vary greatly, ranging from edible with medicinal properties to highly poisonous. Being able to describe and distinguish different plants is key to accurate identification. It can help you understand how different plants progagate, protect themselves and adapt to the environments they favour. To help get you started, this glossary of botanical terms is a short list of common terms describing plant parts and forms, certain qualities of plants, and their life cycle characteristics.

AERIAL PARTS: Parts of a plant located above the ground.

ALTERNATE: Describes leaves growing from each side of a stem but at different heights, not facing one another.

ANNUAL: Describes a plant with a 1-year life cycle.

AROMATIC: Used to describe a scented plant, which can generally be made into essential oil.

AXIL: Junction between a leaf stalk and the stem. **Axillary**, its adjective, means "in the axil".

BASAL: Used to describe leaves growing from the base of a plant (rosette).

BIENNIAL: Describes a plant with a 2-year life cycle, which generally flowers in its second year.

BULB: A plant's round, underground food storage organ.

CAPITULUM: Flower heads characteristic of the Asteraceae family, formed of small flowers tightly clustered together and inserted on the enlarged, flattened stalk called the receptacle.

CAPSULE: Dried fruit that opens by means of pores or splits to release the seeds.

CATKIN: Long, hanging spike of reduced flowers, usually of the same sex.

CLUSTER: Inflorescence with flowers attached by a small stalk to a common axis.

COMPOUND: Describes a leaf which is divided into leaflets.

CORDATE: Heart-shaped.

COROLLA: A flower's set of petals.

DECIDUOUS: Used to describe plants with leaves that fall, generally during cold seasons.

DIOECIOUS: Describes a plant that has male and female flowers on separate plants.

HERBACEOUS: Describes a non-woody plant, which generally has a 1-year life cycle or dies down each year.

LANCEOLATE: In the shape of a spearhead.

LATEX: Liquid in a range of colours (white, yellow or red) characteristic of certain families of plant.

LEAFLET: Each of the subdivisions of a compound leaf.

OPPOSITE: Used to describe leaves that grow in pairs on a stem, opposite each other at the same height.

PANICLE: Inflorescence of some grasses, comprised of small spikes (spikelets) arranged in clusters; it is a "cluster of clusters".

PERENNIAL: Used to describe a plant that lives for several years and flowers and fruits each year.

PINNATE: Used to describe a compound leaf where the leaves are arranged along each side of a common stalk.

RHIZOME: Underground stem that acts as a food storage organ.

SPIKE: Inflorescence formed of small sessile flowers (without stalks).

STAMEN: Male sexual organ of flowering plants.

STIGMA: A flower's female sexual organ.

TRIFOLIATE: Used to describe a leaf with three leaflets.

TUBER: An enlarged storage organ, which is normally a swollen, underground part of the stem.

UMBEL: Inflorescence in which the stalks of approximately equal length grow from a common centre, like the ribs of a parasol.

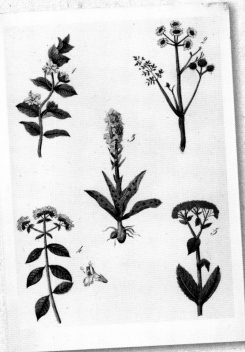

Index of health benefits

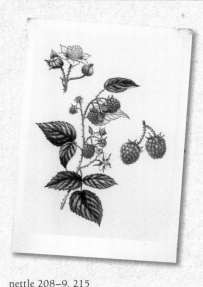

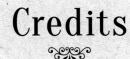

Credits

BOTANICAL PHOTOGRAPHS: © Pierre et Délia Vignes

OTHER ILLUSTRATIONS:
(b: bottom; t: top; r: right; l: left; m: middle)

© **Larousse Archives:** 49r, 127, 179r, 13, 9, 203, 141, 145l, 19, 39b, 31, 109r, 171l, 35r, 181l, 51l, 37r, 107, 43r, 59r, 77l, 191, 165l, 87r, 111l, 55, 135, 89, 195l, 93r, 99l, 113l, 201r, 63, 121, 115r, 115, 139, 61, 167r, 119, 123, 85r, 65, 187, 11, 155l, 71b, 71, 189, 161, 137, 29l, 29, 143, 185, 25, 147, 159, 149, 75, 21, 175b, 79, 193, 7, 27r, 153, 83, 131, 23b, 81, 163b, 157r, 33l, 17, 177l, 199, 47, 101b, 197, 97, 133, 95b, 45, 73l, 15l, 105r, 183, 41, 57, 206, 210, 222, 223

© **François Couplan:** 69, 179l, 181r, 51l, 37l, 43l, 77r, 87l, 111r, 195r, 93l, 113r, 201l, 63r, 27l, 23t, 177r, 105l

© **Pierre and Délia Vignes:** 117r, 49l, 151, 39t, 173, 109l, 59l, 171t, 99r, 85l, 33r, 101t, 95t, 73r, 207l, 207m

Shutterstock: © Ana del Castillo : 167l, 207r; © btwcapture : 171r; © Creative Family: 53; © dabjola: 35l, 181; © David Dohnal: 145r; © FotoLot: 214; © Grigorev Mikhai: 216r; © HandmadePictures: 103r, 209l; © HHelene: 175t; © Ildi Papp: 163t; © kidsnord: 216r; © HandmadePictures: 157l; © Manfred Ruckszio: 33l; © scaners3d: 165r; © Toni Genes: 67; © TunedIn by Westend61: 212

A DAVID AND CHARLES BOOK
© Larousse 2017

David and Charles is an imprint of David and Charles, Ltd
Suite A, Tourism House, Pynes Hill, Exeter, EX2 5WS

Originally published in France as *L'herbier des plantes qui guérissent* in 2017
First published in the UK and USA in 2021

Gérard Debuigne and François Couplan have asserted their right to be identified as authors of this work in accordance with the Copyright, Designs and Patents Act, 1988.

A catalogue record for this book is available from the British Library.

ISBN-13: 9781446308776 paperback
ISBN-13: 9781446380864 EPUB

This book has been printed on paper from approved suppliers and made from pulp from sustainable sources.

Printed in China by Asia Pacific for:
David and Charles, Ltd
Suite A, Tourism House, Pynes Hill, Exeter, EX2 5WS

10 9 8 7 6 5 4 3 2 1

Head of publishing: Isabelle Jeuge-Maynart and Ghislaine Stora
Editor: Valérie de Sahb and Agnès Busière
Publisher: Thierry Olivaux, assisted by Vanina Pialot
Graphic design and layout: Emmanuel Chaspoul

David and Charles publishes high-quality books on a wide range of subjects.
For more information visit www.davidandcharles.com.

Layout of the digital edition of this book may vary depending on reader hardware and display settings.